Sentinel for Health

Sentinel for Health

*A History of the
Centers for Disease Control*

Elizabeth W. Etheridge

UNIVERSITY OF CALIFORNIA PRESS
Berkeley · *Los Angeles* · *Oxford*

University of California Press
Berkeley and Los Angeles, California

University of California Press, Ltd.
Oxford, England

Library of Congress Cataloging-in-Publication Data

Etheridge, Elizabeth W.
    Sentinel for health : a history of the Centers for Disease Control
/ Elizabeth W. Etheridge.
        p.   cm.
    Includes bibliographical references and index.
    ISBN 0-520-07107-7
    1. Centers for Disease Control (U.S.)—History. 2. Epidemiology—
United States—History. I. Title.
RA650.5.E84 1991
614.4′273—dc20   90-24679
                                                            CIP

Printed in the United States of America
9 8 7 6 5 4 3 2

For Deda and Tommy

Contents

Charts

Abbreviations

ACIP	Advisory Committee on Immunization Practices
AID	Agency for International Development
AMA	American Medical Association
APTA	American Physical Therapy Association
BoB	Bureau of Biologics
BOSH	Bureau of Occupational Safety and Health (after 1970, NIOSH)
BSS	Bureau of State Services
CCCD	Combatting Childhood Communicable Disease (AID program)
CDC	Communicable Disease Center; subsequently Centers for Disease Control, Atlanta
CID	Center for Infectious Diseases
EIS	Epidemic Intelligence Service
EPA	Environmental Protection Agency
FA	fluorescent antibody (technique)
FAA	Federal Aviation Agency
FDA	Food and Drug Administration

FRC	Federal Records Center
GBS	Guillain-Barré syndrome
HEW	Department of Health, Education and Welfare (1953–79)
HHS	Department of Health and Human Services
HSMHA	Health Services and Mental Health Administration
ICBC	Interagency Committee on Back Contamination
INH	isoniazid (drug used in treating tuberculosis)
IPV	Salk killed-virus polio vaccine
JAMA	*Journal of the American Medical Association*
MCWA	Malaria Control in War Areas
MMWR	*Morbidity and Mortality Weekly Report*
NCDC	National Communicable Disease Center (CDC before 1970)
NCSH	National Clearinghouse on Smoking and Health
NEJM	*New England Journal of Medicine*
NFIP	National Foundation for Infantile Paralysis (subsequently "the National Foundation")
NIAID	National Institute of Allergy and Infectious Diseases
NIH	National Institute(s) of Health
NIIP	National Influenza Immunization Program
NIOSH	National Institute of Occupational Safety and Health
NLM	National Library of Medicine
NMAV	National Medical Audiovisual Facility
NOVS	National Office of Vital Statistics
ODM	Office of Defense Mobilization
OPV	Sabin oral polio vaccine
OSHA	Occupational Safety and Health Administration
PAHO	Pan American Health Organization
PAS	para-aminosalicylic acid

PHA	public health advisor
PHR	*Public Health Reports*
PHS	Public Health Service
RPR	rapid plasma reagin (blood test for syphilis)
SEP	Smallpox-Eradication Program
STD	Sexually Transmitted Disease Division, Center for Prevention Services
TSS	toxic shock syndrome
VDRL	veneral disease research laboratory
VIA	Villa International Atlanta
WHO	World Health Organization
WNRC	Washington National Records Center, Suitland, Maryland
WPA	Works Progress Administration (1935–43)

Preface

In northeast Atlanta, in buildings of sturdy but unprepossessing appearance, is an extraordinary institution, the Centers for Disease Control. On two sides it is flanked by Emory University, which in 1947 donated the land on which it stands to lure it to the neighborhood. Emory's gift was based mostly on faith that the year-old Communicable Disease Center, as it was then called, would prove to be a stimulating neighbor. CDC was still feeling its way, still spending most of its energy on malaria control. Few could have imagined that it would become a sentinel for health for the nation and the world. In four decades, CDC has justified Emory's faith. The largest federal agency outside the Washington, D.C., area, it has itself become a magnet attracting other institutions. The American Cancer Society built its headquarters across the street just to be close by.

The accident of birth made Atlanta CDC's home. It is descended from a World War II agency established to fight malaria, a disease that ravaged the South throughout the 1930s and threatened the war effort in the 1940s. The South was an ideal location for training troops and producing war matériel, but only if malaria could be kept at bay. This job was assigned to a new unit of the U.S. Public Health Service called Malaria Control in War Areas. There was no room for it in crowded wartime Washington, so MCWA was located in Atlanta in the heart of the malaria zone. At first, MCWA was concerned only with the southeastern United States and Puerto Rico, but before the war was over, its reach extended to California and its mandate to dengue fever and murine typhus.

In 1946, MCWA changed its name and greatly broadened its mission, but stayed where it was. The new institution was the Communicable Disease Center, the first of three names for which its famous acronym has stood. Dr. Joseph Mountin, a visionary leader in the Public Health Service, believed that the public health needs of the states could best be served by centers of excellence, each concentrating on a special area of expertise. There should be one for environmental issues, one for the emerging problems of Arctic health, and one for man's ancient enemy, communicable diseases. MCWA had the structure to handle the latter assignment and the transition was relatively easy. The Communicable Disease Center would provide service to the states and give scientific research a practical application.

For several years, CDC was dominated by engineers and entomologists, but it shifted gradually from an emphasis on tropical diseases with insect vectors to all diseases of zoological origin. Initially, the CDC's laboratory included only parasitology, but as the center's interests broadened, the laboratory grew. It was the first of CDC's divisions to gain a distinguished reputation.

Mountin offered encouragement to all the staff in Atlanta, but at the same time he pushed them impatiently to think and act on an ever-larger scale. He wanted CDC to live up to its name, to encompass all the communicable diseases except those still managed by separate agencies in Washington. A powerful spur to this end was the onset of the Cold War. As the Iron Curtain descended across Eastern Europe and China and the possibility of biological warfare loomed, health officials went on the alert. Outbreak of the Korean War in 1950 underscored the urgency of the situation.

Epidemiology was the first line of defense against enemy germs. When Mountin observed that the nation needed "epidemiological intelligence," he planted the seed of CDC's Epidemic Intelligence Service. Created as an early-warning system against man-made epidemics, EIS became the lookout for naturally occurring ones as well. The disease detectives became famous, and the concept of disease surveillance, which they perfected, became essential to public health practice.

The Communicable Disease Center was established as a field station of the Bureau of State Services, a unit of the Public Health Service, which in the 1940s was part of the Federal Security Administration. Compared to other components of the PHS, especially the National Institutes of Health, it was of only minor importance. NIH, oriented towards research on chronic ailments like cancer and heart disease, was firmly in the twentieth-century mainstream of public health, and it grew rapidly. In comparison, CDC seemed a bit old-fashioned, and for years it was too small to attract much notice. By definition it concentrated on diseases that had declined steadily in importance since the 1920s.

For several years in the early 1950s, the continued existence of CDC was in doubt despite its potentially starring role in the struggle against germs let loose by enemy conspiracy. Two events established its credibility and ensured its survival. The Cutter incident of 1955 (when live virus got into the Salk polio vaccine) and the epidemic of Asian influenza in 1957 demonstrated the value of surveillance dramatically. Threats to dismantle the institution vanished, and CDC began steady growth by accretion. First, the Venereal Disease Branch moved to Atlanta, then the Tuberculosis Branch, giving CDC sole domain over communicable diseases. These two units led a steady procession of public health programs to CDC, which has continued to this day.

The 1960s were a time of rapid expansion for CDC in budget, personnel, and programs. In keeping with President Lyndon Johnson's efforts to build the Great Society, CDC expanded its interests to programs as diverse as family planning and lead-based paint poisoning. It also became involved in projects overseas, the most notable being the campaign to eradicate smallpox. In fact, CDC was the star of the World Health Organization's smallpox crusade; its emphasis on surveillance was the key to that program's success. CDC even played a part in the decade's most dramatic venture, the flight to the moon. It made certain there was no exchange of earth and moon germs.

Inevitably CDC was affected by the drastic reorganization of the Public Health Service in the 1960s and by the subsequent readjustments, which followed like aftershocks for a dozen years. Both CDC's status and name were changed. In 1967, it became the National Communicable Disease Center, and a year later it moved up a notch in the PHS to become a bureau. In 1970, the name was changed once more, to Center for Disease Control, to better reflect the expanding compass of its work and to restore the much-prized initials. In 1973, CDC became, like NIH, an agency of the PHS.

CDC encountered extensive criticism for the first time in the 1970s. The costly campaign to protect the nation against a possible swine flu epidemic plunged CDC into the most difficult days it had ever faced. The epidemic never came, and a massive immunization campaign was abandoned when the vaccine was associated with the onset of Guillain-Barré syndrome. The episode was a chilling plunge into public health as public relations.

By the late 1970s, the most dangerous threats to health and well-being seemed to lurk in environmental and lifestyle issues. CDC's organizational structure, with its separate units for epidemiology, laboratory, and training, was ill suited to cope with problems ranging from Agent Orange to tornadoes, from the dangers of smoking to murder and suicide. Confident that the techniques that had worked against infectious diseases could be applied with equal success to these new challenges, CDC reorganized for efficiency. An *s* was added to the word *center* in 1980 to better describe the structure. The Centers for Disease Control had barely been named when a new infectious disease, subsequently called AIDS, appeared.

Readers may be somewhat puzzled by the numerous changes of name among CDC's major divisions and subdivisions. When the Communicable Disease Center was established in 1946, the various components (there were nine or ten) were called divisions. By 1951, however, these had become branches. The number was soon whittled down to four–Laboratory, Epidemiology, Technology, and Training. Essentially, this was the basic framework of CDC until 1967, when the National Communicable Disease Center came into being. Then all the major units (an even dozen) were called programs. At the same time, the chief became the director. When the Center for Disease Control replaced NCDC in 1970, the nomenclature was changed again. This time the word *bureau* was used to designate laboratory, epidemiology, and so on. In 1980, when CDC became Centers for Disease Control, each major unit was designated as a center. These are subdivided into divisions, which, in turn, are subdivided into branches.

The account that follows traces CDC's history from the MCWA days to the mid 1980s, when the virus that causes AIDS was discovered. At that point, the story of that epidemic becomes so complex it demands separate treatment. CDC, meanwhile, had launched its program to make people healthy by promoting healthy lifestyles, a task that AIDS complicated manyfold. Painting with a broad brush, CDC set health goals for 1990, a reprise of sorts of the ancient search for Utopia. Such an extended reach might have surprised even the visionary Joseph Mountin.

The idea for this study originated in the History Committee of the Centers for Disease Control. Support for it was made possible by CDC and Longwood College, Farmville, Virginia, through the Intergovernmental Personnel Act of 1970. During 1987, CDC supplied me with an office and access to the archives. Donald Hopkins opened doors for me, and many members of the staff, both past and present, generously granted me interviews. I am especially grateful to William Watson and to two former directors, David Sencer and William Foege, who have an encyclopedic knowledge of CDC and the patience to explain it. All three, as well as Jim Bloom, a member of the History Committee, read the first draft and made many suggestions. Alexander Langmuir supplied critiques of two versions of chapter 5. Jackie Meeks, David Rowe, and Jody Golden repeatedly did favors for me, and the Public Affairs Office, especially Don Berreth, Gail Lloyd, Jeanie Daves, and Tom Skinner, helped in countless ways. A display in the CDC lobby prepared by Dennis McDowell and Mary Ann Fenley provided the title for the book.

I am indebted to many librarians, but especially to those at CDC and the Thompson-McCaw Library, Medical College of Virginia; Peter B. Hirtle, History of Medicine Division, National Library of Medicine; and Norma Taylor, Longwood College, who secured materials on interlibrary loan.

Harry M. Marks called my attention to the material on the Cutter incident at the Washington National Records Center. Daniel M. Fox, James Harvey Young, Victoria Harden, Fitzhugh Mullan, and an anonymous reader saved me from many errors of omission and commission. Those that remain are my own. Lynne Withey was a generous editor.

My friends encouraged me to believe that one day this book would be finished. Without my family, especially my sister and brother-in-law, Virginia and Tom Wood, it would not have been. The dedication to them expresses only in part my gratitude.

CHAPTER I

War and the Mosquito

Since ancient times, war has meant malaria, and World War II was no exception. During that struggle, however, marked progress was made against the ancient foe. December 7, 1941, a day President Roosevelt said would "live in infamy," marked the beginning of a new assault on a disease that for centuries had plagued armies the world over. Harry Pratt, an entomologist with the U.S. Public Health Service, knew this instinctively. When he learned of the Japanese attack on Pearl Harbor after a lazy Sunday on the beach, Pratt knew that his south Florida unit would no longer chase the aedes mosquito, vector of dengue and yellow fever. Their new target surely would be the anopheline mosquito, vector of malaria.

The sudden entry into World War II of the United States affected the course of public health, just as it did every national concern. "The MCWA was born that day," Pratt recalled, using an acronym that stood for Malaria Control in War Areas, a government agency created just two months later.[1] Pratt spent the war years at MCWA and the rest of his career at its successor institution, the CDC. In a formal sense, the letters stood for different names over the years, but they were always symbolic of a new and systematic attack on the plagues of the world, ancient and modern.

America's most recent experience with war offered proof enough of the devastation of malaria. Extraordinary measures were taken in World War I to protect both troops and the public from the disease. The U.S. Army vigorously pursued mosquitoes at its southern camps in 1917 and 1918, and the Public Health Service took up the pursuit in forty-three areas around these camps and stations. But in spite of their best efforts and a combined expenditure of more than $5 million, malaria was a problem throughout the war, and more than 10,500 cases were reported. Yet some important lessons were learned: mosquito control was too expensive to be financed locally; the states and the counties played a vital role, but the federal government had to be involved, too.[2]

The early months of World War II focused attention once more on the importance of tropical diseases in wartime, especially malaria. The anopheles mosquito was a worse threat than the Japanese in the Pacific and threatened troops training in the South, which had always been plagued by malaria. "Autumnal fever" discouraged settlement of the region during the colonial period, and during the Civil War, malaria was the major cause of illness in both northern and southern troops. During World War I, the South was the focus of the nation's attack on malaria.

In 1942, there was every reason to believe that malaria posed a threat to the nation's security. The task of fighting it was at once easier and more difficult than in World War I. Advances in technology facilitated the pursuit, but exacted a price of their own. During World War I, it was enough to eliminate mosquitoes from a military base and the surrounding zone over a radius of about one mile, the distance an anopheles mosquito could fly or that persons ordinarily walked. In World War II, the universality of automobiles expanded that radius to thirty miles, a 900-fold increase.[3]

Dr. Louis L. Williams, the Public Health Service's chief expert on malaria, was put in charge of the fight against the disease in the South. A year before the United States entered the war, he was assigned to a liaison detail with the Fourth Corps Headquarters in Atlanta to work with the state health departments, the Army, and the Public Health Service on malaria-control projects on or near military bases. It was Williams's task to keep malaria from spreading to the armed forces from its reservoir in the civilian population. He brought a great deal of experience to the job. He had fought malaria since World War I, his most recent assignment being as director of the Malaria Commission on the China-Burma highway. Colleagues remembered him as a "rare individual of great spirit, professional ability and administrative competence."[4]

In 1941, the incidence of malaria was the lowest since registration had been established in 1910, but the disease was known to occur in five- to seven-year cycles, and the last upswing had been in the mid

1930s. During that decade, the federal government made a massive effort to bring the disease under control. The Works Progress Administration set workers to digging thousands of miles of ditches to drain malaria-breeding sites. In Georgia, where malaria was a particularly difficult problem, two businessmen who later played an important role in making Atlanta an important center for disease prevention also joined in the fight. Preston Arkwright, president of the Georgia Power Company, was concerned about malaria wherever a stream was dammed and a lake created for the production of electric power. In those areas, Dr. Glenville Giddings, Arkwright's son-in-law and a prominent Atlanta physician, organized teams to survey both the mosquito and the human population.[5]

Giddings was the medical advisor of the Coca-Cola Company, whose board chairman, Robert Woodruff, became interested in malaria when he found the disease widespread at Ichuaway Plantation, his hunting preserve in Baker County, Georgia. Woodruff consulted the county health officer, sent enough quinine to treat everyone in the county, and hired two nurses to distribute it. He also made a grant to Emory University to establish a station at Ichuaway to study malaria. It had been in operation for two years when the United States entered World War II.[6]

Dr. Joseph W. Mountin, who directed the PHS's State Services division, had a plan for the emergency. He wanted a national organization to keep the more than 600 military bases and essential war-industrial establishments in the South malaria-free. Teams of physicians, entomologists, and engineers would work together to safeguard "the health of our soldiers, sailors, and workers in defense industries—those who are being trained to do the shooting and those who are providing the guns and materials with which to shoot."[7]

Dr. Williams was relieved of his military duties on February 9, 1942, and told to stand by in Atlanta, ready to establish headquarters for malaria control. The next day Surgeon General Thomas Parran sent a circular letter to all public and state health officials charged with protecting the health of the military. The letter, number seven of a series, referred to a new organization, "National Defense Malaria Control Activities," although the name shortly became "Malaria Control in Defense Areas." A couple of months later, to better conform with the actual facts of the situation, the name was changed to "Malaria Control in War Areas." Circular letter number eight, dated April 27, 1942, made the new name official.[8]

As the man in charge of MCWA, Dr. Williams looked for a suitable headquarters site. Shortage of office space in Washington preempted that possibility. He considered Memphis, then sites in Texas and California to be closer to the war in the Pacific. It was Surgeon General Parran who finally decided that the headquarters would be in Atlanta. Mark Hollis, a PHS engineer from Georgia whom Williams took with him as his executive officer, immediately boasted of victory. "You're a Virginian," Hollis said to Williams. "Let this be the first time Georgia ever got anything over Virginia." It was Hollis who selected space for the agency in Atlanta.[9]

The first offices were modest, just three or four rooms and a bay on the sixth floor of the Volunteer Building on Peachtree Street, but it was enough for the small, sophisticated staff. Although the PHS provided most of the leadership, people were recruited from academe, other federal agencies, and wherever expertise about malaria existed. This expertise was in short supply. All the malaria specialists were snapped up by the Army, Navy, and the PHS in a few weeks in 1940. Thereafter, most of those recruited had to be trained, first at the National Institute of Health, and beginning in 1942, at MCWA. Fewer than 10 percent of the commissioned officers in the Atlanta organization came with any specialized training in malaria control. They learned fast, however, and with no rigid lines of responsibility and no turf to maintain, these outsiders contributed much to MCWA's ability to wage war on malaria. They were a key factor in building the reputation and efficiency of the organization, the first large operational program dealing with domestic health that the Public Health Service had ever undertaken.[10]

From the beginning, engineers and entomologists dominated MCWA. Physicians assessed malaria cases in the field, and parasitologists ran the laboratory, but major emphasis was always on mosquito control, the engineers' specialty. They determined control methods, directed operations, surveyed and designed drainage construction projects, and mapped field activities. Entomologists, first commissioned in large numbers in 1943, provided the necessary expertise on mosquitoes. The wartime need to save time, money, and equipment dictated that temporary measures like larvicidal control take preference over permanent drainage projects.

Innovation was encouraged, especially in the development of equipment. MCWA took over the Henry Rose Carter Laboratory in Savannah, previously owned and operated by that city for malaria control, and began to develop new equipment, materials, and procedures for killing mosquitoes. There were only four or five people in this small lab,

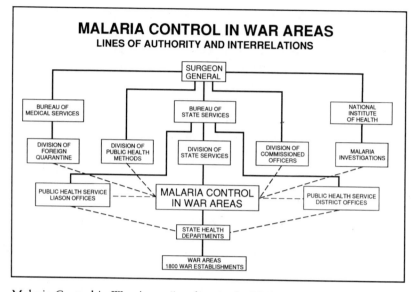

Malaria Control in War Areas (its place in the PHS), 1942–46

but Dr. Samuel W. (Sib) Simmons, who became the lab director in 1944, remembers them as "the finest staff you could ever get. They were handpicked and you could do things then." Simmons loved his work. He got there early, stayed late, and hated to take even Sunday off.[11]

The MCWA staff worked six-day weeks in Atlanta, too. Dr. Mountin's philosophy was that "there was so much work to be done that we could not possibly move fast enough." Initially MCWA's assignment was to control malaria in fifteen southeastern states, Puerto Rico, and the Virgin Islands. The staff was to get rid of the anopheles in areas immediately adjacent to places of military importance: camps, bases, depots, shipyards, factories producing war materials, housing developments where war workers lived, recreational areas for troops, and access highways. In 1942 there were 900 of these "war establishments" to be protected. By 1945 there were approximately 2,000, and MCWA's work had spread westward to California.

These "war establishments" were divided into 250 "war areas," each directed by a supervisor, usually an engineer. An administrator was assigned to each state, and the states, in turn, were responsible for direct operations. The extent to which malaria was a problem could not always be determined. A shortage of medical epidemiologists and the constraints of time prevented the use of conventional methods of measuring malaria prevalence. Eventually, the MCWA staff decided that the presence of anopheles posed a potential hazard even though there were no malaria cases in an area. Malaria control came to mean mosquito control. Vectors should become so scarce that the chance of their transmitting malaria became infinitesimal.[12]

Killing mosquitoes was a labor-intensive task. The WPA provided much of the work force until December 1942, when President Roosevelt ended that program, but malaria control was so important that 3,000 men continued on the job, paid for with other federal funds. They dug 1,274 miles of ditches the first year, using 448,000 pounds of dynamite to speed the job. Still the major emphasis was on larviciding. They used 152,000 pounds of Paris green, a bright green insecticide made from arsenic trioxide and copper acetate, but diesel oil quickly became the larvicide of choice. While Paris green killed only anopheline larvae, diesel oil killed the larvae and pupae of both culicine and anopheline mosquitoes. Oil was readily visible on the water, so its application could be checked. Most of the work was done by men using knapsack and compressed-air sprayers, but large power units on trucks and boats were quickly introduced. In the dense water chestnut–infested areas along the Potomac River, power dusting from airplanes was first used in August 1942. The experiment was so successful that within a year four airplane dusting projects were in operation.[13]

In Puerto Rico, where the principal vector is the *Anopheles albimanus,* the control problem was more complex. This mosquito breeds anywhere there is water—even in hoof prints and car tracks—and transmits malaria year round. It has a flight range of up to three miles, greatly increasing the size of areas to be controlled, some of which were so inaccessible they could be reached only by ox cart. Paris green was used almost exclusively because it would have required the full time use of a tanker to take enough oil to the island. Even so, there were problems of delivery. When German submarines sank cargoes of MCWA's equipment and chemicals, Harry Pratt was certain it was to counter MCWA's efforts in Puerto Rico.[14]

Malaria control also involved education on many levels. Few of the nation's medical schools were then equipped for laboratory study of parasitological diseases, and malaria materials in particular were in short supply. To meet this need quickly, MCWA sent personnel and supplies to the Malaria Investigations Laboratory in Columbia, South Carolina, an adjunct of the National Institute of Health, to make thousands of malaria plasmodium slides for distribution to medical schools.[15]

Not all of MCWA's battles were against the mosquito. As a new-

comer, MCWA challenged other segments of the public health hierarchy, not the least of which were the existing district offices of PHS, each
of which expected to do malaria-control work. There were seven or
eight of these in the South, and Williams thought this was too much
division of authority. As it happened, his brother, Dr. Charles L.
Williams, was head of one of the most important of these, the office in
New Orleans, so Williams and Hollis decided to appeal to him. Bess
Furman, historian of PHS, recounts what happened:

> I had Charles and his staff come over and talk with Mark and me. We came
> to no conclusion. The next week, Mark and I went to New Orleans and
> called on Charles. There came a point in our discussion when I said to him,
> "Visualize your office running this colossal job." He mulled that over—and
> at last answered:
> "You know, if we take over a job of this size, this office will be a little tail
> with a big malaria dog wagging it—and when this war is over all we do here
> will be forgotten and we will have to grow into an office again."
> The District officers expected a fight when they soon met in Washington
> with Surgeon General Parran. Charles was called upon to open the discus-
> sion. He said to them just what he said to me. That ended the meeting.[16]

Other problems were more difficult. A staff of nearly 4,000 people,
ranging from unskilled labor to professional specialists, had to be recruited and trained, a task complicated by draft quotas and high-paying
industrial jobs. The first year there was a 60 percent turnover. To keep
the operation from shutting down, MCWA began in-service training,
making much use of audiovisual materials. This educational program
would have great impact in years to come.

The lack of transportation posed the most serious threat to MCWA's
efficiency. It had 400 bicycles in use the first year, but two-wheeled
transportation was hardly the answer. MCWA needed trucks, and permission to buy them was nearly impossible to obtain. Appropriations
acts prohibited the purchase of new or used passenger-carrying vehicles
without special authorization. There was no prohibition, however,
against interdepartmental transfer of vehicles on a reimbursable basis,
if only they could be found.

The problem was solved serendipitously. On a trip to Washington in
1942, Executive Officer Mark Hollis was having lunch at the Naval Air
Station when he overheard a conversation about the availability of 200
surplus trucks, 60 percent paid for, at Camp Blanding, Florida. Seeing
an opportunity to solve MCWA's transportation problem, Hollis called
Mountin, and together they went to see the surgeon general. Parran
wanted to follow the book and go through the War Department, but

Hollis persuaded him that the direct approach was better. Mountin told him to get two dozen trucks; Parran told him to get as many as he could.

·Hollis went immediately to Florida and soon was in touch with the engineer at Camp Blanding, who happened to be an alumnus of Georgia Tech. He and Hollis, who was a graduate of the University of Georgia, swapped Georgia–Georgia Tech stories for a while and soon reached an agreement on the trucks. There were 250 of them, and the engineer promised to go through, mark the ones Hollis was not to take with an X, and instruct the civilian in charge to let him have the rest. When Hollis arrived at the site, he noted happily that the Xs were there; all he had to do was get the unmarked vehicles off the property that day. A parade of state troopers, many of them off duty, came to help. In a few hours they moved off 123 trucks.

Mountin was astounded when he heard the news and wondered how MCWA would pay for them, but Parran had said to get all he could, and Hollis had simply done his bidding. "It saved us," he later recalled with pride.

A shortage of equipment posed another major problem. MCWA needed tools and shovels. Again Hollis came to the rescue. He had a colleague in Washington who at one time had been with the WPA. Through him he learned that the WPA was unloading its warehouses all over the country. Many government agencies were using the list to order specific items, but Hollis found this process too slow. Why not take a whole warehouse, which was certain to contain thousands of shovels and hand tools? Mountin agreed, and it was done. MCWA thus got its shovels and tools, as well as bonuses like air compressors. With the trucks it already had, MCWA was in business within ten months.[17]

The rather unorthodox way in which MCWA got its trucks and shovels was symbolic of the degree of freedom that existed in the organization. The geographic scope of its operations and the urgency of its mission set MCWA apart from the rest of the PHS. Officials in Washington at the Bureau and Division levels recognized that the Atlanta institution had to have a degree of autonomy and freedom. The immediate result was to eliminate much governmental red tape. This doubtless played a part in the notable esprit that marked the organization from the start. All the emphasis was on getting the job done. Mountin was MCWA's "defense line" in Washington and protected the staff when they did not follow the book.[18] Sib Simmons, who had a long and distinguished career in public health, remembers the freedom of those days during the war, when the "red tape" people were all in the

Army. If Simmons wanted something, he bought it on the market. (Once he found pontoons for a plane on Long Island. "Ship them today," he said. "I'll send you an order.") But as soon as the war was over, Simmons complained, the offices filled up with clerks, and things bogged down.[19] MCWA's distance from Washington—both geographic and administrative—born of wartime necessity, was a legacy long cherished by its much larger successor.

MCWA was but a few months old when the scope of its activities was expanded to include control of the *Aedes aegypti* mosquito, vector of yellow fever and dengue. Although there had been no cases of yellow fever in the United States since 1905, the fear that it might be imported through international air travel was very real, and the nation could expect an epidemic of dengue or "breakbone" fever about once a decade. Before the war, many cities in South America had eradicated *A. aegypti,* and, to protect its investment, Bolivia proposed to the Pan American Sanitary Conference in 1942 that the eradication program be extended to all the Americas.

The United States had to cooperate, at least to the extent of controlling the mosquito, not only to protect the nation's health, but to ensure that South American countries would not quarantine aircraft arriving from infested U.S. cities. The effort to control this most domesticated of mosquitoes was primarily one of education: teaching the public to eliminate the mosquitoes' breeding places around their own homes, like tin cans and old tires. It also involved spraying airplanes on intercontinental flights.[20]

It was Mountin who asked Hollis one day what MCWA would do if dengue broke out in the Pacific:

> I said, "I haven't thought of it."
> He said, "You damn well better think of it! I don't want to know how you do it, or what you do, but do it. Be ready."
> We began to set up some mobile teams. Well, we had a little dengue outbreak at the Key West Base, and . . . had just gotten it done when the Hawaiian epidemic broke. In a matter of 48 hours we had crews, equipment on army transports being flown to Hawaii. . . . We put [Wesley] Gilbertson in charge, gave him a field promotion because . . . the military detachment would be under a captain. He got the job done.

Mountin never took credit for success of the Hawaiian campaign. He answered all queries, "Well, we've got a good team down there."[21]

The 1943 appearance of dengue fever in Hawaii after an absence of thirty years underscored the danger of imported diseases in wartime, so MCWA redoubled its efforts. Working with scientists from the

National Institute of Health, MCWA learned that foreign malarias adapted readily to native anopheline vectors. To keep the situation under control, it extended its control measures from areas adjacent to strategic installations to any place malaria was endemic. It organized mobile units consisting of an entomologist and an engineer with a truck full of supplies and equipment; they roamed the countryside looking for danger.[22]

Just as MCWA expanded its concerns to protection of the civilian population, Louis Williams was ordered to Algeria to prepare for the invasion of Italy. There he renewed his friendship with Dr. Justin Andrews, the Army's chief malariologist and architect of the highly successful anti-malaria programs in Georgia in the 1930s. Andrews spent the war years traveling from one theater of war to the other devising plans of malaria control. In North Africa, Andrews and Williams sat under a palm tree one day and talked about the future. When the war was over, they decided, MCWA should be converted into a permanent agency dedicated to the control of communicable diseases, with headquarters in Atlanta. Andrews had lived in the city and he had close ties to people at Emory University. The combination of talent at Emory and MCWA, they believed, would provide a good foundation for a new kind of health institution.[23]

Williams did not play a major role in bringing these dreams to life. A heart attack kept him from returning to his duties in Atlanta. His older brother, Charles, assumed the responsibility of serving as MCWA director for about six months, but on the first day of the new year, January 1, 1944, Mark Hollis, the procurement genius who had finessed MCWA's acquisition of so many trucks and shovels, became MCWA's director.

Within a few months, MCWA's direction changed entirely. It was not Hollis but the coming of the miracle insecticide DDT in 1943 that was responsible for the shift. DDT (shorthand for dichloro-diphenyl-trichloro-ethane) was surely one of the things Williams and Andrews discussed under the North African palm. Andrews had just heard about it and could hardly believe the incredible stories. The British touted its ability to kill mosquitoes at any stage of the life cycle and to inhibit their reproduction for long periods of time. This seemed too fantastic to be true, and Andrews had his doubts until he tested DDT himself. He used it with great success in barracks and tents as a residual spray, and in Algiers and Naples he used it as a dusting powder to avert a possibly devastating epidemic of typhus (like malaria, a nemesis of war).

Williams became a DDT enthusiast. He believed that if you put DDT on young migratory birds, they would spread the chemical when they stopped at lakes and marshes on their way South.

DDT totally changed the approach to malaria control. From killing mosquito larvae or draining the areas where they bred, the emphasis shifted to residual spraying. It was to test residual-spray formulas and design equipment to apply it that Sib Simmons was recruited to head the Carter Laboratory in Savannah. If mosquitoes could be killed over a period of several months by spraying the walls and ceilings of houses, the attack could be narrowed to a very small segment of the mosquito population.[24]

Early reports were encouraging. At the end of three months, the Carter Laboratory reported that DDT worked. A house could be kept virtually free of mosquitoes for ten weeks or more at a cost of about $2.25. There were problems, however. Two of the solvents used, kerosene and pine oil, smelled bad, and kerosene was a fire hazard. A third solvent, Triton-Xylene, was more effective but was very irritating to the operator. The report noted briefly that DDT was an effective, cheap larvicide costing only one-fifth as much per acre as fuel oil. It was not until much later that it became obvious that there was more than one way to measure cost.[25]

DDT made possible MCWA's most dramatic project, the national malaria-control program that Louis Williams proposed and Congress funded in 1945. State and local health agencies actively participated in this program, designed to protect the general civilian population from returning military carriers of the disease. The first year, sixty-eight counties in nine states participated, and 600,000 homes were sprayed. In the second, there were more than a million.

Residual spraying with DDT was an entirely new approach to malaria control for civilians, one complicated by shortages of transportation, equipment, and trained personnel. District and state supervisory personnel went to Savannah for instruction and, in the tradition of each-one-teach-one, passed along what they had learned. Within two months, 1,200 men were in the field. Word of the magical properties of DDT preceded them. Most people were eager to have their homes sprayed; DDT fought off anything—flies, mosquitoes, bedbugs, fleas, cockroaches. When the program began, the incidence of malaria was at its lowest point in history, so it was difficult to measure the impact of extended malaria control, but those working in the program believed it to be significant.[26]

Two months after the program began, Mountin met with the staff in Atlanta. He listened as they reported on the popularity of DDT. It was so popular, in fact, that state and local health departments were pressured to the point of embarrassment. MCWA depended on the states to select the areas for control, and some awkward situations arose. Mountin issued a timely warning: unless the states were pinned down on their criteria for selecting counties to participate, MCWA would find itself guarding against gnats and cockroaches.

The extended malaria-control program provided MCWA with more money than it had equipment to do the job. Hollis hated to return the money, so he proposed that MCWA furnish the DDT, the chemicals to mix it with, and half the labor if localities would furnish trucks, spraying equipment, and supervision. While the work would not be done as well, it would educate people about DDT, control mosquitoes (and, indirectly, malaria), and buy a lot of goodwill.

Again Mountin issued a warning, reminding Hollis that MCWA had to satisfy Congress, and that Congress hated arbitrary judgment. Whenever demand for a program exceeded the supply, Congress demanded criteria that could be spelled out. Distribute the money among the states, Mountin advised, but have a good reason for it.[27]

Not long after DDT became an important part of insect control, Hollis had a telephone call from Surgeon General Parran. The Public Health Service had been given the responsibility for controlling murine typhus fever at all airfields, and Parran wanted MCWA to handle it. It was a logical expansion of MCWA's activities, and Parran believed that malaria and typhus could be eliminated at once. Hollis had experience in murine typhus control, and he knew a good bit about rats. He knew, for example, that they followed runs, like the coons he had trapped as a boy. From his work in the 1931 typhus epidemic in Dothan, Alabama, he had learned that fleas hitchhike along the runs, jumping from one rat to another. It was only when the flea could not find a rodent that it finally bit a human. He decided that the best approach was to forget the rat and concentrate on the fleas. So MCWA concentrated on rat runs, dusting them with DDT. Typhus miraculously disappeared; Hollis thought it was fantastic.[28]

Operating out of a field station in Thomasville, Georgia, MCWA moved cautiously into a broader typhus-control program, combining it with the spraying of houses for mosquitoes. While Congress approved its efforts, the Bureau of the Budget did not, so MCWA operated in a gray area. Mountin talked about it at the same staff meeting in which he had warned that malaria control could get out of hand and become a campaign against cockroaches. He estimated the cost of the DDT typhus-control program at between $600,000 and $700,000, but the Bureau of Budget refused to approve it on the grounds that the program would be operating in advance of knowledge. When the subject came up at a congressional committee hearing, however, several congressmen thought the malaria and typhus programs were complementary, and urged that work begin at once. Mountin thought they should wait at least until the congressional committee reported. "If it is acted on favorably by the House," Mountin told the MCWA staff, "perhaps next week we can reconcile our position with the Budget Bureau, be willing to be spanked and told not to do it again." Meanwhile, he suggested that they start using some of the malaria money and go to work. "We should study with a vengeance," he said. "We will have to cast out in many directions using a variety of techniques and improve our knowledge very quickly. . . . it is a matter of conscience and . . . I am sure the [Bureau of the] Budget and Congress will be quite insistent on that score."[29]

The House did approve an appropriation for the typhus-control program, and Mountin was ready to recommend that the PHS typhus control unit be moved to MCWA. It meant a transfer of equipment, supplies, and personnel, everything except the chief, Dr. C. R. Eskey, and his administrative staff. Still nothing official came from the Bureau of the Budget, and until it did, the impending transfer was to be kept secret. Within a week, however, it was old news that MCWA had taken over typhus control. George Tremmell, MCWA's administrative officer, announced that the typhus control unit had scooped MCWA on the news. Nearly all the men in the unit knew they were moving to Atlanta.[30]

At the time MCWA took over typhus work, it also moved into the control of other tropical diseases. This was another gray area insofar as the budget was concerned, and Hollis was not convinced that the agency had anything remotely resembling budget clearance for it. All he could get out of Washington was very vague: "We are taking over a program that was started down here anyway." It was a curious state of affairs, stemming from a 1944 resolution of the American Society of Tropical Medicine. With U.S. troops serving in tropical regions, the danger that tropical parasitic diseases would be introduced into the United States was very real. Because most American physicians knew little or nothing about many of these diseases, the society recommended that the Public Health Service develop a program to deal with the problem. Louis Williams, recovering from his heart attack, was assigned this task. An aide, Dr. Paul Weinstein, relieved him of as many duties as possible.

The most immediate concern was to improve the diagnostic capabilities of the nation's laboratories so that tropical diseases seldom seen in the United States would be recognized. At first, the plan was to train returning veterans at university centers, but this scheme was so impractical it was soon abandoned. Weinstein visited several of these centers, from Harvard to the University of California, and found that the pressures of war made the addition of new duties impossible. He approached the National Institute of Health, but it was too oriented toward basic research to take over such an "operational" program. Williams then suggested that MCWA could do the job. It already had a training program in place for its malaria-control workers, and this could be expanded. MCWA was willing, and a tropical diseases education program began. Instead of limiting the program to veterans, however, laboratory directors and technicians already employed by state and local health departments were to be trained.[31]

Weinstein moved to Atlanta to set up the program, and just a month before V-J Day, Dr. Marion Brooke, a member of the faculty of the University of Tennessee Medical School, became program director. By then MCWA had spread into several Atlanta buildings. Brooke's lab was set up in the old Baptist Bookstore at the corner of Baker and Peachtree Streets, where laboratory scientists shared the space with artists and physicians, all of whom were part of the training program. Also in the building were Harry Pratt's insect museum and, in the basement, in a room that must have been a vault at one time, the first library. It consisted of a few bookshelves and a modest selection of books and journals.

Brooke had reservations about moving to Atlanta, even though he was offered a commission in the Public Health Service as senior assistant sanitarian. Only when the Emory University Medical School promised him a job if he did not like it at MCWA did he decide the move was worthwhile. He never regretted the decision. Like the other officers in the commissioned corps who constituted a majority in the Atlanta offices, he proudly wore his uniform to work every day.[32]

All those uniforms awed young Mae Melvin, who joined the staff that summer, a newly minted master's degree in parasitology in hand. She was hired by Weinstein, and the two of them, with Brooke, who arrived shortly, had a "frenzied" time of it setting up the lab and getting ready for the first course.

The new training program amplified work already under way. Dr. Trawick Stubbs, a physician at MCWA, whom Brooke recalls as "a real thinker" and the nearest thing MCWA had to an epidemiologist, had already begun to send out stained slides to state health offices for study. It seemed quite logical to bring laboratory workers from these same offices to Atlanta for formal training.

The first course was held in October 1945. The class was to begin on Monday, and the microscopes did not arrive until Friday. Over the weekend, the microscopes had to be unpacked and assembled, and the last one was barely in place by Monday morning. Twenty-four students from nineteen states and British Columbia attended the six-week course, which had a favorable student-teacher ratio of about four to one. The course was so successful it became a legacy to the permanent agency that replaced MCWA and was repeated over and over again.[33]

Another legacy to the new institution was a ready response to calls for help from the states. The first of these came from Alabama, where there was an outbreak of amoebic dysentery in a mental institution. Brooke joined experts from the National Institute of Health, which had a long history of investigating epidemics, on the investigatory team. They found the source of the problem and recommended a solution. In later years when these kinds of investigations were inseparably linked to the epidemiology branch of CDC, old-timers from MCWA would remind the epidemiologists that these services began in the laboratory. It was obvious that the work of the laboratory would be concerned with more than training, so in March 1946, the laboratory was separated from MCWA's Training and Education Division and set on its own path. This was an important step in the transition of MCWA to a new institution.

Expansion into new areas did not mean that MCWA forgot about malaria. As the war came to a close, the incidence of malaria was so low that it seemed quite feasible to think in terms of eradicating it altogether. Louis Williams first suggested an eradication program in 1943; the next year the National Malaria Society endorsed the concept, and in 1946 the Public Health Service proposed a five-year eradication plan. It was about that time that Justin Andrews was mustered out of the Army and joined the Atlanta group. For Andrews, it was more than a homecoming. It was his North African dream come true. He knew that MCWA was about to be given a greatly broadened mandate.

The Atlanta staff, stimulated by Mountin to think big, were looking ahead even before the war was over. "I don't say it to be throwing any scare into you folks," Mountin told a MCWA staff meeting two weeks after the war was over in Europe, "but we must look forward to the time when the war ends." MCWA had established a pattern that would enable it to move into other diseases. The question was how to encourage the states to move from a position of accepting what was done for them to one of doing for themselves. A staff member suggested that they start with a name change, perhaps to the Office of Infectious Diseases.[34]

Expanding MCWA was not a new idea for Mountin. He hinted at this as early as January 1942, when he wrote that the defense emergency could result in an improvement in civilian health; that after the war, services having to do with improving the health status of the general population could be developed. He wanted several centers of excellence: one in Cincinnati, Ohio, to combat water and air pollution; one in Alaska for the study of Arctic health; and one in Atlanta for communicable diseases. The last would be dedicated to serving the needs of the states.[35] Mountin is generally credited as the man who originated this new categorical approach to public health, the man with the vision, but Surgeon General Parran gave him wholehearted support. Hollis, who served as director of MCWA during the transition, described Mountin as "the real giant in getting the PHS into domestic health problems in the states. He cared not one iota for his reputation or what others thought about his views, but he pressed ahead strongly."[36]

Mountin secured congressional approval for a new center built on the foundation of MCWA, even though no formal act of Congress was necessary. The PHS itself had all the authority it needed to set such a center up as a demonstration project, although, of course, Congress had to fund it. The way was smoothed in the appropriations committees by passing around photographs of MCWA trucks and jeeps, equipped with power sprayers, protecting the South against malaria. Several names were proposed before Communicable Disease Center (CDC) was decided upon. Hollis and Mountin shied away from using the word *institute* in the title: it was too much of a red flag for both Congress and NIH. *Center* was softer; and specifying that it would be concerned with communicable disease narrowed its scope. (Hollis thought it narrowed it too much: it left no room for what he considered the vital study of the environment).[37]

Both Hollis and Mountin anticipated that NIH would probably object to the formation of a possible rival, so they mapped their strategy carefully. At the meeting when the establishment of CDC was to be proposed, they would insist that Dr. Rolla E. Dyer, director of NIH, speak first. They expected that he would set up "straw men" in opposition to the CDC, which Mountin and Hollis would then knock down. Dyer would surely speak of competition for scientists, of overlapping and duplication of work, of politics and appropriations. How could Congress be brought to understand that if a field station were needed, it should not be a field station of NIH? Mountin and Hollis would argue that NIH was concerned essentially with basic research, while the proposed CDC would be concerned with practical service to the states.

The meeting began well. Surgeon General Parran called on Mountin to speak, who in turn deferred to Dr. Dyer. Everyone looked to Dyer in research, Mountin said, and all could learn by listening to him. No one expected Dyer's response: "I've gone over the proposal carefully, Dr. Parran. I don't see anything wrong with it. It's a good idea." He liked the emphasis that CDC would put on disease control, and he approved of its laboratory to support work in the field.

Mountin appeared dumbfounded at such an easy victory. "Well, now, wait a minute," an astonished Hollis heard him say. Mountin then introduced all those "straw men" he and Hollis had thought Dyer would raise. "It wound up," Hollis said, "with Dr. Mountin bringing them up and Dr. Dyer knocking them down! It was amazing! There was Mountin making not the slightest explanation, such as 'I did this to get it all out on the table.' I thought it illustrated completely that Dr. Mountin's whole energy and heart was in the work of getting it done, and he didn't care where he stood in people's minds at all."[38]

In retrospect, it was not surprising that Dyer had no objections to an institution that would emphasize disease control, for this left NIH much freer to pursue basic research, particularly in chronic diseases. Mountin had tried without success to push NIH into more application of health knowledge. Norman Topping, a member of the NIH staff at the time, remembers Mountin as "an abrasive character who wanted things done and wanted them done fast. . . . Joe was resentful that NIH would not take the more practical aspects of control in the states and do something about it. He said, 'By gosh, if you don't do it, I'll do it. I'll take the Bureau of State Services, and we'll do it! We'll do it!'"[39]

With Mountin's push and Dyer's blessing, on July 1, 1946, the Communicable Disease Center began operations.

The Lengthened
Shadow of a Man (1)

The CDC was the capstone of Joseph Mountin's effort to supply state and local health units with the support they needed. It would focus on the traditional concern of public health—communicable diseases—but its approach would be different, its mission broader than anything attempted before.

During World War I, when state health departments were incomplete and local ones almost nonexistent, Mountin learned how vital local support was to maintaining the health of army camps. Commissioned in the regular corps after the war, Mountin served briefly in the quarantine service, but soon was assigned to Missouri, where his job was to encourage local officials to protect public health. There he learned to improvise. "In quarantine," he told Thomas Parran, "we work by the book, but down here there isn't any book, so. . . ." His work in Missouri and later in Tennessee convinced him that state and local communities should take responsibility for public health, but that the PHS should make complex knowledge of science and medicine usable. He spent the rest of his career trying to meet that need.[1]

The far-flung Public Health Service was transferred in 1939 from the Treasury Department to the Federal Security Administration when the Roosevelt administration put under one head all those departments of government devoted to social and economic security, educational opportunity, and health. The PHS had many functions. It provided medical services for merchant seamen, federal prisoners, coast guardsmen, lepers, and narcotics addicts. It conducted medical examinations for immigrants, federal employees, and longshoremen. It administered public health grants to the states and conducted venereal disease and tuberculosis-control programs. It also administered the Biologics Control Act, the cancer program, and intramural research at NIH.[2] Mountin was eager for the PHS to get involved in more and more fields. When he decided someone should be an expert in cancer control, he sent Leonard Scheele, a future surgeon general, to New York to study at Memorial Hospital, and, when the National Cancer Institute had money to spare, got Scheele to establish studies of the epidemiology of cancer in various hospitals throughout the United States. Mountin also initiated a program in heart-disease control and diabetes detection and established the Framingham Center, where important studies of heart disease were made. He wanted the states to have techniques for handling chronic illnesses.[3] On this broad stage, Mountin assigned his newest creation, CDC, the control of communicable diseases, a more traditional role for public health. As a field station of the State Relations Division of the Bureau of State Services, CDC would stand by to help the states. Nothing remotely like it had ever existed before.

CDC did not appear to be very different from its predecessor, MCWA. Mark Hollis still sat in the director's chair, persuaded to stay on for a few months to provide stability for the malaria and typhus programs. After six months, he left. Eager to rise in the Public Health Service, he knew there was no way to put stars on his shoulders at CDC.

His second in command, the deputy officer in charge, was Justin Andrews, just mustered out of the Army, an expert on malaria, and a member of the PHS Scientist Corps. A red-headed native of Rhode Island, Andrews coupled a Puritan commitment to hard work with a flair for the imaginative.[4] He was an extraordinary administrator, and at CDC he had a chance to hone these skills. He had responsibility for day-to-day activities under both Hollis and his successor, Dr. Raymond Vonderlehr, a patriarch who was happy to have someone else handle the details. Andrews brought order, energy, and enthusiasm to the job. He kept his desktop clear by using one top drawer as an in box and another as an out box.[5] This small detail was symbolic of a sense of order important to a new institution.

Andrews hated to waste time, especially in meetings.[6] He wrote terse, precise prose and kept an unabridged dictionary in constant use. He believed both time and clarity were wasted in verbose writing. Aware that the reputations of scientists and scientific institutions rise and fall on the quality of their publications, Andrews insisted that the writing of his staff be as sound and forceful as their research. "You have a tendency to use 'asides,'" he complained to a staff member whose paper he had reviewed. "Frequently these interrupt continuity and weaken the statement. . . . I would sacrifice academic precision to the forcefulness of simple, unqualified expression."[7]

Dr. Vonderlehr, who took over as CDC director in January 1947, was quite different from the scientist Andrews. He was a physician, an old-line officer in the commissioned corps of the Public Health Service who had served at a time when rank had its privileges, when the corps was a guild, when the surgeon general was in his office and all was right with the world. Just as there are cycles in the military when there are prestige services, like battleships, or aviation or submarines, so there are cycles in the Public Health Service when there are prestige units. In the 1920s and 1930s, this was the venereal disease branch, and Vonderlehr was part of it.

The branch was started by Dr. Thomas Parran, who later became surgeon general. Parran brought it to great prominence at a time when some of the most outstanding physicians in the country sought careers in public health. During the depression, the PHS offered relatively high salaries, but this was only part of the reason for successful recruiting. The forcefulness of Parran's character loomed large in the program's success. He made the venereal disease division a kind of boot camp for those who would run all the branches of the service in the years to come. The men he trained were both competent and dedicated. Among them was Raymond Vonderlehr.

Parran and Vonderlehr were close personal friends. They worked together in the 1930s to bring knowledge about venereal disease out of the closet so that the problem could be tackled in a forthright way. Parran's *Shadow on the Land: Syphilis,* published in 1937, recounts the struggle to gain acceptance for using the word *syphilis* in polite company and on the radio. When Parran became surgeon general, Vonderlehr became head of the Venereal Disease Division, one of the most important positions in the Public Health Service. During World War II, however, the Army ran its own venereal disease program, and Vonderlehr, who was critical of the military, lost favor. He was moved out of the service's most elite unit to become director of PHS Region III in Puerto Rico. From there he came to Atlanta. His exile from the center of power did not dim his commitment to the Public Health Service, however, and Vonderlehr brought to his new job the enthusiasm and esprit de corps that he learned from Parran.[8]

Dr. Vonderlehr was a Virginia gentleman, courtly of manner, yet dynamic. His dedication to the corps was absolute, and he protected it absolutely, even to the point of taking young officers to his home and plying them with liquor to see how well they handled themselves. At CDC he set himself the important task of building the kind of esprit that marked the old Venereal Disease Division. "He was what all chiefs of CDC should be," one of those who worked with him recalled years later. Every Friday he made a pilgrimage to the offices and laboratories to see what was needed and what he could do.[9]

It was Andrews who outlined the scope of CDC's work. Its interests would be expanded from tropical diseases with insect vectors to include all those of zoological origin: malaria, amebiasis, the schistosomiases, hookworm disease, filariasis, yellow fever, dengue, certain neurovirologic disorders, various forms of typhus and plague, sand-fly fever, and diverse diarrheas and dysenteries. He considered this heterogeneous collection "eminently sound, sensible, and workable from the standpoints of laboratory diagnosis, epidemiologic investigation, and control operations."[10]

Challenging as the list was, Dr. Mountin was not satisfied. The range of diseases was entirely too narrow. Officially the Atlanta institution was not responsible for control of tuberculosis and venereal diseases, but everything else communicable came within its purview. Whenever Mountin saw references in press releases or in the budget to the CDC's preoccupation with diseases "known or suspected to be caused, vectored, or reservoired by lower animals," he rebuked Andrews impatiently.

"Dr. Mountin was anxious to see his brain child develop as quickly as possible in the direction of laboratory medicine and epidemiology applied to a much broader spectrum of communicable disease than that which was vectored by insects or rodents," Andrews wrote a few months after Mountin's sudden death at the age of sixty-one in 1952. "But the earnest efforts made toward that goal were thwarted largely by the unavailability in 1946 to 1948 of skilled personnel in communicable disease investigation and control, especially with medical backgrounds."[11]

For the first year or so of its existence, CDC did what MCWA had been doing. The staff concentrated on malaria control with an eye to eradicating it entirely. There was some reluctance to use the word *eradication*, however, so it was called simply the "extended program." By 1947 the semantic argument ended and the National Malaria Eradication Program became official. Thirteen states from North Carolina to Texas participated. Mark Hollis told the National Malaria Society that malaria would be wiped out within a few years by the "shoe-leather scientists," who would tramp and tramp until they found an area where malaria still occurred.[12]

Eradication could have been achieved by eliminating all malaria parasites from humans or by annihilating all anopheles mosquitoes, but these methods were too expensive. Instead, the decision was made to reduce both malaria parasites and vectors to the point where general transmission could not occur. This was a joint state-federal venture. CDC paid for spray and provided equipment and experienced personnel; state and local governments paid for labor. The massive spraying campaign was carried out by two- and three-man crews operating from light trucks. If houses were close together, power sprayers were used; if not, the work was done by hand. CDC set up observation stations in three notably malarious areas.

Pursuit of malaria was by far the most absorbing interest of CDC. During the first year of operations, 59 percent of its personnel were engaged in it; during the second, 51 percent. By definition this meant that Engineering was the largest division in the organization, and that Entomology also played a major role. By the time the program ended in 1952, more than six and a half million homes had been sprayed. Cheerful progress reports lent hope that the program would serve as a model for the eradication of malaria in the world. There were skeptics within the ranks of CDC, however, who said that malaria was a "Trojan Horse" that could slip in unawares.[13]

Much of the CDC's most important work was done at field stations and laboratories outside Atlanta. Just before Dr. Vonderlehr assumed his duties as director, Hollis and Dr. Mountin took him on a tour of these stations in Georgia and Alabama. It took them a week to inspect the work being done in Savannah, Thomasville, and the Emory Field Station, all in south Georgia, and at the virus laboratory in Montgomery, Alabama. Savannah was headquarters for the Technical Development Division, which in 1946 still occupied the small Henry Rose Carter laboratory. Much entomology work was done both there and at the Emory Field Station on Ichuaway Plantation in Baker County. Thomasville was headquarters for work on typhus, and the new laboratory for the study of viruses and rickettsia, formerly headquarters for the Rockefeller Foundation's rabies study, had just opened in Montgomery. It was there that CDC began its own rabies work under the direction of Dr. Ernest S. Tierkel.

CDC needed better facilities. Its nine divisions (the large number reflected an institution feeling its way) were cramped. Only the Technical Laboratory in Savannah, which in 1947 moved from the small Carter Laboratory to spacious quarters on Oatland Island, was adequately housed. The Brotherhood of Railway Conductors had built a beautiful retirement home there, one it did not need after the Railway Retirement Act was passed. When the conductors moved out, the WPA and the PHS took over the building. During the war, it was a rapid-treatment center for venereal disease. When CDC acquired it, the main building was converted to laboratory space, and about fifteen more structures were added. From Oatland Island came an incredible flow of information about the life cycle of insects and the best insecticides and equipment to control them, as well as important information on toxicology.[14]

In spite of its poor facilities, the Laboratory Division in Atlanta and Montgomery attracted a distinguished staff. Laboratory Director Seward Miller, a solid, experienced officer in the commissioned corps, was the "pied piper of recruitment," reminiscent of Parran in his heyday. Besides Dr. Marion Brooke in parasitology, there were Dr. Martin Frobisher in bacteriology, Dr. Morris Schaeffer in virology, Dr. Libero Ajello in mycology, and Dr. Philip Edwards, a leading authority on diarrheal organisms. Their distinguished work laid the foundation for much of CDC's success. By the time Miller left to become a regional director of the Federal Security Administration in 1950, the Laboratory Division had five major sections and 225 employees working in laboratories spread from San Francisco to Atlanta and Puerto Rico.

The business of the laboratory, as Miller saw it, was to assist the CDC's Epidemiology Division in emergencies, do research on diagnostic techniques, act as a reference diagnostic center for difficult specimens, and offer training for the states' laboratory technicians. For the first few years, the laboratory experts could concentrate on research, diagnosis, and training, for they got relatively few calls from the minuscule Epidemiology Division. Eventually Epidemiology would spearhead the investigation of communicable diseases, but finding leadership for it was, as Andrews put it, "a most arduous task." The fact that the laboratory was off and running before the epidemiologists got a good start may account in part for the testiness that often marked relations between the two groups in the years to come.[15]

A cornerstone of MCWA was training, and at Mountin's insistence the Training Division expanded its activities in 1945. In ten years, the number of local health departments in the United States had more than doubled, and Mountin knew there were not enough trained workers to staff them. "The states are bereft of personnel," he told Ellis Tisdale, who was hired to direct the expanded program. "We have taken away from [them] their sanitation personnel; they're in the Army or the PHS." The experts in Atlanta, Mountin insisted, had to do something about it: they had to provide practical training in the field.

Tisdale had butterflies in his stomach when he took on the job. A New England native, he did not know how he would be accepted in the deep South, but soon he found himself launched on the "finest experience" of his life. Within two months, he had the first course under way. It was conducted at the county health department in Savannah early in 1946, and it proved so popular it was repeated by popular demand. During the first year, sixty students from the southeastern states, Ohio, Indiana, and Ecuador were trained there. Tisdale next set up a field training station in sanitary engineering in Columbus, Georgia, primarily to serve the needs of the southeastern United States. The idea spread. When Dr. Vonderlehr dropped by the training division one day, he suggested setting up training stations outside the South. Why not New York and New England?

The courses attracted many foreign students. The United States created the Marshall Plan in 1948 to rebuild war-devastated Europe, and in 1949 financed President Truman's Point Four program to assist the underdeveloped world, so it was perfectly natural that some of these nations would look to the United States for help with health problems. Within four years, what had started as a trickle became a flood. More than four hundred visitors from sixty-six different countries came in 1950. For the increasingly popular course for sanitary engineers in Columbus, more than half the trainees came from abroad.[16]

Extensive use of audiovisual material eased the language problems. Even Hollis, who had very little interest in this aspect of the work, admitted the unit did a "fantastic" job. Gale Griswold, of California, just released from the Navy, came to Atlanta to direct the program and turned his corner of CDC into the Hollywood of health films. By 1949 his artists and camera crews turned out fifty moving pictures and filmstrips a year, some of them translated into Persian, Greek, Spanish, or Italian. Their stars were mostly rats, tapeworms, and microscopic organisms.[17]

The Veterinary Public Health Division was added in 1947, with tall, super-confident Dr. James Steele as director. He was commissioned as a sanitarian in the Public Health Service in 1943 and spent most of the war in Puerto Rico. En route to another assignment in the summer of 1945, he stopped by Washington to visit with Dr. Mountin. "Now that the war is over," Mountin asked him, "what are you veterinarians going to do to improve the nation's health?" Steele did not have a ready answer, so the ever-innovative Mountin charged him to come up with a program. "Just stick with diseases," he told Steele. "Stay away from milk and food sanitation problems. That is work for engineers."

Instead of proceeding to his new post, Steele spent the next three or four months in the library of the National Institute of Health drawing up a list of the diseases of animals that impinged on the public health and developing a plan to deal with them. Mountin liked it, set up a veterinary section in Building T-6 at NIH, and put Steele in charge. In recognition of the new importance assigned to zoonoses, the PHS created a new category of commissioned officers for veterinarians. Steele got his new commission a few weeks before his unit moved to CDC in September 1947.[18]

As CDC's work grew, so did the need for more space. In the summer of 1946, the staff learned that the Veterans Hospital at Chamblee, an Atlanta suburb, was available. It was just a row of barracks with ten wards, an auditorium and a chapel, but it had 40,000 square feet of desperately needed space. Lawson Hospital could house the Laboratory Division temporarily until the new building was ready. Everyone was confident construction would begin within a few months. But temporary buildings have an odd way of becoming permanent, and the months of temporary use at Chamblee stretched into years, and the years into decades. In the late 1980s, major portions of CDC were still there.

The durability of the Chamblee buildings may be attributed in large part to the ingenuity of Bob Shackleford, CDC's buildings and grounds genius. He loved Chamblee and always saw to it that the grounds were well kept. When DeKalb County extended the airport adjacent to the laboratories, Shackleford managed to save buildings that would have been demolished. Georgia's Senator Richard B. Russell got them declared surplus property, and Shackleford put a belt around them and moved them out of the way. There was little he could do to mitigate the vibrations caused by planes taking off and landing at the enlarged airport, however, and these created problems for the scientists.

Even with the barracks at Chamblee, there was not enough room, so more space was rented in downtown Atlanta. By 1949 CDC occupied thirty-five buildings in Atlanta, Montgomery, and Savannah. Two years later, some of the Atlanta activities were gathered under one roof in the recently completed Peachtree–Seventh Street Building, a huge 370,000 square foot structure that housed thirteen government agencies. CDC had the entire fourth floor. The white brick, block-long building, with its nine miles of fluorescent light tubing, was dazzling by night, but it was not what CDC wanted.[19]

The staff wanted a building designed specifically for them, and the prospects seemed bright. In 1947 Emory University bought fifteen acres of land on Clifton Road adjacent to the Emory campus and donated it to the Public Health Service. A four- or five-story building, described by the press as the "largest field station of the PHS," was to be built. The price tag was $2 to $4 million. In July 1948, the new surgeon general, Dr. Leonard Scheele, came to Atlanta to accept the property, which was presented by Emory's President Goodrich C. White and the chairman of the Board of Trustees, Charles Howard Candler. The surgeon general promised that "the world's greatest center of communicable disease research and control would be built . . . a health institution of real credit and service to the nation." CDC employees raised a $10 token payment to make the transfer legal.

The gift of land came at the behest of Robert C. Woodruff, chairman of the board of Coca-Cola Company and for many years a member of the Board of Trustees of Emory University. He long had been interested in malaria control. It was Dr. Glenville Giddings, Emory physician, medical advisor to Coca-Cola, and director of mosquito-control projects for the Georgia Power Company, who probably encouraged Woodruff's interest in the Public Health Service and thus brought Emory and the CDC so close together. Giddings knew Mountin well and conferred with him often either in Atlanta or Washington, and he and Mark Hollis, the center's first director, were close personal friends.

Two years after the Clifton Road site was transferred to the Public Health Service, the General Services Administration announced plans for construction of five buildings for CDC. They were the first buildings not related to defense authorized by the government since 1940. The price tag had gone up since the first announcement; the new estimated price of construction was $10 million. Workers at CDC were ecstatic and barely noticed the caveat in the announcement: ". . . if Congress appropriates the money."[20]

The need for more and more space testified to the amount of work under way at the new Communicable Disease Center. To tackle particular problems, various laboratories were established across the United

States. In San Francisco, CDC took over the PHS Plague Laboratory in 1947, and with that acquisition formally acquired an Epidemiology Division. The laboratory director, Dr. Vernon Link, moved to Atlanta as chief of epidemiology. In a quonset hut in Kansas City, work began on histoplasmosis, a disease of particular importance to the Midwest. An old school building in Greeley, Colorado, served as quarters for the study of encephalitis, particularly in the wild bird population. And in Phoenix, Arizona, and Pharr, Texas, a major study on diarrheal diseases was under way, with intense interest focused on the fly. Other specialized studies were done at stations in Wenatchee, Washington; Manning, South Carolina; and Charleston, West Virginia.

The diarrheal-diseases project was unique in that it involved both CDC and NIH. It was designed to learn if flies could be controlled economically without destroying beneficial insects, and what effect that control had on enteric diseases like diarrhea. Because the polio virus had been isolated from flies, there also was an investigation of polio and fly control.[21] Numerous skeptics at CDC urged a measure of caution, since there was no real evidence that flies carried polio, and warned against raised public expectations.

No less was known about polio, however, than about any number of other diseases. To Mountin this was an advantage, not a handicap. "There seems to be a lot of ignorance here," he once said to Steele. "Let's exploit it."[22] Exploitation of ignorance led to many productive programs at CDC. An obvious one dealt with the pesticide DDT. It was marvelously effective, at least until insects developed a resistance to it, but little or nothing was known about its effect on man. With millions of people being exposed to DDT and other poisons, Mountin was convinced such ignorance must be exploited. He assigned the job to the Technical Development Laboratory in Savannah. The toxicology of pesticides was a new field in 1949, and Dr. Simmons did not have anyone especially trained to do the work. As a stopgap measure, he persuaded Dr. Wayland Hayes, who had been working on typhus, to fill in until he could find someone else. Hayes became one of the leading toxicologists of the world, and his replacement never came.[23]

There were no warm-ups for CDC's entry into the field of disaster aid. Multiple explosions in Texas City in April 1947 killed hundreds of people and left the city devastated. Within hours a CDC crew was there to help. "Aid furnished by the Public Health Service . . . may develop a pattern for future assistance in cases of disaster," the minutes of the CDC staff meeting recorded a week later. When voluntary help dispersed after a few days, the county health unit was saddled with heavy problems. The Public Health Service was most needed then. CDC worked in Texas City for seven months, keeping flies and mosquitoes under control as a guard against the outbreak of disease.[24]

Six months after the Texas City explosions, CDC was designated as the PHS agency to administer aid in times of disaster or epidemics. Unfortunately, money to finance this help was in short supply. In 1949 when CDC responded to twenty-one epidemics and disasters—primarily floods—it had but $40,000 in non-emergency funds, hardly enough to stockpile the medical supplies, portable water-treatment plants, spray equipment, and other necessary items. Andrews thought it needed half a million dollars.[25]

With its background in malaria control, CDC may have been better prepared to offer aid in disasters than in epidemics. It did respond to calls for help for diarrheal-disease outbreaks in Mississippi and Alabama, for polio epidemics in Minnesota and Texas, for typhoid fever in Illinois. Many of the calls concerned intestinal parasites, and from the beginning CDC had the laboratory expertise to deal with these. Nevertheless, the PHS's response was uncertain and often delayed. An outbreak of amoebic dysentery in Ohio in 1947 may serve as an example. A request for help went first to the PHS regional director, then to NIH, next to the Bureau of State Services, and finally to CDC. A month and four days had elapsed between the call for help and the response.[26]

Whether in answer to requests for disaster or epidemic aid, the CDC sometimes encountered opposition from better-established wings of the Public Health Service that resented the intrusion of a newcomer. In disasters, it was the regional health director who was most likely to complain. One of them wrote insistently to Vernon Link that all requests for aid should be made to the district director, "who can then determine whether or not his District Office could furnish the assistance, or whether the aid of the Communicable Disease Center was indicated." Link agreed to the demand, but it was a cumbersome system, one that prompted Vonderlehr to complain to Mountin that it would be far better if the center could approach the states directly. As a matter of fact, relations between the CDC and the regional offices were often testy. CDC personnel frequently bypassed the regional offices, even though they were regularly admonished not to do so.[27]

The National Institutes of Health (made plural in 1948) also resented the upstart institution in Atlanta, even though the NIH director, Dr. Dyer, supported it. Representatives of CDC and NIH met to divide up the responsibilities: NIH would do basic research, CDC would help the

HEADQUARTERS ORGANIZATION

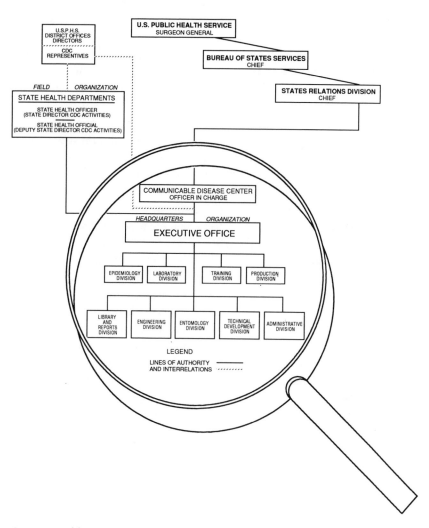

Communicable Disease Center (relationship to the PHS and headquarters), 1946–47

states recognize and control communicable diseases. But the line between the two was not always clear. NIH and its predecessor, the Hygienic Laboratory, had a long and distinguished record of response to epidemics—encephalitis, typhus, Rocky Mountain spotted fever, diphtheria, and pellagra, among others—and some staff members were reluctant to give up fieldwork. Many scientists in NIH's new National Microbiological Institute had served for years as reference serologists and entomologists and continued to do so. NIH used the field, however, only to the extent that it was necessary to support and clarify bench work. The NIH researcher went to the field, not to control disease, but to substantiate his work in the laboratory. CDC's role was just the opposite. Its primary role was to control disease, and the bench would be used as necessary to back that up. This did not mean that CDC's laboratory work would be routine. Andrews recognized that CDC could not do its job without new basic knowledge and must have personnel as gifted and qualified as those at NIH in Bethesda. When CDC hired outside consultants without turning first to Bethesda, the scientists at NIH were offended.[28]

The consultants CDC hired in the spring of 1948, and to which NIH objected, gave advice on how to strengthen the moribund Epidemiology Division. Overwhelmed by the mass of non-medical forces at CDC, no one had succeeded at epidemiology. Mountin reportedly read the riot act to the CDC staff, telling them that if they did not get a competent epidemiologist, CDC would go down the drain. Obviously something stirred the staff to action because at a meeting in late February, they talked about how CDC was to carry out its mission. If they were to advance the knowledge of the transmission, animal reservoirs, and methods of control of communicable disease, delineate areas where control was needed, and evaluate the results, then "a lot more time and effort had to go into the planning of the program." They needed help. The consultants met for the first time in Atlanta in April to discuss psittacosis, ornithosis, poliomyelitis, diarrhea and dysentery, encephalitis, typhus control, and malaria epidemiology.

Meanwhile, the Epidemiology Division wrote job descriptions and established positions in grades high enough to attract those scarce persons with training and experience. "It is going to be very difficult to employ such people as these," the minutes of the staff meeting record, "as there aren't very many, and they all have jobs. The only possibility is to make the assignment here more attractive than the one they now have, and entice them away from someone else. The Division is attempting also to recruit young medical officers interested in the field of epidemiology for the regular corps to do the leg work and gain experience so that eventually—in five or ten years from now—well qualified and capable personnel will be available." The Statistical Branch had to be expanded, too, for epidemiology and statistics are the twin pillars of a single science.[29]

It took many months, but the search paid off. More than a year later minutes of the CDC staff meeting reflected a decidedly upbeat mood:

> Dr. Langmuir is coming with CDC in charge of Epidemiology Division sometime in June.
>
> Dr. Miller commended Dr. Serfling, recently appointed in Temporary Charge of the Statistical Branch of the Epidemiology Division, on the excellent work he is doing in the Statistical Branch.
>
> The first one of our series of short courses for laboratory directors was begun this morning at Lawson.
>
> Dr. Morris Schaeffer is to be placed in charge of the Virus and Rickettsial Branch Laboratory at Montgomery, Alabama. He will report for duty in June.[30]

All the news was good, but the first item, noting the impending arrival of Dr. Alexander Langmuir, signaled a watershed in CDC's development. Epidemiology would become the hallmark of the institution, and Langmuir's name synonymous with the aggressive pursuit of disease. He came to Atlanta at a fortuitous moment. The institution was young and there was no set pattern of doing things. Langmuir himself was well trained, aggressive, and organized, and like Mountin, who became his close friend, he knew how to operate when and where there were no ground rules. In the long run, his influence permeated not only CDC but medical schools and medical practice. In the short run, he cut the waiting time for sending CDC epidemiologists into the field from the anticipated five to ten years to only two.

It was Justin Andrews who persuaded Langmuir to come. Andrews taught at the School of Hygiene and Public Health at the Johns Hopkins University before he became malariologist for the state of Georgia in 1937. Langmuir was an associate professor there in 1949, teaching double sessions and, as he put it, "using his capital of experience and not going anywhere." His friends thought he was crazy to go to CDC, a place they viewed as peopled by "a bunch of broken-down malariologists, [with] a non-medical dominance." It was the last place in the world to go. Langmuir saw it quite differently. "Andrews," he said, "took me up the mountain and showed me the promised land."

Langmuir admired many things about the Atlanta institution. He liked Andrews, whom he credited with being the imaginative creator of CDC and its effective leader. He admired the spunkiness of the place. Even without an epidemiologist, it had a program of epidemic aid to the states, and it had multiprofessional teams already at work on big problems like encephalitis. The laboratory was well staffed and through its training and reference diagnostic programs provided excellent service to the states. CDC was breaking out of the malaria tradition of World War II to become an organization to aid states in control of communicable disease. "The range of opportunity, the potential was obvious," Langmuir recalled, "and with my considerable self confidence, I had no trouble going."[31]

A few months after Langmuir's arrival, the Association of State and Territorial Health officers held its first annual conference at CDC. They learned what CDC—the "combat division" in the war against communicable diseases, Surgeon General Scheele called it—could and could not do for them. It could help the states with emergencies, provide diagnostic help for difficult cases, and offer training. Dr. Reginald M. Atwater of the American Public Health Association pledged the association's support for the Atlanta institution and announced that CDC would help prepare future editions of its widely acclaimed report, *The Control of Communicable Diseases*. It was Langmuir's first opportunity to meet the men on whom much of the success of his efforts would depend. He talked about communicable diseases, and he reeled off those that had been substantially eliminated, those on which much progress had been made, and those that still posed a threat. He also explained what epidemiology is: the study of the factors that determine the balance between the host and the parasite. Infectious disease exists because neither the host nor the parasite can destroy the other. They have achieved an unstable biological balance. Epidemiology is concerned with the factors that cause this balance to fluctuate, the object being to provide a scientific basis for altering those trends in favor of man.

Before the conference was over, the state health officers agreed that the Public Health Service and the American Public Health Association should study the diseases that were reportable and make recommendations on additions to or deletions from the list, and that the PHS should establish morbidity requirements for notifiable diseases. Langmuir got permission to call a meeting of the state epidemiologists in the spring to talk about the fundamental importance of reporting communicable diseases.[32]

The state epidemiologists gathered in Atlanta the following April. Although few of them had any training in epidemiology, they were an independent and self-reliant bunch and Langmuir deliberately built up their self-esteem. He gave them the responsibility of deciding what diseases should be reported. They argued back and forth on whether rabies, for example, should be included, since it was a disease of animals. Eventually, they decided that it should. "But it was their decision," Langmuir recalled, "and that made all the difference." The Atlanta meeting was the first of many. After 1950, the state epidemiologists gathered every two years to go over the list.[33]

When the epidemiologists were brought into CDC's orbit, Mountin's plan for an institution that would be of service to the states was complete. Langmuir thought it brilliant. "The chief epidemiologist related to the state epidemiologist; the chief of the lab branch related to the chief of the state lab branch; the technology branch related to engineering services; the training branch to training service. Each had a critical line of communication in an orderly form." Passage of the Public Health Act of 1966 made the cycle of communications complete. It provided that regional health directors of the PHS (who had not faded away) have access to governors of the states. They made a formal visit once a year to discuss problems. CDC funneled its proposals to the governors through the regional directors. According to Langmuir, "[It was] long-term planning, nicely structured. When we paid attention, it worked beautifully."[34]

Langmuir received a warm welcome at CDC, and he began work at once. He was convinced that malaria already had been eradicated, but CDC was still spraying DDT in thirteen states and the program had a $7 million budget. Not everyone agreed that malaria no longer posed a threat. Entomologists insisted that a barrier against malaria be maintained, but Andrews agreed with Langmuir; malaria had diminished to the vanishing point. In 1947 Andrews had initiated a program of malaria appraisal to evaluate progress towards eradication of the disease. He assigned medical and nurse epidemiologists to check each case, a task in which they were soon drowning because of the huge number of cases reported. Most of these cases came from only a few physicians, however, a clue that false reporting, not the spread of disease, was at work.

Langmuir proposed a different approach. He had been on the staff but six months when he wrote a memo suggesting a surveillance program paid for with malaria funds. A team of four would be assigned to each state: an epidemiologist, a nurse epidemiologist, an engineer, and an entomologist. The epidemiologists would investigate and evaluate every malaria case. When they found one that definitely could be confirmed by laboratory diagnosis, the entomologist and the engineer would be brought in to mount appropriate control programs. Langmuir recalled the memo as "crucial." It dealt with engineers and entomologists on an equal basis with medical personnel, but it moved CDC away from their dominance and towards an emphasis on epidemiology.

CDC was indeed cutting its staff as malaria operations were reduced in scale. Wesley Gilbertson, an engineer who served as CDC's executive officer, told Langmuir later that the staff supported his project because they knew he could not get the necessary medical epidemiologists. That proved to be true, but nine nurses were assigned to epidemiologic studies, and the program went forward.

Langmuir was confident that most of the reported cases of malaria were bogus, but he did not say it too loudly. Andrews knew it, too. CDC had entrenched personnel doing what had at one time been intelligent, but that time had passed.

Malaria-surveillance teams were assigned full-time to Mississippi and South Carolina, and for part of the year in Georgia, Alabama, Arkansas, and Texas. They investigated as many of the reported malaria cases and deaths as they could, and gathered information of epidemiological significance: How frequent were attacks? Had the victim been out of the country to malarious areas? Had there been recent transfusions? What treatment was given? A copy of the team's report went to state epidemiologists to confirm each case and source of infection.[35]

There was a startling 91 percent drop in the incidence of malaria in the United States from 1945 to 1949, but the figures were misleading. Langmuir and Andrews attributed the drop entirely to a new method of reporting instigated in 1949. Instead of physicians' reporting the number of cases of malaria they had seen—an easy diagnosis—they had to supply names. In 1950, Langmuir's appraisal and surveillance teams could find only fifty-five positive cases. Of these only nineteen were not wholly and adequately explained as relapses, transfusions, or clearly imported cases. They occurred singly. The teams had to go back to 1942 to find an instance when two or more cases of malaria appeared in relation to each other, the ultimate test for determining an endemic presence.[36] In the 1930s, a hundred thousand cases of malaria were reported annually in the United States, and that figure was probably low. By 1945, malaria for all practical purposes had mysteriously disappeared, probably before the massive efforts to control it got under way.[37]

The successful malaria-surveillance program had an important, carefully devised administrative angle to it. In his original memo, Langmuir suggested that when there was no more malaria to investigate, the teams should be available to investigate any kind of epidemic. As a matter of fact, the nurses on the first teams were already looking at other diseases: leprosy in Louisiana and Florida, polio and dysentery in New Mexico, histoplasmosis in Kansas, typhus and conjunctivitis in south Georgia.

"It was quite subtle," Langmuir said. "Budget-wise, it was legitimate. It expanded our program without any real authorization other than the fact that [the teams] were just there and they are supporting the states in the tradition of CDC." This basic concept was folded into the Epidemic Intelligence Service when that important unit was created a year later.[38]

The work of the malaria appraisal and surveillance teams was the first use of surveillance as applied to a disease in public health. Until those first teams went out from CDC, *surveillance* in public health meant watching persons who had been in contact with certain serious diseases like plague or smallpox or syphilis to detect the first symptoms so that the patient could be isolated. Beginning in 1950, the term was applied to specific diseases rather than to individuals. The methodology included systematic collection and constant evaluation of relevant data, and their dissemination to all who needed to know. The purpose was to improve the control of disease. It would work when well-informed officials, supported by an understanding public, took corrective measures.[39]

When Langmuir tried to set up a similar program for typhus, he was temporarily stymied by entomologists who claimed that surveillance was not an epidemiological function. Ultimately, Langmuir's will prevailed. Surveillance was established in the Epidemiology Division he headed, first for malaria and then for many other diseases. It was the cornerstone on which CDC's mission of service to the states was built.

CHAPTER 3

The Disease Detectives

The Cold War lent a sense of urgency to CDC's role. In 1949, when the United States lost its nuclear monopoly and communist armies triumphed in China, CDC tackled biological warfare, an exotic new threat to health. As the designated agency to respond to disasters and epidemics, the fledgling Atlanta institution was hardly ready for the day when germs became weapons, even though its new epidemiology chief knew more about biological warfare than anyone else in the Public Health Service. Alexander Langmuir raised the topic with state health officers when they met at CDC in October 1949. Sabotage of food and water supplies, he said, was the most likely mode of attack.[1] Epidemiology was surely the first line of defense, but this, unfortunately, was not a strength of the state health departments, and it barely existed at CDC.

Just two months later, the National Security Resources Board decreed that the nation must develop measures to cope with all types of enemy attack, including conventional bombing and bacteriological or chemical warfare.[2] CDC promptly ordered planning reports from leaders in every division. Some of these, though solidly based on the successful MCWA experience of World War II, were seriously out of date. The entomologists suggested that insect-borne diseases could be combatted by deploying men about the country equipped with hand-pumped spray cans of insecticides. The experts in typhus control were confident that their rat-control specialists, already assigned to the states, were sufficient to any emergency. The laboratory staff, more aware of new threats to health in the Cold War era, had little confidence that the nation could be ready if an attack came. How could blood studies be done of all those exposed to nuclear attack? How could all the milk, food, and water be checked for pathogens? How indeed? To make the best use of its own limited personnel, CDC again sought expert advice from consultants. They came from twenty states.[3]

In a war emergency, the shortage of epidemiologists certainly would be critical. Just how critical was demonstrated early in 1950, when CDC could not supply even one person to do an investigation requested by the Environmental Health Center in Cincinnati. Certainly, CDC was not ready to take over all the epidemiological work of the PHS, as Mountin wanted it to do, much less deal with anything so frightening as biological warfare. Building an effective epidemiology unit at CDC was an obvious priority, but Langmuir's first effort at recruitment was disappointing. On a trip to the West Coast in the spring of 1950, he found only five prospects, four of whom were "green" interns. He netted but two "genuinely interested but totally untrained" physicians.[4]

The outbreak of the Korean War in June 1950 meant that planning for a wartime emergency gave way to action. President Truman ordered all budgets scaled down, with defense items getting priority. At CDC, two lists were prepared. Under *defense* the staff put control of communicable diseases around military areas, epidemiologic intelligence, and laboratory technological studies. Everything else—including malaria, diarrheal studies, and rat control—went in the *non-defense* column, although a bit of creative thinking could place most of these programs in broad defense-related projects. Because CDC's position in "the firmament of defense" was poorly defined, no one was certain how war would affect the institution. Partial mobilization might bring no more than a straight budget cut, but total mobilization could change CDC's role significantly. Would it be cut off from Washington and operate autonomously? If the Office of Vital Statistics proved unequal to the task, might not CDC be given responsibility for morbidity and mortality reporting?[5]

Signals from Washington indicated that CDC's role would become more important. Dr. Charles L. Williams, chief of the Bureau of State Services, sought congressional approval for the Public Health Service to function on a broad front, as it had done in World War II, and he told Vonderlehr that more activities would be transferred to Atlanta. Williams thought CDC needed a name more nearly descriptive of its new role, perhaps Preventable Disease Center. The suggestion particularly pleased Justin Andrews, who had long wanted the word *preventable* in the title. Although new responsibilities came, CDC kept its name. Mountin decided it was unwise to change it "when we are trying

to feature defense measures against communicable diseases, both natural and induced." Williams, too, backed away from his proposal,
citing the "present confused emergency situation."[6]

"Induced" communicable diseases, of course, meant biological warfare. "What we need is an epidemic intelligence service," Dr. Mountin
blurted out one day, thus labeling a unit destined to have a major
impact on the course of epidemiology. The name had a covert ring to it,
entirely appropriate for the wartime emergency. Inherent in it, however,
were "administrative inconsistencies," which Langmuir and others
noted but "no one had the temerity to point out." For reasons not hard
to follow, recruitment problems vanished: doctors were liable to be
drafted for military service as of July 1951. In a single week in early
September 1950, many applications for active duty in the commissioned
corps, with preference for epidemiologic assignment, arrived at CDC.[7]

Major General A. C. McAuliffe, the chief chemical officer of the
Department of the Army, wrote urgently to Surgeon General Leonard
Scheele in October 1950 about the vulnerability of the United States to
biological warfare, particularly against the civilian population. Biological agents in the environment could not rapidly be detected; the techniques for specific identification of agents were too slow and complicated. Nor was there sufficient knowledge on how to treat those
exposed to agents of biological warfare to curtail illness, prevent deaths,
and lessen the possibility of secondary spread. He wanted the Public
Health Service to assume responsibility for research that would provide
answers in the shortest possible time.[8]

The possibility of biological warfare became general knowledge in
the scientific community in December 1950 when the Executive Office
of the President issued *Health Services and Special Weapons Defense*, a
manual that stated categorically that "an enemy could employ . . .
biological warfare against us effectively." The manual, to which Langmuir contributed, cited two forms of possible attack: the creation of
clouds of pathogenic aerosols over cities and the contamination of water and food supplies by sabotage. The first would produce large numbers of casualties in urban areas; the second would target specific
groups. Publication of the manual set off a bitter debate in health
circles.

The public learned about biological warfare from *What You Should
Know about Biological Warfare*, a pamphlet issued by Federal Civil
Defense Administration, which listed botulinus toxin and the agents
causing plague, typhus, cholera, smallpox, tularemia, brucellosis, an-

thrax, and glanders as possibilities. Hundreds of infectious organisms are smaller than five microns—about the size of a red blood cell—the upper limit of particles that can reach the alveoli in the lungs. All these organisms could be used for airborne attacks, and opportunities for contaminating food and water supplies were even greater. Long familiarity with typhoid fever and the epidemic of amebiasis that spread from the Chicago World's Fair of 1933 were reminders of the ease with which malicious contamination could occur.[9]

No super germ was necessary to create havoc. Diseases that had bothered man from "Adam to the atom," as Langmuir put it, were quite enough. But what kind of defenses could be mounted against warfare in which every dairy or food factory needed protection? Besides inoculations, the best defense seemed to be early detection of airborne attacks through a kind of health radar network. A perpetual worry was the possibility of panic in the populace. When a rumor started that the Birmingham, Alabama, waterworks had been poisoned—and "The Communists did it"—it was hard to calm people down.[10]

Sorting out biological-warfare assignments among the various units of the Public Health Service—CDC, NIH, and the Environmental Health Center—was not complete until the spring of 1951, by which time CDC had appointed a committee on biological warfare and had begun research.[11] For ten years the Department of Defense had engaged in biological-warfare work, and it provided funding for some of CDC's work. Air-sampling devices were set up in Atlanta, Chamblee, Savannah, and New Orleans to get a base line against which the introduction of harmful agents in the air could be measured. CDC envisioned a grid of these air-sampling stations in strategic areas, each operated in conjunction with a local air-pathogens laboratory. The rapid identification of pathogenic microorganisms and viruses in those laboratories was a more difficult problem: work that once took days had to be done in hours. The final segment of the project was assigned to the epidemiologists. They would correlate the findings of air-monitoring with observed human illnesses.[12]

In Langmuir the CDC had a man ideally suited to seize the opportunity. He was an experienced epidemiologist, a member of the inner circle of those mapping strategy for defense against biological and chemical warfare, and he was creative. He knew how to take what might have been a handicap and turn it into an opportunity. If the Korean War meant that CDC must give priority to defense-related activities, then he would build an organization that, while initially for defense, could be converted later to a panoply of peacetime uses. Dr. Theodore Bauer, CDC's chief in the early 1950s, recalled that Langmuir came to CDC with the express purpose of training young men to take their places in health departments and in academia. He could have been tripped up at any time, "but he had big strong legs and big shoes and he just walked over and got what was necessary to do it."[13]

Langmuir was born in Santa Monica, California, in 1910, moved to New Jersey as a child, and entered Harvard University at the age of seventeen, where he majored in physics. He was influenced by his uncle, Dr. Irving Langmuir, a physicist and chemist who won the Nobel Prize for chemistry in 1932. Uncle Irving assured him that physics was more fundamental than chemistry, Langmuir's preference, and, for him, an easy subject.[14] He did not like physics—"the advanced mathematics was just impossible"—so he took enough pre-medical courses to get into medical school, having determined to become a physician. In his sophomore year, he was elected president of the Harvard Liberal Club, which, though dying, still hosted many speakers. Among them was Margaret Sanger. From the day Langmuir heard her speak, he was a devotee of the concept of family planning as a means of improving the quality of life.

Another speaker Langmuir heard at Harvard was Dr. George Bigelow, commissioner of health in Massachusetts, who talked not about careers in public health but about an epidemic of septic sore throat and scarlet fever in nearby Lynn. Langmuir was fascinated by Bigelow's presentation and sought his advice. He was the first student Bigelow had met in years who was interested in public health. Study medicine, Bigelow told the young man, then, in this specific order, find a good internship, get some experience, and train in public health.

It was the midst of the depression. To save money, Langmuir looked at medical schools in the New York area and chose Cornell University. Upon graduation, he interned at Boston City Hospital. That part of his life he remembers with intense satisfaction and would live over again without change. Following Bigelow's advice to the letter, he got a job in New York State working with Dr. Edward S. Godfrey, Jr., the commissioner of health and a "paragon of the shoe-leather epidemiologist." Langmuir joined Godfrey's program for epidemiologists in training, and after a couple of years went to Johns Hopkins University to study public health.[15]

Wade Hampton Frost, father of epidemiology in America, and for many years on loan from the Public Health Service to teach at Johns

Hopkins, died the year before Langmuir arrived, but the epidemiology course Langmuir took had been designed by Frost and was well taught by Kenneth F. Maxcy. Langmuir relished the statistics course taught by Lowell Reed, who had the ability "to make a difficult subject perfectly clear." Thanks to his physics undergraduate major, he was well prepared in college mathematics and found the statistics course "superb." Margaret Merrell, who directed the statistical laboratory work when Langmuir was a student, remembered how Reed would drop by a student's office, chat about what he was doing, and put ideas into the student's mind in such a way that he sometimes thought they were his own.[16] Merrell used the case-control study method, which Langmuir later used with the epidemiologists he trained.

After graduating from Johns Hopkins School of Hygiene and Public Health, Langmuir returned to New York State as an "indentured slave" and learned the terrible problems of being a regional health officer, persuading the local people to do what officials in Albany dictated. "It was a job I would not wish on a dog." But he got some valuable experience, including an epidemiological investigation that greatly accelerated his career. There was an epidemic of five polio cases, and as part of the investigation, Langmuir collected many specimens from people in the community. They all turned out to be positive for polio, the first proof by laboratory methods that polio had a large proportion of inapparent infections. The epidemic created much excitement, and some of the nation's leaders in public health, including Albert Sabin (whose name later became a household word), came to see for themselves.

Langmuir's career got another lucky break when on a visit to his Uncle Irving he met Dr. John Dingle, a member of the Armed Forces Epidemiological Board. They hit it off, and before the United States entered World War II, Langmuir was serving as a consultant to this board. Dingle was leader of the group; they turned out many papers. At the end of the war, when Dingle and the others went en masse to Case Western Reserve University, Langmuir withdrew and joined the faculty at Johns Hopkins as an associate professor of epidemiology.

It was then that he was introduced to the arcane world of biological warfare. Dr. Kenneth Maxcy, his mentor and former teacher, was a member of the Department of Defense's Committee on Biological Warfare, and Langmuir was the alternate. When Maxcy retired, Langmuir became a full-fledged member of that committee, and after 1949 he served on the Army Chemical Corps's Advisory Council as well. For both assignments, he had high-level security clearance, higher than that granted the surgeon general. He came to know most of those engaged in biological warfare work, including General McAuliffe, but the work was so secret he could not discuss it with his scientific colleagues. After a time, the secrecy began to chafe, and Langmuir was among those pushing to bring the unspeakable topic into the open.[17]

The idea for the Epidemic Intelligence Service came out of a meeting at the Public Health Service in July 1950. Langmuir had gone to Washington at the request of Dr. J. O. Dean for talks on biological warfare. Dr. Mountin was there, as were a number of others. Of prime importance was how to detect masked biological-warfare attacks, something very difficult to do without better morbidity reporting. If absentee records from schools and industries were tabulated, these might give a clue to an attack, but not without a competent epidemiological investigation. Langmuir insisted that epidemic reporting as well as routine case reporting should be encouraged. The idea was well received, and within a few hours there was "common agreement . . . that the basic need was the development of strong epidemiological investigation of all types of epidemics occurring anywhere in the nation."[18]

The next day, July 18, the surgeon general's staff meeting approved the idea of "epidemiological intelligence," and Dr. Dean began preparing a budget for this and other civil defense activities to be presented to Congress. Asked how much he needed, Langmuir suggested that they begin with six positions at higher levels to form the nucleus of a training team. More could be added later. Many more professional positions would be required in the laboratory services, because effective epidemiological intelligence required substantial laboratory support. He believed the doctor draft would offer at least a partial solution to the personnel problem, and he had no doubt that reasonably competent medical graduates with one or two years' experience could be turned into epidemiologists.[19]

CDC's first opportunity to test its response to a hypothetical biological-warfare attack came with a naturally occurring polio epidemic in Paulding County, Ohio, in September 1950. Polio was often mentioned as a possible biological-warfare agent, and the Paulding County epidemic had the potential to serve as a prototype for wartime intelligence investigations. A mobile team visited each case and determined the circumstances surrounding it. Water, food, and milk supplies were surveyed, a census made of the insect population, and specimens for virus isolation and antibody study collected. Before the investigation was over, a team of thirty men and women, half of them from CDC, half from Ohio, descended on the two small townships affected. There were entomologists, surgeons, nurses, statisticians, clerks, engineers, virologists, and a veterinarian.[20] It was the world's first epidemiological survey of polio.

The team was led by Dr. Ralph Paffenbarger, only three years out of medical school but a veteran of the CDC staff who had worked on polio investigations in Texas. His team was large and unwieldy, but obeying orders, they checked everything. They began with the patients and moved on to family members, pets, and livestock, taking blood samples from all. There were so many blood samples that an Ohio health officer predicted it would take months in the laboratory to analyze them all. The CDC team also trapped insects and mice, tested water supplies and milk, and gathered food and sewage to be analyzed later. A statistician plotted a map of all the minor illnesses in the area.

For two weeks they made their headquarters in the city hall, stumbling over each other and the press, who came in large numbers to witness this high drama in health. The *Paulding Progress* described the investigation as "shoe-leather detective work," which might not lead directly to the criminal but could conceivably turn up enough clues to add up to something. *Life* called its story "On the Trail of an Epidemic."[21] When the investigation was over, the epidemiologists did not have any clearer notion of why Paulding County had been singled out for a polio epidemic than they had had before they went, but they did have some knowledge about what worked and what did not in an epidemiological investigation. Thirty people were far too many to send. It was better to send only one, who could summon help if needed.

Langmuir had a three-point plan for guarding health during the Cold War: research on airborne infections, development of an epidemic intelligence service, and training in biological-warfare defense. He would recruit young medical graduates, train them, and assign them to strategic areas throughout the country—in infectious-disease labs or in departments of preventive medicine—with their first responsibility to official health agencies. He hoped to strengthen the whole communicable-disease program and revise national morbidity reporting. He would work with existing official agencies, which had the clear responsibility in the event of a biological-warfare attack. To transfer this responsibility to some other agency would cause violent administrative and political repercussions to no good advantage.[22]

Twenty-three young men, all physicians except one, made up the first

Epidemic Intelligence Service (EIS) class. Some were recruited from the spontaneous applications that came across Langmuir's desk. Others came in response to a letter sent to medical schools and schools of public health. One or two came from within the ranks of CDC itself, including Ralph Paffenbarger. The class reported to Atlanta in July 1951 for six weeks of training. Faculty from the School of Hygiene and Public Health at Johns Hopkins University taught the first course. When Langmuir asked his alma mater for help in training the epidemiologists, he said, "I want them to be challenged to the maximum of their capacity and to work harder than they ever have before. I believe their youth, high scholastic standing, evident enthusiasm and the subject matter will make this possible."

Langmuir planned to call in consultants, too, and talked informally with several of them, including Dr. Karl F. Meyer, an expert on psittacosis and plague; Dr. Albert Sabin and Dr. W. McD. Hammon, authorities on polio; and Dr. James Watt, an NIH specialist in infectious diseases. "While such men can add zest and glamour to the course, I believe strongly that the course will be most effective if we can provide the consistency of a well-organized curriculum which can be achieved only by having one or more competent persons who have full responsibility for it."[23]

Johns Hopkins sent a staff of three to teach the first course: John Hume, public health administration; Philip S. Sartwell, epidemiology; and Abraham M. Lilienfeld, biostatistics. They used the traditional Johns Hopkins case-control study method. The course was strictly academic and set a precedent for years to come. After the first year, the teaching staff came from within CDC and often included EIS officers who had been students only the year before. The adage that one learns more as a teacher than as a student applied to epidemiologists, too. Training the new EIS officers proved the most rewarding aspect of Langmuir's career.[24]

Epidemiology is an ancient discipline, which has borrowed from other fields of study.[25] Hippocrates observed that the proper investigation of medicine involved a study of the seasons, the winds, the waters, the situations of cities, the habits of the people. In biblical times, people learned to isolate those with contagious diseases, a practice that anticipated by many centuries the germ theory of disease. Epidemiology spread its roots through the Middle Ages and the Renaissance and began to come into its own in the seventeenth century, when the value of statistics in studying matters of life and death was demonstrated. The

Englishman John Graunt collected mortality statistics for the City of London and in 1662 constructed the first known life table. Over the next century, as mathematical principles were refined and extended, the idea of using control groups to study disease emerged. In the most famous of these controlled experiments, John Lind learned that eating citrus fruits would cure scurvy. Sir Isaac Newton's discovery of the law of gravity and of the natural laws that govern the movement of the planets around the sun stimulated a search for the natural laws of health and bolstered an interest in public health and preventive medicine. The French Revolution, which culminated the Age of Enlightenment, advanced the cause of health by making it possible for the first time for people from the lower classes to become leaders in medicine. Among them was Pierre Charles-Alexandre Louis, one of the first modern epidemiologists.

Louis emphasized the importance of statistics in medicine and taught *la methode numerique* to his students; among these was William Farr, who introduced the numerical method to England. Farr developed England's national vital statistics system, producing a model eventually used throughout the world. His work earned him the title of father of vital statistics. Farr and his colleague, John Snow, were members of the London Epidemiological Society, founded in 1850 for the specific purpose of determining the etiology of cholera. In 1854 Snow, a London physician, stemmed a cholera epidemic in London by removing the handle from the Broad Street pump. The wisdom of this dramatic action was confirmed by his statistical study of cholera victims and the sources of their water supply. Those who got their water from the Southwark and Vauxhall Company were many times more likely to have cholera than a quite similar population in the adjacent district, which secured water through the Lambeth Company from sources further upstream. Snow's success implied that a "cholera poison" was transmitted through polluted water, although identification of the causative microorganisms, *Vibrio cholerae*, was several decades in the future. British advances in epidemiology were paralleled in the United States by studies of health conditions in New York and Massachusetts.

In the late nineteenth century, the cause of public health took a giant leap forward with proof of the germ theory of disease. Discovery of the organisms that cause disease and development of a method of proof provided a rational scientific basis for health policy. Public health workers gave American health policy its epidemiologic cast in the early twentieth century. Charles V. Chapin, health officer of Providence, Rhode

Island, brought the science of epidemiology into the modern world by insisting for nearly half a century that the findings of Lister and Pasteur be incorporated into it. The giant among American epidemiologists was Wade Hampton Frost, loaned by the Public Health Service to Johns Hopkins University in 1919, where he organized the world's first academic department of epidemiology. When Rockefeller Foundation began to provide funding for schools of public health, epidemiology had the academic base it needed to make an impact on public health.[26] Langmuir, beginning his career at CDC in 1949, stood on the shoulders of these giants.[27] He had portraits of three of them—Farr, Snow, and Chapin—on his office wall. They were constant reminders of the need to keep ahead of communicable disease.

From the first, the EIS course emphasized statistics. Lilienfeld believed that quantitative reasoning was a major thread in the epidemiologic fabric. He quoted Farr, who said, "The death rate is a fact; anything beyond this is an inference." Statistics gives epidemiology a scientific tradition. Langmuir's definition of epidemiology encompassed this tenet. "[T]he basic operation of the epidemiologist is to count cases and measure the population in which they arise."[28]

At the end of the course, the EIS officers were given assignments. Some went to the states, some to universities where research of particular importance was under way. Some remained in the Atlanta office or went to CDC field stations; others did malaria surveillance, funds for which supplied almost half the EIS budget. All were on call to go wherever there was an epidemic. It was an attempt to recapture "some of the old and vital spirit of William Farr," who believed that natural laws governed the occurrence of disease, and that these laws could be discovered by orderly epidemiological inquiry.

EIS officers were always liable to give an account of themselves. Langmuir suspected that Richard Prindle, a member of the first EIS class who was assigned to the Phoenix City-County Health Department, might be more interested in research than in shoe-leather epidemiology, so he asked Dr. Karl Meyer, a distinguished researcher at the University of California and a great supporter of CDC, to stop by Phoenix and check on him. Meyer, a large man, bounded onto a porch in a poor Mexican-American neighborhood calling, "Where the hell is Prindle?" He promptly crashed through the floor, but he found Prindle on the job drawing blood. Meyer wrote Langmuir a glowing note: even Prindle was doing reasonable shoe-leather epidemiology. A shoe with a hole in it became the symbol of the EIS, proudly emblazoned on the EIS tie.[29]

The EIS was born out of a concern about biological warfare. Its first emphasis was thus on infectious diseases, the thrust of most epidemiology in the early 1950s, but within a year its work spread to other areas. At the first EIS Conference in Atlanta in the spring of 1952, all but one of the two dozen papers presented concerned infectious diseases. The lone exception was about a leukemia cluster in Ridgewood, New Jersey, EIS's first venture into chronic epidemiology, a field that would become increasingly important. The spring EIS conferences provided postgraduate training for officers already at work and an introduction to the program for new ones coming in. The 1952 conference set the pattern of those that followed: a series of ten-minute papers on work done during the year, followed by ten minutes of rigorous questions from the floor.

For the first months of EIS's existence, every epidemic call to CDC required consultation with the epidemiologists at NIH, who, despite a marked shift towards basic research, only reluctantly left the field in which they had scored brilliant successes for a half century. CDC countered NIH opposition by pointing to its charge to serve the states in the control of communicable diseases. Asked if they would accept responsibility for answering all epidemic requests, NIH officials replied, according to Langmuir, "Certainly not. Only the interesting ones." CDC, however, would respond to any request. During the months when epidemiological investigations shifted gradually from Bethesda to Atlanta, Langmuir was in frequent telephone contact with the director of the National Microbiological Institute. To keep everyone informed, a simple administrative device, the Epidemic Aid Memorandum, was created. The day a request for help came in and a team organized to respond, an "Epi 1" memo was sent to officials with a "need to know." The mailing list, originally quite small, eventually swelled to more than two hundred. When CDC began to answer nearly all epidemic calls, "Epi 1" continued to be a valuable communication and education tool.[30]

Prompt response to calls for help in epidemics became the EIS trademark. "State health officers were astounded to find bright, young, responsive epidemiologists in their offices the next morning, or even sometimes the same day that they called," explained Langmuir. "Each epidemic aid call was an adventure and a training experience, even the false alarms." During 1952, the first full year of EIS work, the corps responded to more than two hundred calls for aid. An internal report called their efforts "prodigious."[31]

Many of the EIS investigations were high drama, and they attracted much attention from the national press. The *Saturday Evening Post* described the EIS officers as "Dr. Langmuir's Indians," who went door to door tracking down deadly disease germs on foot. Sophisticated readers of the *New Yorker* were introduced to shoe-leather epidemiology in 1957, when Berton Roueché wrote the first of a number of exciting accounts of EIS adventures.[32]

Langmuir reveled in the excitement of working with the bright young men (and later women) in the EIS, "[better] than any school of public health ever will have. . . . They are tip-top. . . . This is a hell of a lot more fun than dealing with the complexities of an academic situation." For the EIS officers, the experience was a challenge. As fast as Langmuir could, he sent them to investigate an epidemic. "[We] throw them overboard. See if they can swim, and if they can't throw them a life ring, pull them out, and throw them in again. . . . These men become different. As soon as they have met one epidemic problem and licked it, they are as different as they can be. Fifty per cent of them stay in the field."[33]

The EIS had an enormous impact on CDC. Ever-larger classes came in. Composed mostly of young medical officers, they were assigned to an increasing variety of assignments. Dr. Philip Brachman, a member of an early class, who eventually became director of the Bureau of Epidemiology, saw EIS as an "octopus" whose tentacles reached everywhere. Another early graduate, who later became director of CDC, called it the "backbone" of the organization. "You don't often see the spine, but it still supports the body," Dr. James Mason explained. "In the early days of CDC, it was really epidemiology, Langmuir, and the credibility of the EIS that brought a relatively small, obscure communicable disease center into a national light where it could grow and be appreciated. Instead of CDC becoming part of another organization, other organizations became a part of CDC."[34]

CHAPTER 4

Building the Temple (1)

In the early 1950s, the possibility that CDC would be dismantled and merged with NIH was very real. Mountin's death deprived CDC of its strongest supporter in Washington, and Justin Andrews was worried enough to write a long letter to his new boss at the Bureau of State Services. The Preventable Disease Center (as he hoped the Atlanta institution would be called) should be continued for four reasons, he wrote: to watch for the reappearance of ancient, but rarely seen, diseases like smallpox and diphtheria; to distribute the latest information on disease control to those who would apply it; to look for better methods of fighting communicable diseases; and to become involved in international health. Better health anywhere in the world paid dividends in America. Andrews thought CDC should be not only maintained but expanded. One day, he predicted, it would be "the temple of applied medico-biologic science in public health in the same sense that the National Institutes of Health has become the Olympus of all fundamental science in public health."

CDC had changed since 1950. In obedience to Mountin's plan, laboratory and epidemiology work were much more important. Whether pursued independently or in cooperation with NIH, projects in medicine and science dominated the institution. Changes in the staff reflected the shift of emphasis. When Andrews joined MCWA early in 1946, only seven medical officers were on duty, four of whom left shortly. Six years later, when he succeeded Vonderlehr as director, there were sixty-three.[1]

From a modest start in parasitology in 1947, CDC's laboratories had become well known for distinguished work on enteric bacteria, and the virus and rickettsia laboratory in Montgomery fast gained a national reputation. In 1950 Dr. Seward Miller, the laboratory director, moved on to a higher position in the Federal Security Administration, but he left behind an eminent staff. In bacteriology, Dr. Philip Edwards and Dr. William H. Ewing had world reputations for their work with salmonella and shigella respectively, and scientists from around the world came to work with them. Only a fraction of their time could be spent on research, however, for CDC was a service institution, and even the most renowned scientists did diagnostic work for the states.

At Chamblee, the laboratory specialists also trained workers from state laboratories and checked the accuracy of their work, just as they had since MCWA days. The Montgomery laboratory supplied training in a field where none had existed before. The world's first training course in diagnostic virology was held there in 1949. Designed for state lab personnel, it soon attracted students from universities and foreign countries as well. At all CDC laboratories, workers devised new techniques and evaluated old ones, always with an eye to improving the quality of testing in the nation's laboratories. Their aim was to simplify, speed up, and standardize many key tests.[2]

They did their work under the difficult conditions imposed by makeshift physical facilities. The clinical pathology laboratory, housed in a remodeled transportation building in Atlanta, was the best of the lot. Other laboratories in the Atlanta area were located at the old Lawson General Hospital, a series of temporary wooden structures connected by covered corridors. Hastily built during World War II, they were intended for only brief occupancy. When Dr. William Cherry came to CDC to work with Dr. Edwards in 1951, his first impression was that the people were great, the facilities terrible: freezing cold in winter, burning hot in summer. In Washington, when the temperature reached the nineties, government workers were sent home, but not in Atlanta. In the 1950s, CDC approved air-conditioning only for experimental animals and delicate equipment, not for people. Mae Melvin liked the roominess of the labs at Chamblee—they were so much larger than the quarters at the Baptist Book Store—but when the July heat beat down, she longed for winter, forgetting for the moment the cold air that came through an eight-inch hole in the floor, covered only with a paint bucket, directly under her microscope table. Whenever a hard freeze was forecast, Jim Paine of the management office, and Jim Pritchett, the maintenance supervisor at Chamblee, turned on all the taps to keep the pipes from freezing. At least once, the drains froze, water backed up and spilled on the floor, and workers were greeted with a sheet of ice the next morning. Even when the weather was mild, the laboratories' shortcomings were everywhere evident. Areas in which dangerous organisms were handled daily were divided by partitions that did not reach the ceiling. Cockroaches were omnipresent. With great effectiveness, the staff blasted these unwelcome tenants with bug bombs brought from home, simultaneously killing colonies of mosquitoes used in research.[3]

Conditions at the virus and rickettsia laboratory in Montgomery were, if anything, worse than those at Chamblee. Earl Arnold, the sanitary engineer who was assistant director in Montgomery, was charged to do something. After two years' effort, conditions were still so deplorable that a review committee recommended that all training activities be suspended until the physical facilities were improved. "Trainees should not be allowed to observe a staff working under these conditions."[4]

In Montgomery, a frame building provided office, laboratory, and experimental animal space. It was neither rat nor insect proof, and there were serious ventilation problems. The insecure cages were hard to clean, and the monkeys frequently escaped. One of them fled to the nurses' quarters at nearby Gunter Air Force Base and hid between the roof and the ceiling; a pursuing caretaker crashed ingloriously into the quarters below.

It took Arnold several years to design new facilities, get the buildings constructed, and equip them. The task was complicated by the fact that everything, including the buildings, had to be portable. This meant either barracks or quonset huts, and the Montgomery laboratory had both. Proper equipment for a laboratory on the cutting edge of diagnostic virology often could not be purchased. Much gadgeteering took place.

Unique conditions called for unique solutions in personnel as well as in equipment. At Montgomery, the officer-of-the-day system was instituted, a novelty in the PHS at that time. It was the OD's job to round up escaped monkeys, keep the laboratory's freezers at the post office and bus station supplied with dry ice, and do any other onerous job that popped up, all without compensation or reimbursement for expenses.[5]

Dr. Ralph Hogan, who replaced Miller as director of the laboratories in 1950, longed for a new building where all the laboratory work could be consolidated. It would serve a double purpose: provide superior space needed for high-quality work and give the center itself a much-needed sense of longevity. Plans were made, but as the years passed and no money was appropriated, Hogan despaired that it was "love's labor lost."

Hogan was as concerned about the program of the laboratories as he was about the facilities. Far too much time was spent on routine diagnostic work, far too little time on research that could improve the methods of disease control. To turn things around, he had to improve relations with the states and secure the cooperation of the state laboratory directors, some of whom wanted nothing to do with CDC. They would accept monetary help from the federal government but not advice. Eventually, Hogan lured forty of them to Atlanta with a training session on typhus and while they were there persuaded them to form the Association of State and Territorial Laboratory Directors. While most were cooperative, the dissenters were reluctant and vociferous. It took Hogan a long time—seven or eight years—to gain their confidence. He helped them when he could, and told them no when he could not. Ultimately, he was so successful in developing a relationship with the states that when he asked for voluntary retirement in 1961, the chief of CDC asked the surgeon general, unsuccessfully, to deny the request lest that relationship suffer.

While streamlining services to the states, Hogan streamlined work within the laboratories. He installed a central system to order media and other supplies and to wash glassware. He set up one laboratory whose responsibility it was to make diagnostic reagents and standardize them, and he began to breed the laboratories' own animals—primarily mice—to get a standard group that would react identically to scientific tests.[6]

What could not be standardized were relations with other branches of CDC. From the first, Ralph Hogan and Alexander Langmuir clashed. Some tension between the laboratory and epidemiology units was inevitable, and this tension was exacerbated by the very different work styles of these two men and their opposite personalities. Langmuir believed that nothing save Hogan was impossible. If something had never been done before, all the more reason to begin at once. Hogan, a cautious man, never committed himself unless he was certain he could deliver.

A decade after Hogan left CDC to become Florida's public health officer, an EIS officer assigned to work with him described the former laboratory director as "a fantastic person, a bit of a gray ghost, tending to blend with the furniture and other people in the crowd."

He is an incredibly patient listener, and philosophically analytical beyond belief. However, he won't tell you anything unless you ask him. . . . [He] is to the laboratory branch at CDC what Alex Langmuir is to the Epi program. He built it, organized it, and saw it through its first growing pains. . . . He is a good guy and has an interesting streak of conservatism. . . . Ralph's first reaction to a question is always "no" because he reasons that you can say "yes" after you have said "no" without making any enemies, but it is very difficult to do it the other way around. He will never make a promise he can't keep, and he will keep every promise he makes.[7]

The clash between Langmuir and Hogan began during the polio epidemic in Paulding County, Ohio, to which Langmuir dispatched a large staff. He wanted an equally large representation from the laboratory, but Hogan refused. He sent only two people; he wanted to establish the existence of an epidemic before he committed himself. Even if the epidemic were real, the specimens could be collected and sent to Atlanta by air, where the work could be done much more efficiently. Hogan considered it pointless to transport a large laboratory to the spot. The "gray ghost" thought of Langmuir as something of a "showman [who] wanted to put on a show anywhere he had a possible outbreak for all the publicity it was worth." Langmuir interpreted Hogan's refusal to go along with the demands of epidemiology as "violently hostile." Seward Miller had seen the function of the laboratory branch as one of offering support to epidemiology, but Hogan insisted there was no budget to support the epidemic studies. To Langmuir, Hogan was impossible.[8]

Hogan, like Vonderlehr, came out of the Public Health Service's elite Venereal Disease Division, and this may have contributed to his difficulties with the dynamic epidemiology chief. Langmuir did not get along well with Vonderlehr and considered him weak, an assessment shared by no one else at CDC. When Vonderlehr was director of the Venereal Disease Division, long before he came to Atlanta, he created a career-development program for young officers like the one Parran had used so successfully, which may also have been a model for Langmuir's EIS program. William Watson, who began his career in PHS in the Venereal Disease Division and later rose in the ranks of CDC management, explains the friction between Langmuir and Vonderlehr this way: "Langmuir was not in the corps and in those days there was a limit to how far you went in the PHS unless you were in the corps. . . . [Vonderlehr] was in charge and let Langmuir know it. Vonderlehr . . . was a Patton, a ball of fire."[9]

Langmuir got along very well with Justin Andrews, and when Andrews succeeded Vonderlehr as director of CDC, Langmuir apparently pressured the director for some changes in the laboratory. Not long after the polio outbreak in Ohio, Dr. Vernon Link, deputy director of CDC, paid Hogan a visit to ask if he would be willing to transfer, saying that not everyone was satisfied with his work. Hogan inquired who was dissatisfied. "No one in particular," Link replied, "but we'd like to appoint Ralph Muckenfuss as laboratory director." To Hogan this meant that Langmuir wanted to have his friend directing the laboratory. He promised Link he would get back to him.

Within the week, Hogan went to Washington to consult with Dr. Otis Anderson, chief of the Bureau of State Services, who expressed surprise that anyone wanted Hogan to leave and assured him that he wanted the laboratory director to stay. Hogan returned to Atlanta, never mentioned his visit to Link, and nothing further was said. Over the years, Hogan and Langmuir came to some accommodation of their attitudes. As Hogan explained: "Dr. Langmuir's approach needed some attenuation and so did Ralph Hogan's. These were growing pains. You could expect a difference of opinion."[10]

The ascendancy of laboratories and epidemiology at CDC meant streamlining other activities, and a new organizational plan was worked out. Engineering and entomology were combined to form the Vector Analysis Branch in 1951, the same year that Veterinary Public Health was merged into Epidemiology. An imaginative organizational chart depicted CDC as a mosquito.[11]

Within a year or two, the organization was further streamlined, the number of branches being reduced to four. Training and Audio-Visual became simply Training; the Vector Analysis Branch and the Technical Development Laboratory were merged into the Technology Branch. With Epidemiology and Laboratory, these constituted the basic units of CDC for years to come.

Creation of the Technology Branch was the most important of these changes, and Sib Simmons moved from the laboratories in Savannah to take control. It was part of CDC's survival plan. Chris Hansen, a talented sanitary engineer who had come to MCWA with Mark Hollis, was executive officer in 1953 in charge of planning. He explained the changes to Simmons: before CDC could get the appropriations it needed, it had to convince Congress that communicable diseases were still a threat, and that positive steps could be taken to prevent them. The epidemiological method, backed by laboratory participation, offered

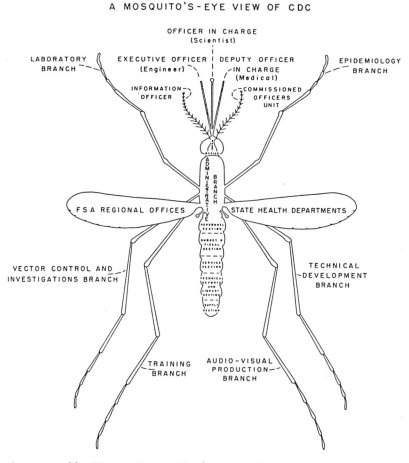

A MOSQUITO'S-EYE VIEW OF CDC

Communicable Disease Center, Headquarters Organization (as mosquito), 1951

the most promising approach, and the Technology Branch had to streamline itself and alter its program to fit CDC objectives. CDC was ordered to cease all its malaria- and typhus-control work, those massive spraying operations under way for a decade. The Thomasville Field station and all malaria and typhus surveillance were transferred to Epidemiology. The personnel of Technology Branch would be greatly reduced.[12]

Simmons moved to Atlanta and began the hardest work of his life.

He had to reduce a staff of five hundred by half and get rid of many vehicles from the organization's MCWA days. Much heavy equipment and hundreds of cars were scattered around the United States, and CDC's four-story warehouse was filled with shovels, jacks, outboard motor boats, and bicycles, all of which had to go (most of the vehicles were transferred to the states).

Cutting personnel was painful. Operational people were not needed anymore; chemists and physicians were. Inevitably, feelings were ruffled, and in the 1950s there was a ready ear in Washington to listen to tales of such possibly un-American activities as disposal of government property. Senator Joseph McCarthy was told that CDC was mishandling materials. It was not the first time that CDC had come under the watchful eye of the senator from Wisconsin. In 1950, a dozen CDC consultants failed to meet the requirements of the Loyalty Investigation Code. For CDC, the Cold War was a two-edged sword. It gave the Atlanta institution the important job of guarding against biological warfare, but also subjected it to intense scrutiny.[13]

The Training Branch changed its emphasis in the 1950s. Ellis Tisdale, the sanitary engineer and educator who joined MCWA staff in 1945, was still in charge, but he moved away from teaching vector control to something much broader. He organized courses that enabled states to train their own health workers at centers scattered around the nation; foreigners continued to flock to Atlanta. The film studios at Chamblee produced more films and filmstrips than the rest of the Public Health Service combined, and these were used to train both U.S. and foreign health workers.[14]

The shift of emphasis towards epidemiology changed the work of CDC's field stations, too. At the Newton Field Station on Ichuaway Plantation, operated jointly with Emory University, work on malaria continued. Data were accumulated and malariologists trained just in case an outbreak of malaria occurred. The Korean War made this more than a remote possibility. Some returning veterans brought malaria with them and every relapsed case was a site of possible infection. The work at the Newton Station was a good example of Andrews's first principle justifying CDC's existence: the nation must be vigilant against the reappearance of diseases believed to be conquered. While watching out for malaria, the Newton Station also studied other diseases. Scientists used blue jays and crows to study the filarial worms that cause filariasis; they trapped and studied many different kinds of mosquitoes; and they worked on the ecology of snails, hosts for the parasite of schistosomiasis, a disease as important in global public health as malaria.[15]

The field station in Phoenix, Arizona, became headquarters for the study of diarrhea and other possibly fly-borne diseases, including polio. When Langmuir joined the CDC staff, work on polio was well advanced, most of it concentrated on flies as possible carriers. In five American cities, including Charleston, West Virginia, and Phoenix, Arizona, programs were under way to determine if rigid fly control would ward off polio epidemics. Langmuir considered this "the most primitive kind of plan." He immediately changed its orientation, illustrating another of Andrews's principles: that new methods of disease control must be developed. The fly-control studies had a budget of several hundred thousand dollars, which could be used more effectively. Langmuir proposed a "Gallup poll of diseases" in Charleston, Phoenix, and Topeka, Kansas. His investigators would look for influenza, diarrhea, dysentery, common colds and respiratory diseases to try to find out how, when, and why these diseases began and spread, and if that spread preceded outbreaks of polio. With budgetary legerdemain, he quickly converted the funds for fly control to positions in the Epidemic Intelligence Service. At Phoenix all the enteric pathogens associated with diarrhea—bacterial, parasitic, and viral—were studied. Eventually the Phoenix station became the major center for the study of hepatitis.[16]

The Kansas City Field Station, formerly called Midwestern CDC, came under control of the Epidemiology Branch. Encephalitis had been studied there for several years before Langmuir appeared on the scene, and that project was one of the things that appealed to him most. It already had a sizable budget and a multiprofessional group approach. Langmuir decided to move the work to Greeley, Colorado. The Technology Branch had work on encephalitis under way, too, at its Logan, Utah, station. When the Logan and Greeley stations were combined in the late 1950s and put under Simmons's control, Langmuir was not happy. "There was bitter competition there between Simmons and me," Langmuir recalled. "They gave me $50,000 for more EIS officers as a token. I did not like it, but that is what happened. It was one of the more critical crises of the period which I survived."[17]

Simmons was always able to hold his own with the forceful epidemiology chief, pushing into epidemiology's domain in such fields as encephalitis and hospital infections. When staphylococcus infections became a problem in the nation's hospitals, Simmons decided immediately it was a technical problem and his forces moved right in. He knew that it was also an epidemiology problem, but the Epidemiology Branch did not move fast enough. When Epidemiology decided belatedly that it should be concerned with hospital infections, Simmons had a ready retort: "Yes, you should have been in it last year. We are in it now." Simmons's success in holding his own may be attributed in part to his budgetary genius. He always came to budget sessions with three budgets. If one was not accepted, he reached in his pocket and produced another.

David Sencer, a later center director, described this period of accommodation and change at CDC as one of "multiple fiefdoms—one for Langmuir, one for Hogan, one for training, one for engineers, another for doctors. Everybody was trying to establish his own thing."[18]

While branch chiefs within CDC jockeyed for position, the existence of the institution itself was challenged. This worried Andrews, who told his staff that CDC had to maintain good relations with every public health unit—the Bureau of State Services, the National Institutes of Health, the Environmental Health Center, the regions, and the states. "It is imperative that we be well thought of," he said. With some logic, he pointed out that both NIH and CDC worked for the Public Health Service and should complement each other.

Andrews was blunter about CDC's notoriously bad relations with the regional health offices, which usually referred to the CDC as the "rich relatives." "It is entirely our fault that these relations have not flourished," Andrews said. "The Regions are here to stay. We should seek their advice when we start something new." As for the states, he repeated what had become gospel at CDC. "We exist to serve the states. No communication exists which can ruin us quicker than from the states to the Surgeon General." When a CDC person was assigned to the state, he became for all practical purposes a state employee. Andrews considered it the surest path to ruin to go to a state and discuss transfer of personnel without informing the state health officer.[19]

Dr. Theodore Bauer, who became CDC's chief in October 1952, inherited from Andrews the task of promoting peace within CDC and fending off attacks from without. He did it at a time when there were demands to reduce the size of government and no institution was spared, especially if it had not yet established its credibility. Like Vonderlehr, Bauer came out of PHS's Venereal Disease Division and had been singled out by Surgeon General Parran for special attention. Most of his training was in venereal disease, specifically syphilis. In 1948 he became chief of the Venereal Disease Division, where he presided over the slashing of its huge budget. The effectiveness of penicillin as a rapid treatment for venereal disease made it no longer necessary to maintain the twenty-six government-operated VD hospitals. It was Bauer's job to dispose of them and all their equipment. The experience readied him for the trimming operations in store at CDC. If he had any doubts that the Atlanta institution was in for some difficult days, he quickly learned differently. Lunching with Surgeon General Scheele soon after his appointment was announced, Bauer mentioned that CDC needed a new building. Scheele bluntly rejected the idea.

Bauer's first year in Atlanta coincided with the beginning of the Eisenhower administration, and there was much sentiment in Washington to reduce the size of government. CDC's budget of $6 million was cut by a third, so draconian measures were necessary. Many of the cuts came in the reorganization of the Technology Branch, when several hundred entomologists and engineers were declared surplus. If CDC had not already been committed to change its orientation towards epidemiology, it would have had to invent the need. Before the year was out, Bauer announced the withdrawal of all personnel from the regional health offices and from the states, most of whom were vector- and rodent-control specialists. Also victims of the appropriations cut were the polio and diarrhea fly-control projects.[20]

Bauer knew that CDC had a fine staff, the leadership of the branches being so strong that strength itself posed a problem. It meant a duplication of effort and a lack of coordination. Some epidemiologists developed their own laboratories; some laboratories developed their own epidemiology. Difficult as it was to get the staff to work together, keeping CDC from being dismembered was harder. Even a small incident was threatening. When a clinical pathology laboratory was established at Atlanta's Grady Hospital, CDC was allowed to use it and in return did diagnoses too complex for the hospital to do itself. When a local clinical pathologist fell into disrepute with the hospital, he raised the issue of the propriety of the federal government's practicing clinical pathology. The College of Pathologists subsequently passed a resolution that the laboratory be closed. The matter was investigated by the surgeon general and Congress, and for six months rattled the foundation of CDC.[21]

The greatest satisfaction Bauer found in his work was keeping CDC from being thrown out of the Public Health Service. The administration did not understand why CDC was important, and the PHS offered little help. Preoccupied with a growing interest in research and the subsequent expansion of the National Institutes of Health, neither the surgeon general nor the deputy surgeon general had much interest in what went on in Atlanta. Congress was more supportive. While it was concerned that CDC might duplicate the efforts of NIH, it nevertheless looked with favor on the work being done in Atlanta. Bauer and his successors learned quickly that it was much easier to get money from Congress than it was to get support from the Bureau of the Budget or even from the Public Health Service. In Congress, Representative John Fogarty of Rhode Island and Senator Lister Hill of Alabama, both Democrats, chaired the congressional appropriations committees, and were always friendly toward CDC. It was not unusual for Congress to raise the budget for public health as much as 30 percent, to the chagrin of the Bureau of the Budget.[22]

Bauer was excited about the work done at CDC. At Savannah, a talented staff worked on insecticides to determine both their effectiveness against insects and their toxicity to man. Flies were the first to develop a resistance to DDT, and the tools of the atomic era were used to determine how "super-fly" developed. Using radioactive flies and a Geiger counter, the scientists found that some flies converted DDT into harmless DDE, dichloro-diphenyl-ethylene. Flies also changed their habits to lessen their exposure to insecticides, resting on floors rather than the ceilings and walls, which were more likely to have been sprayed, and staying still instead of walking about. Admitting that flies had won the battle against insecticides, the Savannah scientists called for a return to such older methods of fly control as elimination of breeding places.[23]

More disturbing was the increasing resistance of mosquitoes to insecticides. By 1952, salt marsh mosquitoes were highly resistant to DDT. To Simmons, who was chairman of WHO's Committee on Insecticides, this signaled a threat to world health and he called for increased vigilance. He warned that the practical application of insecticides was too far ahead of fundamental research.[24]

Chief among the fundamental research projects at Savannah was the study of the toxicity of pesticides to man. Nothing much was known about this, and at Dr. Mountin's insistence, work began on this problem in 1951. The Food and Drug Administration favored CDC's expansion into the field.[25] Congress was interested, too. The first public debate on the safety of DDT took place before the House Select Committee to Investigate the Use of Chemicals in Food Products in 1950–51. Named for its chairman, James J. Delaney of New York, the

Delaney Committee was more concerned with the fluoridation of water and the use of chemicals in cosmetics, but it did take up the problem of DDT. In answer to fruit growers who protested any possible ban on the popular insecticide, the Department of Agriculture transferred $50,000 to the PHS for a study of toxic residues on fruits and vegetables. The work was done at the small CDC lab in Wenatchee, Washington.

Dr. Wayland Hayes of the Savannah laboratories did the only extensive studies of DDT in man. His work showed that although DDT was stored in fatty tissues, there was little indication that it was harmful. In human beings, as in flies, much of the DDT degraded into DDE. Although Hayes doubted there were any materials harmful to one form of life and totally harmless to man, he defended the safety of DDT for the next twenty years. Simmons supported him. "It began to look as though the amount of stored toxic material in fat was a lot less dangerous than we had thought," he said in 1952. "We think now there is very little indication that DDT is harmful. . . . It is used by the thousands of tons throughout the world, and if there is any danger from it, except where it is used promiscuously, we do not know about it." Parathion, he warned, was a different matter. It was much more toxic than DDT.[26]

Nothing was said about insecticides and the environment. Rachel Carson's *Silent Spring* had not yet been published. More than three decades later, Simmons defended the use of DDT. So long as it was used for malaria control there were few problems. It was when DDT was used in agriculture that trouble followed. It washed into streams and was toxic to fish and wildlife. "We could have used it in disease control without any ecological effects," Simmons insisted.[27]

Almost every part of CDC was engaged in preparation for a possible biological-warfare attack, with Langmuir whipping up interest by citing American cities like Atlanta and Pittsburgh as ideal targets. Half the nights in Atlanta were "reasonably favorable" for biological warfare. On those nights, germs would be kept close to the earth and would remain in a relatively stationary spot for minutes or hours. In Pittsburgh, Langmuir listed the most likely biological-warfare agents: undulant fever, rabbit fever, parrot fever, typhoid fever, cholera, botulisms, and pneumonic plague, the latter being one form of the dreaded "black plague" that wiped out a third of Europe in the fourteenth century. But, he added, "don't get panicky; get prepared." CDC would help. One of the twenty stations it set up around the country to watch for epidemics, including biological-warfare attacks, was in Pittsburgh,

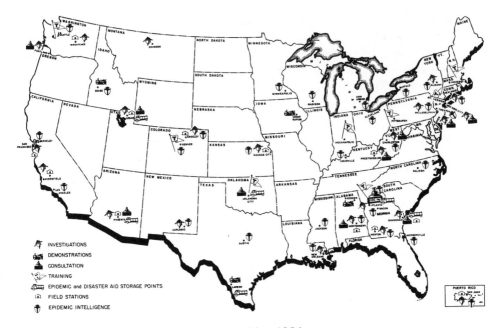

Communicable Disease Center, Activities, 1956

where Dr. Paul Wehrle was in charge. Wehrle was a member of the first EIS class and was then assigned to the University of Pittsburgh School of Public Health. There was effectively a BW lookout station wherever an EIS man was assigned.[28]

In the laboratories, the chief concern about biological warfare was how to shorten the time required for identification of airborne pathogens from two days to a few hours. Scientists from CDC went to Fort Detrick, Maryland, to determine the effectiveness of air-sampling devices and to develop new ones. They took daily air samples at Savannah, Chamblee, and Montgomery, and in January 1953, they moved the experiment to downtown Atlanta. News of CDC's air-sampling work spread beyond the Iron Curtain. A picture of an air-sampling machine atop a Savannah building was picked up by a newspaper in East Germany, which captioned it "criminal research." About 85 percent of the work done on airborne pathogens at the technical development laboratory on Oatland Island was defense-related.[29]

Much of CDC's most interesting work in the 1950s was done at the virus and rickettsia laboratory in Montgomery. Before Dr. Morris Schaeffer was named director of the laboratory in the summer of 1949, it had been used primarily to process specimens, but the new director oversaw exciting projects in polio, psittacosis, encephalitis, and Q fever. He recruited an excellent staff, including scientists, technicians, and the "best secretary I ever had—Robbie Kelso." Their team effort produced such remarkable work that the laboratory soon had a national reputation for excellence. Schaeffer knew they had succeeded when representatives from the virus laboratories at Walter Reed Hospital and the University of California came to see what they were doing.[30]

Of particular interest was its work on eastern equine encephalitis, a deadly strain that might be used in biological warfare. The Montgomery laboratory isolated the virus from mosquitoes and subsequently found antibodies in birds. Determining the relationship between birds, mosquitoes, mammals, and humans was done mostly at the summer field station at Greeley, Colorado. It was at Greeley, in fact, that the disease was first associated with wild birds. A wildlife research biologist, Dr. Clarence A. Sooter, working with George Thompson and Virgil Miles, specialists in mosquitoes and mites, set out to find where the encephalitis virus lived between epidemics. They found it in the blood of wild birds—baby red-winged blackbirds and baby magpies—and in mites taken from the nest of an English sparrow. The birds themselves were unaffected; they acted only as carriers. The workers at Greeley took blood samples from the birds and shipped them to Montgomery to be injected into mice. If the virus was present, the mice died. The virus could then be recovered.[31]

The work at Greeley was supervised by Dr. Thomas Aidan Cockburn of the Kansas City Station. By the spring of 1951, he was unhappy with the laboratory work done at Montgomery and began a series of protests that rattled the walls in Atlanta. Cockburn wanted eight mice used for each test instead of four, and he questioned the accuracy of the Montgomery laboratory's work. He asked Langmuir to transfer him to some other duty and wrote Andrews that he must have his own lab. A year after these complaints, Cockburn wrote a paper entitled "Encephalitis in the Midwest." It went for review to Schaeffer, who had serious objections to both the first and second drafts. He said it was "lengthy, rambling, and diffuse" and offered little that was new. Schaeffer did not want to be listed as a joint author.

The clash between Schaeffer and Cockburn was so great that Deputy Director Vernon Link thought it would never be resolved and probably damaged the reputation of CDC. Langmuir believed that enough data had been assembled for publication, and that as an interbranch activity, the paper should be prepared jointly. The Laboratory Branch insisted that it did not participate in the planning; it only processed specimens for Epidemiology. Link blamed the rift between Cockburn and Schaeffer for the difficulties between Hogan and Langmuir. The attempt at joint publication was to try to "gain cooperation between two individuals who apparently have vowed not to be nice to each other. It may be doomed to failure."[32] To achieve joint planning in fact as well as on paper, Link suggested that a field laboratory be set up at Greeley, and ultimately that was done. Part of the virus laboratory was moved from Montgomery and the work expanded from summer to a year-round operation.[33]

At Montgomery, Schaeffer set his staff to the serious work of determining the relationship between birds, mosquitoes, and the eastern equine encephalitis virus. Dr. Donald Stamm, a veterinarian, looked for the year-round reservoir of the virus. Using a Japanese mist net, he trapped birds in the Louisiana bayou, bled them, and released them. He captured some birds as many as eight times and followed the development of the antibodies. He learned which birds were a good source of the virus, which ones readily infected mosquitoes, and which mosquitoes were most significant.[34]

The fieldwork was important, but it was dwarfed by the work done in the Montgomery laboratory by entomologists Roy Chamberlain and Dan Sudia. They were gadgeteers who made nearly everything they needed for their research. Eventually they were able to say which birds produced a virus at a high enough level to infect mosquitoes, and how often mosquitoes needed a second blood meal to transmit it.[35]

With increasing frequency after the first EIS class went into the field, calls came to CDC for help with epidemics. The national rage for parakeets made psittacosis, a disease carried by psittacine birds, a problem. When the government dropped its ban on interstate transportation of these birds in 1952, psittacosis spread rapidly. So many cases of psittacosis appeared in New Jersey that the state banned the sale of birds, and the Quarantine Service asked Schaeffer to take the birds for testing. He got more than he bargained for: 5,792 birds were delivered to him.[36]

Psittacosis was not limited to birds kept as pets but affected turkeys and poultry as well. In Texas, two hundred workers in a turkey-processing plant developed pneumonia after contact with infected birds. When Bauer and Jim Steele visited the plant, they found that workers were exposed to the aerosol infection when they beat off the feathers. They knew that turkeys from the plant had been shipped all over the

United States, and a decision had to be made to recall them or not. As a matter of fact, hundreds of the birds were on their way to Korea to provide Christmas dinner for the troops. Was turkey ornithosis transmissible through food? What would be the effect on troop morale if there were no turkey for Christmas? There was no evidence that psittacosis was transmitted through food, and after consulting with the FDA, they let the turkeys go. Still Steele was nervous. The military promised to maintain intensive surveillance, and throughout the holidays Steele listened to the radio for news of parrot fever among the troops, news that fortunately never came.[37]

Bauer also remembered the rabid bats. In 1953 a child in Florida was bitten by a bat subsequently found to be rabid, the first ever identified in the United States. The news created a great stir. Within a few months there were other accounts of encounters with rabid bats, including a lively story about one in a Pennsylvania tavern. There was immediate concern about the millions of bats in the nation's caves, particularly at Carlsbad Caverns. Was it safe to go there? Dr. Kenneth Quist, an EIS officer assigned to Texas, and George C. Menzies, an entomologist from the Texas Health Department who had once been on the CDC staff, began a study of Texas caves, their bats and their insects. What they learned was horrifying. Menzies developed rabies and died, even though he had not been bitten. It was the first evidence that the rabies virus could be transmitted by droplets. For weeks, as the incubation period dragged by, Quist did not know if he, too, would be a victim.[38]

Aerosol transmission of rabies had to be proved conclusively, a job that fell to Dr. Denny Constantine, an EIS officer and, like Quist, a veterinarian. For five years he worked with coyotes and other animals in Texas caves and finally got the proof he needed. Animals placed in cages so secure the occupants could not possibly be bitten died of rabies. The frightening news had to be handled carefully. A low key announcement in September 1961 let the world know that "under special conditions in a bat cave," rabies could be spread through the air.[39]

Histoplasmosis was another airborne infection CDC studied in the early 1950s. The disease was important because of its close relationship to coccidiomycosis, a potential biological-warfare agent. Dr. Michael L. Furculow of the Kansas City Station proposed the study of this little-known disease, which was believed to be highly fatal. Caused by a fungus that grows on tree bark and in the soil, it is found chiefly in the Midwest and is sometimes called Mississippi Valley disease.[40]

An epidemic of histoplasmosis in 1955 at a school in Mountain

Home, Arkansas, brought Dr. Tom D. Y. Chin and three others to the scene from the Kansas City Station. At first they suspected psittacosis because so many sick children came from a class whose parakeet, Liberace, appeared to be as sick as the children. An autopsy of Liberace revealed no trace of psittacosis, however, and blood tests of the children were positive for histoplasmosis, not parrot fever.

But what made the children sick? Dr. Furculow led this part of the investigation and finally determined that the infectious agent came from a load of coal taken from an old strip mine. By the time he got to the mine, however, a winter storm had weakened an overhang and dropped it in the pit. Further investigation was impossible. Furculow had never seen a likelier place for the soil fungus *H. capsulatum*, but he could not prove it. Subsequently, he did prove that histoplasmosis was not a rare disease at all, that fully 80 percent of the population of Missouri had been exposed. Anyone could pick it up from hollow trees, caves, chicken coops, storm cellars, and silos. He estimated that thirty million people living west of the Appalachians had had the disease, and that half a million more were infected each year. Its symptoms mimicked many other diseases—influenza, typhoid, septicemia, leukemia. Discovery of its prevalence solved the mystery of why so many people with serious calcification of the lungs tested negative for tuberculosis. An international mystery was solved, too. Tingo Maria Fever, a strange malady that struck visitors to the Cave of the Owls in Tingo Maria, Peru, proved to be histoplasmosis. A CDC mycologist, Dr. Libero Ajello, found *H. capsulatum* in the droppings of the cave-dwelling oil bird.[41]

Successes in the laboratory and in the field were building blocks for Justin Andrews's "temple of . . . public health" and were in the best tradition of public health practice. In Washington, however, the emphasis had shifted to research, Surgeon General Scheele's chief interest and the forte of NIH. President Eisenhower's replacement of the Federal Security Administration with the Department of Health, Education and Welfare in 1953 was part of this trend. In the new era, politics would play an ever-larger role.[42] CDC would have to prove itself.

CHAPTER 5

Establishing Credibility

Two major health crises in the mid 1950s ensured that CDC would survive and grow. The increasing incidence of poliomyelitis early in the decade and the Asian flu pandemic of 1957 gave the Atlanta institution an opportunity to prove itself. In a five-year period, CDC moved from a position of relative obscurity in public health to one with major responsibilities for epidemic control.

Polio was the most feared disease of the 1950s. From a low level in 1938, the number of cases steadily rose. By 1952, polio had reached truly epidemic proportions—more than fifty thousand cases—and more children died of it than of any other infectious disease.[1] At the same time, some of the mysteries of polio were being stripped away, and there was hope that a safe vaccine might be developed. This was the goal of the National Foundation for Infantile Paralysis (NFIP). Basil O'Connor, a former law partner of the nation's most famous polio victim, President Franklin Roosevelt, spurred on the effort. To finance the necessary research, he asked the public to send dimes to the White House in honor of the president's birthday. Thus began in January 1938 the March of Dimes.

In the next fifteen years, there were three major scientific breakthroughs: isolation of the virus in tissue culture, identification of one dominant serological and only two subordinate types of the virus (subsequently labeled Types I, II, and III), and the demonstration of viremia as an essential element in the development of the disease in a person. These three discoveries ensured the development of the vaccine, which was achieved by the spring of 1955.[2]

Polio was one of the first diseases to which the Communicable Disease Center turned its attention. In the late 1940s, its expertise in entomology was called on to control flies during a polio epidemic in New Jersey, while in the Rio Grande Valley the staff quickly turned their attention from dysentery to polio when a major outbreak occurred there. Fly-control studies yielded few results, but they provided young professionals with field experience.[3]

As polio incidence increased in the 1950s, interest developed in trying gamma globulin, a blood extract containing antibodies, as a polio preventive. This was a project of Dr. William McD. Hammon, professor of epidemiology at the University of Pittsburgh, a longtime friend of Alexander Langmuir's. Discovery that polio virus circulated in the blood made this an especially promising avenue of research. Langmuir was skeptical, but he agreed to assign an EIS officer, Dr. Paul Wehrle, to assist in the work. The first gamma globulin field trial was conducted in Provo, Utah, in 1951 during an incipient epidemic of polio. Wehrle participated in this test and at similar field trials in Houston, Texas, and Sioux City, Iowa, the following summer. All three tests indicated that gamma globulin afforded marked protection for at least five weeks.[4]

Public pressure mounted for a larger gamma globulin program, and Basil O'Connor, who loved big mass programs with their attendant publicity, was eager to respond. Local chapters of NFIP were deeply involved in the project. There was only one major problem: gamma globulin was in short supply. Most of it was reserved for use by the military to combat measles and hepatitis among troops fighting in Korea. For the nationwide test of gamma globulin's effectiveness against polio, some of that supply had to be pried loose. President Eisenhower ordered the Office of Defense Mobilization to determine how the limited supplies of gamma globulin should be allocated, and it, in turn, asked the National Research Council, the action agency of the National Academy of Sciences, for advice. CDC became part of the picture when the chairman of the council's Division of Medical Sciences, Dr. Keith Cannon, invited Langmuir to participate.[5]

Langmuir felt strongly that all state health officers should be included in such a national program and that CDC, which had primary responsibility to aid the states in control of communicable diseases, should play an important part. He and Dr. William Clark, an associate in the Epidemiology Branch, proposed that 20 percent of the gamma globulin allocation be distributed to states for use among household contacts of polio cases. A complicated formula was worked out based on the number of cases of polio in a state over a five-year period.[6]

O'Connor was not happy about Langmuir's "butting into his domain," and Surgeon General Leonard Scheele was worried about anyone crossing the powerful leader of the NFIP. Although Langmuir's plan prevailed, the surgeon general directed Langmuir to go to O'Connor and make peace.

"I went in the company of Ted Bauer, then the chief of CDC and David Price, then the deputy surgeon general," Langmuir remembered. "At a luncheon at the Bankers Trust Company in Wall Street, I talked [over] my views with Mr. O'C. Everybody seemed awfully nervous but me. I just talked [over] my views. At the end of the luncheon, Mr. O'C. said, 'I'll give you $50,000 to prove yourself wrong.'"[7]

The NFIP subsequently made a grant of $51,164 to the American Physical Therapy Association to defray the costs of physical therapy services for the study. This money largely paid for a sixty-day muscle evaluation of all cases of polio in the nationwide study. The therapists used the standardized abridged system of muscle grading developed by Dr. Jessie Wright, director of the D. T. Watson School of Physiatrics in Leetsdale, Pennsylvania. Dr. Wright, the "guru" of physical therapists, had been instrumental in developing the rocking bed widely used in rehabilitation of polio patients with mild respiratory muscle paralysis.

With this "blessing of sorts" from O'Connor, CDC organized an advisory committee to plan the study, and many of the leaders in polio research accepted an invitation to join. The committee had seventeen members. Among them were Hammon; Dr. Thomas Francis of the University of Michigan; Dr. Albert Sabin of the University of Cincinnati; Dr. John R. Paul of Yale University; and a physical therapist, Dr. Lucy Blair of the American Physical Therapy Association. State health officials were also represented. The prestige of this committee, which met often in Atlanta, was a major step in getting CDC into what Langmuir calls "the big time" of public health.[8]

The committee recognized that rigidly controlled studies were an impossibility in 1953, but much could be learned from well-defined descriptive epidemiological data. It put together a two-part study: a detailed study of each epidemic where gamma globulin was given, and an investigation by physical therapists of all household cases. CDC asked for cooperation from state health officials and got an enthusiastic response. Forty-one states and four cities, representing 90 percent of the population of the United States, participated. The data were carefully analyzed and compared with past epidemiological experience in the country.

A temporary unit—the National Gamma Globulin Evaluation Center—was set up in Atlanta with Professor Abraham Lilienfeld of Johns Hopkins University as director. Nearly all the resources of the Epidemiology Branch were thrown into the work. Twenty EIS officers, eight nurses, and six statisticians set to work assessing gamma globulin.

Participating states watched closely for polio. If an epidemic occurred, local health officials administered gamma globulin in the community and determined if its use modified the severity of the disease or altered its spread. The work was made more difficult by a shortage of gamma globulin. A third of the nation's supply was gone by late July, when the study had barely begun. Wherever polio appeared, there was almost certain to be a demand for more gamma globulin than was available. That summer health departments did mass inoculations of gamma globulin in twenty-three communities in thirteen states and sent their reports to CDC for analysis.[9]

In January 1954 the whole committee on evaluation of gamma globulin met in Atlanta to go over the report word by word. The most valuable finding came from the work of the physical therapists who had investigated all the household cases, carefully separating polio cases from those caused by ECHO viruses, which mimic polio but do not cause permanent paralysis. It was this study that established the standard criteria for assaying residual paralysis. Unhappily for O'Connor and others who had such high hopes that gamma globulin's effectiveness in preventing polio would be proved, the study did not demonstrate its usefulness as a community prophylaxis. Neither did it significantly influence the severity of paralysis that developed among contacts of polio cases. Hammon could not endorse the report, and O'Connor pledged that the NFIP would again make gamma globulin available for mass inoculations in the summer of 1954. The study had a greater impact on the history of CDC than it did on the fight against polio. The stature of the Atlanta institution as a force in public health was greatly increased.[10]

Gamma globulin offered the first hope for preventing polio, but it was only a stopgap measure until a vaccine could be developed. Work was under way in several laboratories. At the University of Pittsburgh, Dr. Jonas Salk, financed by NFIP, began work on an inactivated polio vaccine in 1951. At three other laboratories, including the CDC's virus and rickettsia laboratory in Montgomery, scientists worked on an attenuated polio vaccine.[11]

Morris Schaeffer was excited about the polio work in Montgomery.

At the lab, where so many specimens were sent for diagnostic tests, scientists spent part of their time making tissue culture of polio virus more efficient, but their most exciting work was developing an attenuated vaccine. Schaeffer and Dr. C. P. Li worked on it. Li, a refugee from China, had successfully transmitted Type III polio virus to mice before he came to Alabama, a feat previously possible only for Type II. His job at Montgomery was to accomplish the same thing for the far more prevalent Type I. Within a few months, he achieved success through intracerebral inoculation of the Mahoney strain. His accomplishment sharply reduced the cost of research. A mouse cost thirty cents, a monkey from twenty to twenty-five dollars. Eventually Li and Schaeffer produced a weakened strain of the Type I virus that was not virulent for mice, monkeys, or chimpanzees, yet would grow in tissue culture. Believing they were on their way to developing an oral polio vaccine, Schaeffer and Li and several lab workers volunteered to take the virus. As they had hoped, the weakened virus multiplied in the gut and was excreted. They then inoculated the excreted virus into the nervous systems of chimpanzees and rejoiced when the animals showed no ill effects. Li and Schaeffer were certain enough about their work to give their vaccine a name. They called it LSC—*L* for Li, *S* for Schaeffer, and *C* for the third of four strains of virus with which they worked. They did not know then that the drama attending the introduction of Salk vaccine would prevent them from ever doing the definitive tests on LSC.[12]

The Salk polio vaccine was ready for testing in the spring of 1954. On April 26, children in the first, second, and third grades in communities throughout the country lined up to get a shot of either the killed-virus vaccine or a placebo. They were the first of more than half a million children who participated in field trials sponsored by the NFIP to test the effectiveness of the Salk vaccine. By June all the shots had been given and the tedious process of observing all these children began. The important job of analyzing results went to Dr. Thomas Francis, Jr., a pioneer in the fields of microbiology and immunology, who commanded the respect of the scientific community. To ensure objectivity, Francis refused to look at any of the data until they were all collected, and he said nothing at all about the results until every scrap of data had been analyzed.

The Francis field trials took place during an epidemic year for polio, the third worst in America's history. There were 38,476 cases, half of them paralytic. CDC participated in the trials in several ways. Langmuir

served on the advisory committee, twenty EIS medical officers and statisticians collected data, and the Montgomery laboratory was one of a
dozen or more enlisted to do the lab work. The Public Health Service,
however, distanced itself from the Salk trials lest the vaccine prove
unsafe. In 1954 it took no official position on the relative safety of the
vaccine.[13]

Dr. Francis announced the result of the trials to an audience of
leaders in medicine, virology, and public health in Ann Arbor on April
12, 1955, the tenth anniversary of the death of President Roosevelt. The
NFIP insisted that no hype was intended, but the anniversary height-
ened the inherent drama. The auditorium was packed with scientists
and television and newsreel cameramen. The nationally known television figures Edward R. Murrow and Fred Friendly were there. Francis
read his report in a monotone, and there was reasonable dignity, but
this was not the case in the pressroom. Reporters scrambled for copies
of the report and broke the release time. As Francis was talking, Dave
Garroway of the National Broadcasting Company announced the results: the field trials had proved the effectiveness of the Salk vaccine—
about 70 percent against Type I and 90 percent against Types II and III.
Church bells rang, sirens sounded, and "Thank you, Dr. Salk" signs
appeared in store windows.

Seated next to Langmuir at Ann Arbor that day was a statistician
from Harvard, Professor William Cochran. As Francis completed his
report, Cochran turned to him and said, "The size of the sample—
200,745 children—was barely large enough." That observation, tinged
as it was with doubt, may have been an omen of things to come.
Francis's report was followed by a luncheon for the visiting scientists.
As Langmuir walked into the hall where lunch was to be served, he
heard most of the prominent people in polio research being paged on
the public address system. They were to go at once to a designated room
at an Ann Arbor hotel.[14] The group composed the panel of experts who
were to advise Mrs. Oveta Culp Hobby, secretary of the Department of
Health, Education and Welfare, on whether or not the vaccine should
be licensed.

The meeting was hurried, but the government had to make an immediate decision. It could no longer distance itself from the Salk vaccine
trials. Until the vaccine had the approval of the Laboratory of Biologics
Control at NIH, it could not be licensed, and that action depended on
the recommendation of the experts gathered in Ann Arbor. As Secretary
Hobby and Surgeon General Scheele stood by in Washington in front of

television and newsreel cameras, they kept an open telephone line to Ann Arbor. The committee had no time to examine the report, and so they accepted Dr. Francis's interpretation on all points, including one that would take on great significance in just two weeks' time: that there was no evidence that a larger number of paralytic cases occurred during the first few weeks after the beginning of the program among those who received the vaccine than among those who did not.[15] After two hours of deliberation, they approved the report, recommended licensing the vaccine, and Mrs. Hobby signed the papers before the newsmen, who flashed the news to a waiting world.

Distribution of the vaccine began immediately, the NFIP having months before provided $9 million to pay manufacturers to produce a vaccine not yet licensed. The NFIP also set initial standards for distribution of the vaccine. It would go to children in the first and second grades and those who had received placebos in the trials. Dr. Jonas Salk administered the first shot the very next day to ten-year-old Randy Bazilauskakas.[16]

Allan M. Brandt has observed that development of the polio shot typified the culture of the 1950s as the moon shot did a later era. "The image of the scientist-hero, unhampered by government intervention, held great appeal. . . . The vaccine became a perfect cause for an age in which ideology was suspect." In the atmosphere of the Cold War, the Salk vaccine was "an affirmation of American scientific and technological progress, [and] was viewed as a triumph of the American system."[17] Until the vaccine was licensed, the government's role in the process had been relatively small. That would change.

The CDC staff prepared for the announcement well before April 12 and developed major plans for national surveillance of poliomyelitis. They anticipated two problems: the possible failure of potency in the vaccine and the confusion caused by other diseases that simulate the symptoms of polio. They considered and discarded the problem of vaccine safety. That, after all, had been the concern of the Francis field trials.

Within two weeks, elation and certainty about the Salk vaccine turned to doubt. On the evening of April 25, word came to CDC of a Chicago baby, inoculated with the Salk vaccine just nine days earlier, who had symptoms of polio. Langmuir promised that an EIS officer would be there the next morning. On Tuesday, April 26, another EIS officer in Napa Valley, California, called to say that a recently inoculated four-year-old child had polio. At two o'clock that afternoon,

Langmuir flew to Washington for a previously scheduled meeting on rationing the short supplies of vaccine. But when he got there, four more polio cases in California vaccinees had been reported to the Biologics Control laboratory at NIH. An emergency conference was assembled at the National Institutes of Health. All six victims had received vaccine produced by the Cutter Laboratories in California. In each case, paralysis had first appeared in the inoculated limb.

The meeting began at 7:30 in the office of Dr. James Shannon, deputy director of NIH, and lasted until four o'clock the next morning. Those present included Shannon; Dr. William G. Workman, director of the Biologics Control laboratory; Assistant Surgeon General David Price; Dr. Victor Haas, director of the National Institute for Allergy and Infectious Diseases; two other officials from the Laboratory of Biologics Control, Drs. Roderick Murray and Karl Habel; Langmuir; and an EIS officer, Dr. Richard Seibert. The cases were not easily explained. Several different production lots were implicated, although all the detailed production protocols were in order. The intervals between inoculation and paralysis—four to nine days—seemed short. The children might have been naturally infected, but epidemiologists recognized the ominous signs of a common-source epidemic and feared that many more cases would follow in a predictable wave.[18]

The group could not reach unanimous agreement. So much public goodwill was at stake that some wanted to wait. There were calls to the California Health Department and to the Cutter Laboratory. Surgeon General Scheele was alerted to the problem about 3 A.M., and the meeting at NIH ended about an hour later. Large-scale vaccination clinics using the Cutter vaccine were to begin in Los Angeles within a few hours.[19]

At 8 A.M. on April 27, Dr. Haas and Dr. Workman put through a conference call to several authorities on polio—Drs. H. J. Shaughnessy, Thomas Francis, William McD. Hammon, and Joseph A. Smadel—seeking their advice. They all agreed that the surgeon general had to do something, although, like the group the night before, they differed on the degree of action. Hammon recommended caution in using the vaccine; Smadel thought that to discontinue its use would would be fairly stringent. Haas asked them to serve on an advisory committee. After the conference call ended, it was Deputy Surgeon General Price who spoke to Scheele again and recommended withdrawing the Cutter vaccine. Scheele agreed and immediately requested Cutter Laboratories to recall all outstanding lots of the vaccine pending further inquiry. Meanwhile,

California State Health officer Malcolm Merrill on his own initiative decided to cancel the Los Angeles clinics. Inoculation programs continued elsewhere in the United States, however, using vaccine produced by other manufacturers. Haas called Jonas Salk to break the news; Price called the NFIP.[20]

The meeting to discuss distribution of the vaccine, which had brought Langmuir to Washington, went on as scheduled. Representatives from many national organizations were there, and Langmuir was among the speakers at the morning session devoted to a review of polio and the vaccine's potential. Surgeon General Scheele opened the afternoon session with the startling announcement that Cutter Laboratories had withdrawn all lots of its vaccine from distribution. He insisted, however, there was no real problem: the PHS was just playing it safe. "We don't think that this particular thing should slow down the vaccination program," he said. He urged his listeners to make it clear to their constituencies that the Salk vaccine was good, that there was nothing wrong with the program under way in the United States. To an earnest question from the floor on the adequacy of vaccine testing, he was not prepared to answer. "[A]ll we can say is . . . it will be studied carefully, and if it proves that our standards aren't adequate surely we will improve the standards."[21]

That day two more cases of polio in vaccinees were reported from Idaho. On Thursday, April 28, the top staff of the surgeon general met and for hours tried to decide what to do. Langmuir was there and argued repeatedly for a national surveillance system, but Scheele would do nothing without clearing it first with Basil O'Connor, and he seemed reluctant to do that. The meeting disbanded about 5:30 P.M., and Langmuir, totally dejected, returned to CDC's office in the HEW Building. In about twenty minutes, Mary Ross, a public affairs officer, appeared with a press release the surgeon general wanted to issue immediately. It announced the establishment of the polio surveillance program at CDC, with Langmuir in charge. He was dumbfounded.

"I asked her what had happened," he recalled. "It was clearly not the decision of the group I just left. She smiled and said, 'The SG has a whole room full of national news reporters he must meet with now. He asked me what he should say. I replied by showing him a news release I drafted in the late afternoon, because what you were saying made the most sense and the SG had to say something.'"[22]

With this authorization by press release, Langmuir that day organized the poliomyelitis surveillance unit, thus implementing a plan de-

veloped at CDC the month before. Forty-two epidemiologists would
track polio and report on each case. Surgeon General Scheele described
the unit as "'epidemic intelligence' in the sense of intelligence in
battle."[23]

On Friday, April 29, there was a top secret meeting of representatives
from PHS, state health departments, and universities at NIH.[24] By then
the Cutter incident had become quite urgent, and there was no sense of
the reassurance Surgeon General Scheele had tried to convey in public
just two days earlier. As the meeting began that Friday, Scheele was at
the White House discussing the problem with the president. All day this
ad hoc committee on poliomyelitis vaccine pored over the problems
posed by cases of paralytic polio in vaccinees. Langmuir explained how
surveillance worked; Sabin suggested testing the inactivation of the
virus at more frequent intervals, and Sebrell agreed that if that was the
course to be taken, NIH would begin construction on a new building
within two days and get however many "hundreds of thousands of
monkeys" it would take. Enders proposed that the inoculation program
be suspended. If another producer's vaccine produced even two or three
more cases, he said, "we should have to abandon it." It was this suggestion that created the most spirited debate. NIH director Sebrell was
reluctant to take that course until absolutely necessary. "We haven't got
there yet," he said. To that Langmuir responded, "Then you will have
a disaster on your hands. This is a big enough disaster anyway. But
everything . . . points that there is something about the Cutter vaccine
. . . and nothing about any other vaccine yet that makes any sense."[25]
The statement was made behind closed doors. Nobody used the word
disaster in public.

Polio surveillance seemed to offer the most positive response to the
crisis, and Langmuir returned to Atlanta to direct it. State and territorial health officers were asked to designate a poliomyelitis reporting
officer to send detailed information to CDC, and everyone was kept
informed through poliomyelitis surveillance reports, the first of which
appeared on May 1, just three days after the unit was organized. It
reported twenty-two cases associated with Cutter vaccine and three
associated with a different brand.[26] The reports appeared daily for five
weeks and weekly thereafter for the remainder of the poliomyelitis
season. They contained the descriptive data on each vaccine-associated
case. More than two hundred people were on the mailing list, including
those who contributed the data. It was a valuable two-way communication. With the steady flow of carefully evaluated case reports, it soon
became apparent at CDC and to all who read the Surveillance Reports

that the problem lay in the Cutter vaccine and not that made by other companies.

Reports of cases came flooding in. Idaho was hit particularly hard. Twenty-two cases occurred there among vaccinated children, all of whom had taken the Cutter vaccine. Announcement of any case caused public concern, but those that appeared among contacts of inoculated children were especially frightening. The first two of these occurred in Atlanta, and the surveillance unit knew about them at once. Just two weeks after the unit was established, a Knoxville woman visiting in Atlanta was hospitalized with bulbar polio. Her two children had been inoculated twenty-six days earlier with the Cutter vaccine. The next morning, Langmuir's secretary told him about a neighbor of hers who had been rushed to the hospital with bulbar polio and died several hours later. Her baby had been given a Cutter shot four weeks earlier. "It was a remarkable and fortuitous coincidence that both of these cases occurred in Atlanta where only a little of the involved brand of vaccine had been used," Langmuir observed. He got permission to cable the state health officers about the possible danger. At 3 P.M. on a Friday, the message was hand-carried to the telegraph office. A bit later a call came from the telegraph operator. The message was awfully scary, he said. Should it go out? Indeed, Langmuir was scared. He saw a possibly uncontrolled spread of the epidemic.[27] Langmuir expressed his fears at a meeting in Washington at which Tom Rivers, chairman of the Scientific Research Committee, NFIP, was present. Rivers differed sharply with him:

"Alex," I said—although not in these words, "you are just a damn fool. Nothing like that is going to happen. I don't care if ten kids have polio or a hundred kids have polio. There has never been a man-made epidemic among humans, and I don't think there is going to be one this time." Well, we argued the point. . . . You know how it is when two bulls lock horns—each bull thinks that he has won. . . . For the record, we never had that epidemic that Alex was so afraid of.[28]

The information gathered in Atlanta was funneled immediately to Washington, where the surgeon general met, sometimes around the clock, with his advisory committee assembled to monitor the situation.[29] At 4 A.M. on May 7, acting on the committee's advice, Scheele announced a suspension of the Salk vaccine program until the safety of the vaccine could be assured. "We have been guided . . . by a continuing flow of detailed information" from the polio surveillance unit at CDC, he explained.[30]

The timing of Scheele's announcement did little to inspire confidence, but the next day the surgeon general sought to reassure the public by announcing that vaccine production would be monitored for safety on a plant-by-plant basis. He hoped that vaccination could be resumed shortly. It took some time to determine just what had gone wrong at Cutter Laboratories. Initially, investigators found nothing, but in late May live virus was detected in vaccine produced by Cutter, thus confirming the epidemiological evidence provided by polio surveillance. The virus had been protected from deactivation by a precipitate that formed when too much storage time elapsed between filtration and starting the formaldehyde treatment. NIH ordered a complete review of the manufacturing process and ultimately required an extra filtration during the course of formaldehyde inactivation to remove the clumps. As the investigation proceeded, batches of vaccine found to be safe were released piecemeal to complete the vaccination programs for first and second grade schoolchildren. Otherwise no vaccine was available until the following November.[31]

Inevitably, the fight against polio became a political issue. Despite the plan-ahead efforts of the NFIP, there was not enough vaccine to go around, a shortage Mrs. Hobby attempted to explain with an incredible statement: "No one could have foreseen the public demand for the vaccine."[32] The day after the vaccine was licensed, the HEW secretary revealed the administration's proposal to spend $28 million to vaccinate poor children. Senator Lister Hill of Alabama, who exercised much control over health matters, declared that no bill would be passed that limited the vaccine to the financially needy. "We don't believe in the pauper's oath," he declared.[33] The Cutter incident added a complicated medical problem to a sticky political situation. From the time the first Cutter cases appeared until May 6, Mrs. Hobby made it plain to the surgeon general that the administration did not want any more post-inoculation polio cases on its political doorstep. When the program was suspended, President Eisenhower suggested that public pressure to make the vaccine available probably caused scientists to "shortcut a little bit." Democrats called for action to straighten out the mess. When Mrs. Hobby continued to oppose free distribution of the vaccine to schoolchildren, the furor became so great she resigned as HEW secretary. Dr. Sebrell also resigned as director of NIH, but he insisted that there was no connection to the Cutter incident; he had told Surgeon General Scheele months earlier that he planned to retire.[34]

CDC turned the scarcity of vaccine into an opportunity for evaluation studies. Before the inoculation program was suspended in early May, few plans had been made to conduct controlled studies of the effectiveness of the vaccine. The number of vaccinated children would have been too large to select adequate control groups. But as vaccine supplies dwindled, a unique opportunity emerged. Ten times as many children received one inoculation in 1955 as in the Francis field trials the year before, so a really broad-scale evaluation was possible. Many states were eager to cooperate, and EIS officers were assigned to them. Information was gathered from eight and a half million vaccinated and unvaccinated children. Weeks before laboratory tests confirmed that the vaccine was safe when produced under rigid controls, surveillance proved both its broad effectiveness and its safety. Key to the national evaluation was that vaccine in the spring of 1955 was restricted to first and second grade schoolchildren. During the epidemic summer of 1955, these children were markedly spared compared with those both older and younger.[35]

At the meeting of the American Public Health Association in Kansas City in November, Langmuir reported results of CDC's surveillance of polio. He had nothing but good news. There would be no polio epidemic in 1956 if the limited supplies of Salk vaccine were spread out, one shot to each child. The vaccine was 75 percent effective; paralytic polio struck the unvaccinated from two to five times as often as the vaccinated. The vaccine itself was perfectly safe. "Since the middle of May when a complete revision of safety standards . . . was adopted, no epidemiological evidence has come to light that tends to render suspect any lot of vaccine of any manufacture." The *New York Times* reported that the health officers were "obviously impressed" and that there was a "renewal of last April's optimism about the vaccine's future." The newspaper described Langmuir as the nation's "leading medical intelligence officer," but lowercased his home base: communicable disease center.[36]

A few days after the meeting in Kansas City, Langmuir was in Stockholm to report on polio surveillance to a world conference on the Salk vaccine. His appearance added to the list of things making CDC more visible. In retrospect, it was apparent that the Cutter incident was a turning point in the history of the Atlanta institution. The extensive surveillance program required a bigger budget, always a help in achieving recognition, and the value of the Epidemic Intelligence Service was apparent. The importance of competent viral diagnostic services in the public health movement was clearly demonstrated and CDC led the way to accomplish this. On the basis of just six cases of polio in children who had been inoculated with vaccine from a single manufacturer, a serious but specific problem was pinpointed. Extensive surveillance provided ample confirmation that the Salk vaccine was effective in field use. By the summer of 1956, confidence in the Salk vaccine was restored, and so many children received the shots that the detailed controlled studies of the previous two years were no longer possible. There were only half as many cases of polio in the United States as the year before.[37]

Good surveillance of polio depended on accurate and widely available diagnostic laboratory services. The responsibility for helping those laboratories engaged in polio diagnosis was given to CDC. The work was complicated by the presence of "orphan viruses," which cause diseases that look suspiciously like polio but are not. The NFIP proposed that these be named ECHO viruses because they are enteric, cytopathogenic, and human as well as orphan. None was affected by the Salk vaccine. The ever cautious Ralph Hogan said the ECHO viruses made it difficult to prove just how effective the Salk vaccine was. He thought it would be years before a final report could be made. When CDC's director, Theodore Bauer, asked Congress for a supplemental appropriation for research on the new viruses, he estimated that a third of the "polio" cases of 1955 were not polio at all but something else entirely.[38]

Soon after the Cutter incident, Dr. Li left the Montgomery Laboratory for the Division of Biologics Standards at NIH, where he continued his efforts to develop a live polio vaccine. In Montgomery the careful watch of the chimpanzees and humans who had taken LSC, the attenuated Type I poliovirus, continued. After a year and a half, they all demonstrated a satisfactory antibody increase. The scientists had equal success with an attenuated Type III poliovirus.[39] Original difficulties with the Salk vaccine, however, especially the political implications of possible vaccine failure, made caution advisable in proposing an oral vaccine for humans. After the Cutter incident, the Montgomery lab was asked to stop working on the oral vaccine altogether. Its strains of the attenuated virus—LSC—were sent to Albert Sabin and others working in the field. It was a signal contribution by CDC to the oral poliovirus programs.[40]

In the early summer of 1957, CDC shifted its emphasis to influenza as it became apparent that a pandemic was at hand. In the spring Dr. Maurice R. Hilleman, a physician at Walter Reed Hospital in Washington, D.C., spotted a filler in the newspaper reporting that 250,000 residents of Hong Kong had a flu-like illness. The number was so large he knew that it must be some new virus; U.S. military personnel would surely be affected. He contacted army research laboratories in the Far East and asked for throat washings from servicemen. Within seventeen days, he had specimens from Hong Kong, Japan, and Malaya, and all checks pointed to a single conclusion. The virus was strikingly different from any influenza A virus recovered before. He noticed the World Health Organization headquarters in Geneva, which received similar reports from Melbourne and London. WHO's International Influenza Center for the Americas was the Montgomery laboratory of the CDC.[41]

By late May 1957, most of Asia was in the grip of flu. There were millions of cases and thousands of deaths. Health officials believed that it began somewhere in China in February and spread to Hong Kong, where it was first noticed in refugees from the mainland. From there it swept all of Southeast Asia, Japan, northern Australia, and India. WHO expected it to spread around the world.[42]

In June, cases of influenza were reported in the United States, first among the crews of Navy ships docked at Newport, Rhode Island, and shortly thereafter in California, where the liner *President Cleveland* arrived at San Francisco with 96 cases aboard. On June 26, the epidemic leaped to the Midwest when 100 delegates from California chartered a railroad coach for a trip to Grinnell, Iowa, to attend an international church conference. Some of them were sick en route. The college where the conference was held normally accommodated 800 students, but there were more than twice that many delegates. They came from forty-three states and several foreign countries. On arrival the California delegates, in a true spirit of togetherness, were systematically intermingled in double-bunked dormitory rooms among the remaining 1,600 with predictable results. Within a few days there were 200 clinical cases of influenza. The conference ended abruptly. The separate delegations, well seeded with infection, returned to their homes, disseminating the new strain of virus throughout the country.[43]

CDC's epidemiologists were alerted for emergency field duty in mid June, and all the laboratories cooperating with the WHO International Influenza Center for the Americas in Montgomery were put on guard. In early July, Dr. Leroy Burney, who had succeeded Scheele as surgeon general, sent a message to CDC: "Tell Alex to set up surveillance for influenza as he did for polio."[44] Langmuir immediately offered the services of the EIS to the Montgomery laboratory and to Schaeffer, who enjoyed much status among those doing influenza research. The resulting influenza surveillance unit was a joint operation of CDC's Epidemiology and Laboratory Branches. One of its first jobs was to warn health officials in the hometowns of those who had attended the Iowa conference. The first formal influenza surveillance report was issued July 9. Twice a week during the summer and once a week after the epidemic got under way, reports regularly went to about a hundred persons, but by widespread demand, the mailing list was soon expanded to two thousand people directly involved with influenza control. The two-way flow of information made it possible to offer advice that helped stem the tide of the epidemic.[45]

In August, the country got a preview of what could be expected when schools opened in the fall. Outbreaks of flu in Tangipahoa Parish, Louisiana—where the schools opened early in August so that students might have time off the next spring to pick strawberries—spread quickly to the entire population. The next outbreak occurred in nearby New Orleans. When more cases occurred in Mississippi, again just after the schools opened, the pattern seemed clear. An epidemic could be expected nationwide with the opening of schools in September.[46]

Influenza is an elusive and potentially deadly disease, for which biomedical research has been unable to propose, even in theory, a permanent solution. There are four groups of influenza viruses, labeled A through D, with only strains A and B being important in the United States, where the A strain poses the most serious threat. It is believed to have caused the great influenza epidemic of 1889 and the pandemic of 1918. Certainly it was responsible for the epidemics of 1934 and 1947. The influenza virus, chameleonlike, changes the surface proteins on its coat (designated H for hemagglutinin and N for neuraminidase), and whenever this happens the influenza vaccine must be changed, too. Sometimes virus undergoes a "drift," and the change is slight. Sometimes the change is marked, and a "shift" occurs. When the latter happens, the population has little, if any, immunity. The new virus might attack a few people and go into hiding, or it might spread until an epidemic, or even a pandemic, occurs. This is what happened in 1957. The virus was the A2 strain (H2N2), but laymen knew it simply as Asian flu.[47]

Since the new strain was identified so early, there was time to put a national plan of control into action, and the Public Health Service took a position of active leadership. The pharmaceutical manufacturers rushed to manufacture a vaccine based on the new Asian strain. The

American Medical Association, the American Hospital Association, and the state health officers began an educational program for health-care workers to prepare them for the emergency. Surveillance began at CDC. President Eisenhower asked Congress for half a million dollars to fight the disease, half for diagnostic tools to be distributed to the states and localities, half for surveillance. Part of the money provided for more EIS officers.

The march of influenza across the country was plotted exactly. In July, there were only sporadic outbreaks. By October, nearly every state in the union reported influenza in half or more of its counties. By early November, 82 million Americans had been ill, losing 282 million days to disability. No state was spared in December. The day after Christmas, the surgeon general announced that the first wave of influenza was passing but a second might be on the way.[48]

CDC's influenza surveillance unit gathered information from counties, industry, newspaper accounts, and the *National Health Survey,* a weekly report from 700 American households across the country. It also calculated the number of excess deaths from influenza and pneumonia from data supplied by the National Office of Vital Statistics. In dealing with tens of millions of cases, simple narrative reports of epidemics and outbreaks prove to be a better measure of spread than reporting and counting individual cases.[49]

The Montgomery laboratory was a major source of information to the surveillance unit. As WHO's International Influenza Center for the Americas, it worked with more than a hundred others around the world observing respiratory disease outbreaks and was the country's most comprehensive influenza-testing laboratory. One of its jobs was to determine if the vaccine was potent enough. The only thing comparable to it was the World Influenza Center in London. Dr. Keith Jensen directed the influenza work in Montgomery; he operated a typing service to catch virus variations and antigenic changes.[50] One of the dangers was the development of a more virulent strain of Asian flu. Specimens poured into the laboratory from outbreaks in the United States. Newly isolated strains were sent to other laboratories in the Americas so that they could provide more diagnostic antigens and antisera.[51]

Manufacturers rushed to supply the vaccine on which curbing the epidemic depended, but they never quite made it. It was difficult to produce a monovalent vaccine specifically keyed to Asian flu and at the same time manufacture polyvalent vaccines for general use. Asian flu was well seeded before the new vaccine was available in large quantity.

Before it could be released to the public, it had to be tested for safety and potency. CDC personnel, both in Atlanta and Montgomery, volunteered for the tests, and so did prisoners at Atlanta's Federal Penitentiary. A brand-new EIS officer, H. Bruce Dull, was put in charge of tests at the prison, and he spent much of his first six months on the job there. Because the epidemic went into a second wave in the early months of 1958, the prison study proved quite productive—"the most contributory of all that were done," as he put it—because it provided an opportunity to test the effectiveness of the vaccine. It was 80 to 90 percent effective in the first round and slightly less so the second time around. More important, the protection lasted into the second wave of the epidemic.[52]

Almost immediately there was a huge demand for what was described as a "mere dribble" of vaccine. The armed forces were first in line, and then doctors, nurses, other health care workers, and those in essential industries. In Washington, President Eisenhower was inoculated. In England, Queen Elizabeth and Prince Philip received their flu shots before leaving for a visit to the United States and Canada. Elsewhere, the distribution did not always go as planned. In California, the 49ers professional football team and the football squads at the University of California and Stanford got flu shots, as did the clerks at Dun & Bradstreet, but not police or firemen. As the sales manager for Merck, Sharp & Dohme, one of six pharmaceutical houses making the vaccine, explained, "You got twenty-five people wanting apples and you got one apple. So who gets the apple? The guy who's got his hand out first." A spokesman for another, unnamed pharmaceutical firm explained why there was a shortage. "It's simply a matter of economics. We can't make any more vaccine because there's just no more space in our facilities, no more equipment to be had, or eggs to be bought or personnel to process it." Eventually forty million doses of the vaccine were distributed.[53] Columnist Jack Anderson quoted unnamed government doctors in September as saying that the Asian flu scare had been exaggerated to sell vaccine. Karl Meyer, long-time consultant for CDC and an authority on epidemic disease, was also skeptical of the wisdom of mass inoculations. He asked what induced this near hysteria, this public demand for vaccine manufactured only for emergency purposes. New York City's health commissioner, Dr. Leona Baumgartner, agreed with him. She thought the flu strain was too mild to urge mass immunizaton. Something was obviously wrong with the distribution system, however. In

December, after the first wave of the epidemic peaked, the American Medical Association moved to establish a code of practice that would regulate future distribution of important therapeutic products like the Salk and Asian flu vaccines.[54]

From the two waves of the Asian flu epidemic in 1957–58, much was learned about the nature of influenza. The first wave struck particularly hard at teenagers, probably because they experienced the highest contact rate of any segment of the population, far surpassing the number of contacts of the housewife, her preschool children, or her husband at work. The consolidated high school was certainly a factor in spreading the disease. Many students rode to school on buses where there was a closeness that exceeded that of household contacts. The unique second wave of the epidemic occurred throughout the country in the early months of 1958. This provided new information vital to formulating a policy for the distribution of scarce vaccine. The traditional index of an influenza epidemic is excess mortality, which, in 1957, occurred during the first wave in November. Beginning in January, there was another wave of excess deaths almost as great as the first. But no schools closed, and many fewer people were absent from work. An examination of death certificates provided a clue to this phenomenon. The deaths occurred most often in those people above the age of sixty-five. They had less contact with the world than younger people and so were not exposed to influenza as soon as those with many social contacts, but when the virus struck, these older people were much more susceptible. When the excess deaths of 1957–58 were added to those from the influenza epidemic of 1960, the total came to 86,000, two-thirds of whom were sixty-five or older. These 86,000 excess deaths provided confirmation for the recommendation that the aged and chronically ill should receive an annual influenza shot.[55]

The Asian flu epidemic did much to enhance the image of the Communicable Disease Center. Jensen was named one of the ten Outstanding Young Men of the Year by the U.S. Chamber of Commerce; Langmuir made his debut on national television—a first for CDC—as a guest on Dave Garroway's "Wide, Wide World" to explain the origin, spread, control, and outlook of Asian flu. The *New York Times* uppercased Communicable Disease Center.[56] Only a half dozen years earlier, the continued existence of the fledgling institution had been in doubt. In its response to the polio and influenza crises, however, CDC proved its value in the control of epidemic disease. Dr. Tom Rivers, chairman of

NFIP's Scientific Research Committee, who clashed with Langmuir during the tense spring and summer of 1955 when the safety of the Salk vaccine was in doubt, was often asked, " 'Did anything good come out of the Cutter incident?' My answer is always, 'Yes, the Polio Surveillance Unit at the Communicable Disease Center in Atlanta.' I don't know of anyone . . . who works in the field of polio research who hasn't in one way or another been indebted to them."[57]

CHAPTER 6

Building the Temple (2)

In the spring of 1957, there were two tangible signs that CDC was making progress towards becoming the "temple of public health" that Justin Andrews envisioned. CDC's new chief, Dr. Robert J. Anderson, wore the star of assistant surgeon general on his shoulder, marking him as the highest-ranking officer yet to head the agency. More important was the transfer of the PHS's elite Venereal Disease Division to Atlanta, for this established the pattern by which CDC would continue to grow.

Surgeon General Leroy Burney was at Dr. Anderson's side for his first meeting with the staff. The new chief warned against complacency at a time when four million youngsters a year had measles and outbreaks of encephalitis could be neither anticipated nor controlled. Surgeon General Burney had a larger vision. Broaden your thinking to include environmental issues and chronic diseases, "the real killers of America," he urged the 1,224-member staff. Have the courage "to bump [your] heads and make some mistakes."[1]

Like his predecessors, Vonderlehr and Bauer, Anderson had been trained in the Venereal Disease Division, but for a decade before his transfer to Atlanta, he had been in the Tuberculosis and Chronic Diseases Division, having served most recently as its chief. He wanted to move the tuberculosis program to Atlanta with him, but higher PHS officials ruled against it, lest CDC be overwhelmed.[2] That move had to wait for another three years.

To ease the transfer of the Venereal Disease Division to what seemed like the outer fringes of society, its director, Dr. Clarence A. (Larry) Smith, was named CDC's deputy chief. William C. (Bill) Watson, Jr., Smith's second in command in Washington, remembered how hard the move was. Families and lives were disconcerted. Atlanta was a southern town, civil rights was a hot issue, and the question of the survival of the public schools was still in the air. Those with children were worried. Even worse was the sense of loss that the move to Atlanta brought.

"Here was this proud old program that had been the largest thing in the PHS not too many years before that, now being subsumed into that upstart young outfit in Atlanta that nobody had ever really heard much about at that point," Watson said. The two units had about the same number of people and almost equal budgets: CDC about $5 million and the venereal disease program about $6 million. There was bound to be friction. "We probably did not engage in the most seemly kind of conduct towards CDC," Watson admitted.[3]

Moving the division headquarters had little effect on venereal disease workers in the field, those assigned to the regional health offices, but most members of the Washington office resigned rather than comply with orders. Only about a dozen were willing to come. In retrospect, it was obvious that the reluctance of many people to move was one of CDC's strengths. The Atlanta institution grew primarily by absorbing other units of the Public Health Service, but every time another unit moved in, about 90 percent of the old staff stayed behind. Watson, who in time would become one of the most significant of CDC's leaders, said, "CDC had the best of both worlds, the experience that had gone before and the opportunity to start over."[4]

It was the surgeon general who decided to move the venereal disease program to Atlanta, and in those days when the surgeon general made a decision, the Public Health Service complied with no argument. The move had been in the works ever since the venereal disease research laboratory (VDRL) had been moved to Chamblee from Staten Island several years earlier. Vonderlehr got space for the laboratory in the old Lawson General Hospital. The VDRL staff feared that their laboratory would be broken up and absorbed into the laboratories of CDC—a self-fulfilling prophecy—but it took several years for this to happen. Dr. Sidney Olansky, director of the VDRL at Chamblee from 1950 to 1955, recalled the pride of workers in the Venereal Disease Division. They were "the most dedicated group of all—competent and dedicated." The enthusiastic leadership of Parran, Vonderlehr, and Bauer "translated down."[5]

The VDRL did distinguished work. During World War II, Dr. John Mahoney recaptured penicillin from the urine of military patients and used it for the first time to treat syphilis. The results were almost magical, and penicillin soon became the standard treatment for syphilis. Before moving to Georgia, the VDRL laboratory developed the best serologic test for syphilis—the eponymous VDRL test. The rapid plasma reagin (RPR) blood test for syphilis was developed after the move to Chamblee and was first used in the spring of 1957. It was both fast and accurate, and it made immediate treatment possible. A second laboratory for venereal disease research did not move to Atlanta, but remained at the University of North Carolina in Chapel Hill. As part of the venereal disease program, however, it, too, came under the aegis of the Atlanta institution.[6]

The transfer of the Venereal Disease Division to Atlanta had a profound effect, mostly beneficial, on CDC. Besides representation in the regional offices, the move brought two important innovations to CDC's activities: a grant program and a new kind of employee, public health advisors. Grants to the states for public health care were authorized by Title VI of the Social Security Act of 1935, the first federal money made available to the states for health since World War I. At the insistence of then Surgeon General Parran, about 10 percent of the first allocation of $8 million went to venereal disease control. Passage of the National Venereal Disease Control Act in 1938 put the federal government at the center of the nation's fight against venereal disease. It provided federal grants to the states for programs approved by the Public Health Service.[7] The Venereal Disease Division administered these grants and brought that authority to CDC.

Just as important as grants in CDC's future were the public health advisors (PHAs). In 1948 Dr. Johannes Stuart, an economist in the VD division, came up with a pragmatic solution to a difficult problem. The division had trouble hiring health workers, since the civil service lists were filled with people who could not do this special work. Stuart persuaded his boss, Lida J. Usilton, that bright young college graduates could be trained to interview venereal disease patients, track down their sexual contacts, and persuade them to get treatment. She was skeptical, but Stuart was persuasive and in the summer of 1948 six young men just out of college were hired on an experimental basis to work on Maryland's Eastern Shore. Half would make their careers in the Public Health Service. Among them was Bill Watson.[8]

The PHAs were in keeping with an idea of Joseph Mountin's. In one of his last public speeches, Mountin had called attention to "the need for auxiliary and nonprofessional workers. . . . inspectors, aides, technicians and others who perform many of the routine operations in this country, and who could be relied upon to provide the bulk of services in less highly developed countries."[9] Prescient though he was, Mountin could not have foreseen the importance of the public health advisors.

At first, appointments could be made only for a short term, but within four years Stuart managed to smuggle the program into the civil service. He obtained permanent positions, first for disabled veterans and later for all those in the program. He hired the first advisors mostly on intuition; there were no tests. Watson was interviewed by Stuart himself. They talked for an hour, and a couple of weeks later Stuart offered Watson a job in Maryland. From the beginning, a PHA was expected to be mobile. Watson moved three times in two years, but in the process advanced from a position as VD investigator through several intermediate steps to become the chief assistant to the director of the venereal disease–control program in South Carolina. Eventually he moved to the headquarters in Washington. The work was not easy, but there was esprit de corps, and once in, a person became a member of the club.

Advisors were assigned to the states, where they organized teams to track down venereal disease county by county. Vigorously applying "contact epidemiology," a traditional approach to communicable disease, they interviewed VD patients and searched out their sexual contacts. They also attempted mass blood-testing, sending teams to churches, bars, and general stores, onto street corners, and out into the country to urge people to be tested for syphilis. They worked primarily with rural blacks, often through the churches, which remarkably showed no sign of resentment. The object was to find as many victims as possible and treat them in outpatient facilities.[10]

The program succeeded perhaps too well. In 1953 the Eisenhower administration proposed the elimination of the venereal disease program of the PHS on the grounds that the job had been done. Advocates of venereal disease control managed to save the program, but it was cut almost in half. The proven value of the public health advisors was not lost, however. When venereal disease control moved to CDC, the public health advisors came along, too. Many of them were already stationed in the regional offices or in the states where their very first assignment put them in contact with patients. Ideally, they did not lose the personal touch as they advanced. The PHAs got to know the state and local health departments that were CDC's main constituents well, and they would be important to much of CDC's success, particularly in the immunization campaigns launched in the 1960s. Many PHAs came to be among CDC's top managers.[11]

With the addition of public health advisors to CDC's cadre of employees, all the basic elements for building the temple of public health were in place: the experts in the laboratory who yearly became more distinguished, the epidemiologists (EIS officers who stayed on the staff), able managers, and PHAs who brought with them a set of attitudes, beliefs, and abilities that proved to be crucial to an institution dedicated to service.

Addition of the Venereal Disease Division to CDC had so many advantages that little, if any, heed was paid to a relatively obscure long-term research program the division brought with it. In Macon County, Alabama, in and around the county seat of Tuskegee, the division had studied untreated syphilis in the male Negro since 1932. The study thus was a quarter of a century old when, by absorption, it became a CDC program. In 1955, the arrest of a black woman named Rosa Parks for refusing to give up her seat to a white person on a Montgomery, Alabama, bus brought an obscure Baptist minister, the Reverend Martin Luther King, Jr., into the national spotlight. He was the most eloquent spokesman for the Montgomery bus boycott, which ignited the massive push for civil rights across the South. But if anybody at CDC put these two Alabama events together—the Tuskegee experiment and the bus boycott—and saw trouble ahead, he said nothing. The Tuskegee experiment, set up to study complications that develop in the final stages of syphilis, continued for another fifteen years before the inevitable explosion came (see chapter 17).[12]

If the VD unit was insensitive to the civil rights movement, it was keenly aware of the rising tide of syphilis and gonorrhea across the nation. Dr. William J. Brown, who came to CDC as head of the Venereal Disease Branch in 1957, declared war on VD, particularly in teenagers and young adults, aged fourteen to twenty-five, who accounted for more than half the cases. He did not know why the dragnet had failed or what social forces might be at work, but he knew that more money was needed. He agreed with Deputy Chief Smith, who asked Congress for $100,000 for research to develop an immunizing agent.[13]

Meanwhile, there was a new technique, if not a new weapon, to use in the fight on venereal disease: the cluster method of control. Hall County, Georgia, was the first to bring syphilis under control through this technique, which involved questioning not only the infected person's contacts but all those people thought by contacts possibly to have been infected. This new approach may have contributed to the drop in the syphilis rate, which reached the lowest point ever in 1958, but it could not keep the rate down. Venereal disease rose rapidly in 1959 and 1960. Dr. Brown took to the stump to try to slow its advance. By the spring of 1960, VD rates were up 42 percent, and in cities of a million or more population, the increase was more than 100 percent. Brown blamed physicians who did not report syphilis cases, thus making it impossible to trace contacts.[14]

The social dimension of disease complicated the fight against polio, as it did against venereal disease. In the fight against polio, CDC redoubled its efforts. E. Russell Alexander, a former EIS officer, returned to Atlanta to become chief of the polio-surveillance section. He arrived just in time to chart a sharp increase in polio in 1959, the worst year since the introduction of the Salk vaccine. There were more than twice as many cases of paralytic poliomyelitis as the year before, nearly all of them in preschool children from lower economic groups who had not received the standard four shots of vaccine. The pattern of the disease had changed. Instead of attacking children aged five to nine, many of whom had been immunized, polio was concentrated in the very young, particularly among the poor, wherever they lived.[15]

CDC was involved in the long and bitter controversy over the merits of the killed-virus vaccine of Jonas Salk and the oral vaccine developed by Albert Sabin. Langmuir served on a six-member advisory committee on live poliomyelitis vaccine appointed by the surgeon general in the summer of 1958, which investigated the new oral vaccine, consulted with the pharmaceutical industry, and established standards leading to licensure.[16] This government involvement was in sharp contrast to the virtual hands-off stance that had preceded the testing of the Salk vaccine. After a meeting of the committee in November 1958, Langmuir reported to his staff on the oral vaccine trials under way. Dr. Herald Cox, of Lederle Laboratories, tested his vaccine in Colombia, Uruguay, and Minnesota; Dr. Hilary Koprowski, of the Wistar Institute, in the Belgian Congo and New Jersey; and Dr. Albert Sabin, of the University of Cincinnati, in the Soviet Union, Sweden, Poland, and Czechoslovakia. Little goodwill existed among the three. Langmuir feared that the live vaccine tests were already out of hand, that another Cutter incident might be in the making somewhere. "It is a mess of a situation, complicated and confused. The whole question of what is an attenuated strain is a wide open question. The fears of the Public Health Service have been more than justified and we will wait a long time before there is clearance for . . . use in this country."[17]

The use of oral vaccine was a radical departure in preventive medicine because its effects spread beyond those originally vaccinated. The attenuated virus multiplies in the intestinal tract and is excreted. This is both an advantage and a danger. If the excreted virus remains stable, it can provide protection against polio even to unvaccinated people in a community. If it reverts to the virulence of the wild strain, it can be a threat to public health.[18]

The committee's task was to evaluate results of laboratory and field research closely. Sabin kept in touch with Langmuir and pushed for the widest possible use of his oral vaccine *"free of charge* to all pre-school and school age children, and as many adults as possible in the shortest possible time." The committee was cautious, and in 1960 it recommended more field trials. Lederle Laboratories, anxious to protect its $13 million investment in research and equipment, arranged for large-scale trials in Minnesota and Florida. For the trials in Dade County, Florida, Langmuir was the only outside consultant. They began at the University of Miami and then moved out into the community to health clinics, schools, business offices, special centers, and private physicians. Lederle provided 520,000 doses of free vaccine. Langmuir was astounded at the response. Acceptance of the Cox strains fooled everyone, including the people in Miami. Ninety percent of the school population received doses of the vaccine.[19] Meanwhile, the Sabin strain was tested on fifty to sixty thousand schoolchildren in Cincinnati in trials sponsored by the County Medical Society and the local health department. Langmuir was impressed enough with the Sabin strain to consider sponsoring tests in New York State. He wrote confidentially to the chief of CDC that he had "been converted" at the meeting of the American Epidemiological Society. In May 1960, Langmuir and Albert Sabin were half of the U.S. team that attended a joint American-Soviet meeting on poliomyelitis in Moscow.[20]

The surgeon general approved use of the Sabin vaccine in the United States on August 24, 1960, but added that the Salk vaccine would continue to be used. There were some problems with the live vaccine. The number of doses and their spacing had not been determined, and neither had any restrictions been placed on the vaccine's use. To resolve these issues, the surgeon general appointed a large advisory committee composed of representatives of the medical and public health professions and the general public. It met at CDC in January 1961, a subtle recognition of the institution's increased stature in the world of public health. The session was lively.

Surgeon General Burney presided, flanked by Drs. Sabin and Salk. Basil O'Connor of the National Foundation for Infantile Paralysis was also present. The committee members sat at four tables, and observers and the press sat on chairs lining the walls. In general, one reporter noted, the discussions were carried on in a "calm, gentlemanly way. Nobody has screamed or pounded a shoe on the table." Salk said that the problem with his vaccine was not "vaccine potency, but vaccine use." Sabin stressed the convenience of an oral vaccine. The hottest words at the meeting were exchanged between Sabin and Dr. R. N. Barr, representing the Association of State and Territorial Health Officers. Sabin blamed the long delay in making the oral vaccine available in the United States on a lack of leadership. "That's a damned insult," Barr countered, but no retraction was made. The committee recommended a fourteen-point program: seven points dealt with increased use of Salk shots, five with the best use of the Sabin vaccine, and two with research and international polio control. The oral vaccine would go first for epidemic control, second to infants and preschool children, and third to those population segments least well protected.[21]

The Sabin vaccine was not widely available for the polio season of 1961, so CDC's staff determined to use the weapons they had. They launched an intensive campaign to boost use of the Salk vaccine, which they called "Babies and Breadwinners," hoping to reach the two elements of the population least likely to have been vaccinated. A pilot demonstration program, involving much hoopla, was conducted in Columbus, Georgia. Ministers touted the campaign from the pulpit, and it was front-page news. The vaccine was flown in by plane, presumably to add drama. Vaccination booths were set up on the sidewalk, and the new jet injectors were used. Children got to ride the fire truck; breadwinners got free loaves of bread. CDC hoped to make Columbus the best-vaccinated city in the nation and apply the techniques learned there to other communities. The American Medical Association backed the effort. A "how-to" booklet told how other communities could do the same thing. The idea did not catch on.[22] By the time the effort was well under way, the Sabin oral vaccine was gaining acceptance. Virtual elimination of poliomyelitis would come with virus-laden sugar cubes.

There was a time when the CDC staff felt that someday they would work themselves out of a job, that once the communicable diseases were conquered, there would be nothing more for them to do. But as one disease appeared to be on its way out, another came into prominence. In the late 1950s, one of the emerging disease problems was hepatitis. EIS officers answered emergency calls whenever sporadic outbreaks occurred, sought out the source of infection, and in the short term encouraged the use of gamma globulin, the best-known treatment for the disease.[23] This work was the beginning of an exciting thirty-year pursuit of the mysteries of Type A, infectious hepatitis, and Type B, serum hepatitis. No one knew then that the work would be one of CDC's greatest success stories, or that it would provide a thread affecting the evolution of the institution itself.

Leptospirosis was another disease the investigation of which affected the course of CDC's evolution as an institution. Langmuir took advantage of the study of this ancient disease of animals to get a small separate laboratory for the Epidemiology Branch. In Jacksonville, Florida, a bacteriologist, Mildred Galton, and a small staff began work on leptospirosis and salmonella in 1954. Within three years, they found more than two dozen new leptospiral serotypes, bringing the number to more than sixty. Except for the Division of Veterinary Medicine at Walter Reed Hospital, this small lab was the only one in the United States working on leptospirosis.[24]

At this time the study of salmonella was a major activity in CDC's Laboratory Branch. Dr. Philip Edwards, a giant in the field of salmonella research and possessive about his specialty, was interested only in the human aspects of salmonella, however, and raised no objection to the studies under way in Florida. Rather, he cooperated beautifully with Mrs. Galton, and together they led the nation in leptospirosis research. Neither did Ralph Hogan object to the laboratory in Florida, although he and Langmuir continued to swap barbs when they met for the regular meetings of the joint subcommittees overseeing investigations of various diseases. "Langmuir and Hogan did not agree on anything," Alan Donaldson, assistant chief of operations, wrote his boss after one of these sessions.[25]

When economy dictated that the Florida lab be closed, Mrs. Galton and her staff moved to Atlanta. Suddenly, the Epidemiology Branch had a leptospirosis and salmonella lab at Lawson General Hospital. It was not long before the work expanded to include staphylococcus. During the crisis of staphylococcal infections in hospitals in the late 1950s, André J. Nahmias, an EIS officer who liked to work on staphylococcus, carved out a bit of bench space for himself in the leptospirosis laboratory.

Administratively, it was very difficult. Langmuir wanted more and more space and the authority to do what he was already doing. The long-awaited new building for CDC was under construction, and he was determined to have laboratory space in it. Philip Brachman, one of the first EIS career officers, would come back only if he got a laboratory for his work on anthrax, and Langmuir used that as a wedge. The fact that CDC's future depended on recruiting doctors put him in a "unique and powerful spot." After the annual EIS dinner, he pounded away at CDC's chief: "We have got to have laboratories. We have got to have laboratories. 'Carthago delenda est.'" Daily he pressed his case with Ross Buck, CDC's chief of facilities planning, who, conveniently, was in his car pool. He also courted the engineer-architect of the building, who obligingly included a big space for epidemiology. For a time the space was empty, but within a half dozen years the Epidemiology Branch had "a very marvelous lab." Ironically, relations with the Laboratory Branch improved as a result. When the epidemiologists brought back interesting specimens from the field, someone in the Laboratory Branch would ask, "Oh, can I have a little of that?" More fruitful relationships developed.[26]

At first the epidemiologists were careful to request help from the Laboratory Branch when they had an epidemic call, but staff members of the latter often were too busy to comply. They had too many research projects under way, too many diagnoses to do for the states, too many diagnostic reagents to prepare. Supplying these reagents was one of the laboratory's chief jobs, since these often were not available commercially.

Whether the specimens for diagnosis were funneled to the Laboratory Branch or the Epidemiology Branch, they most likely came by mail, about 40,000 a year. The whole CDC staff was thrown into a state of consternation in the early fall of 1958 when the U.S. Post Office considered banning the shipment of biologic agents through the mail. The ban was sparked when a plane landed in Baltimore with a leaky vial of live polio virus. Although nothing untoward happened, the airlines asked the Post Office to change its regulations so that they could refuse shipment. The medical world was alarmed, said that these materials must be made available, and cited the flu epidemic as the best recent example. The Bureau of State Services said that without air transportation, there would be delays of days or even weeks; patients who could have been saved would die.[27]

To make the PHS's argument more compelling, CDC rigorously

tested its own cardboard containers. Navy fliers bombarded the Naval Air Station at Chamblee, adjacent to the CDC laboratories, with well-padded packages containing vials of colored alcohol. When dropped from 1,500 feet at speeds of 160 miles an hour, the vials were unbroken. Packages were subjected to slow and explosive decompression and were bounced on paved runways. One was put under a hydraulic press at Georgia Tech and subjected to thousands of pounds of pressure. The packages withstood every test. "The tests came out far better than we expected," Dr. John F. Winn, Jr., chief of the diagnostic reagent section of the laboratory, commented somewhat dryly. The Post Office, deluged with complaints, postponed an immediate decision and the crisis ended.[28]

Hogan took much pride in the quality of work done in the Laboratory Branch. The patient work of Dr. Edwards on salmonella and of Dr. William Ewing on shigella made it possible to track down the cause of outbreaks of enteric diseases that caused "horrendous degrees of illness in the United States and around the world." Edwards and Ewing carefully typed these organisms and put them in their proper niches so that it was possible to follow an epidemic and get it under control. They did phage typing of salmonella, prepared typing serums for shigella, evaluated commercial serums, and typed *E. coli,* the cause of so much infantile diarrheal disease. At first they worked only for the states, but it was not long before their work became international in scope. They had close relationships with centers in Copenhagen and London, and their laboratories became the WHO reference centers for shigella and salmonella. "We had the reputation of being very good," Ewing recalled. They examined material sent to them from all over the world and sometimes went to investigate outbreaks themselves. Their book on salmonella and shigella typing, *Identification of Enterobacteriaceae,* was used around the world. Its red cover made it informally known as the "Red Bible" or the "Red Devil." A fourth edition was published in 1986.[29]

In the mid 1950s, the Laboratory Branch developed a new, accurate, and much faster way of diagnosing specimens. Morris Goldman, a meticulous and innovative scientist who headed the intestinal parasite laboratory, picked up an idea at Johns Hopkins University, where he went for further study. He wanted to distinguish *Entamoeba histolytica,* the agent of amebiasis, from non-pathogens, and it occurred to him that if he could stain the pathogens red and the non-pathogens blue, diagnosis would be much easier. While at Hopkins, he studied with

Dr. Albert H. Coons, who had used fluorescent material to label streptococcus antibodies in his research on rheumatic fever at Harvard in the 1940s. Since blue fluorescence is common in mammalian tissues, whereas green is rare, Coons decided upon fluorescein isocyanate as the tagging material. His work had no immediate practical application and was interrupted by World War II.[30]

When Goldman completed his work at Johns Hopkins and returned to CDC, he successfully stained *E. histolytica,* but this did not immediately develop into a real analytic tool. Almost a year passed before the technique was picked up by others, and then the work mushroomed. Dr. William Cherry found the first practical use for the fluorescent technique. He became interested in the process when Hogan assigned him the job of shortening the time required to identify organisms that might be used in biological warfare from weeks to hours or even minutes. Cherry moved into Building 22 at the Chamblee Laboratory and with Dr. Max Moody set to work. They took the fluorescent techniques Goldman had used with parasites and applied them to bacteria antibodies. They identified the pathogens that cause brucellosis, salmonellosis, plague, tularemia, anthrax, and meliodosis. Even when contamination made identification difficult or impossible with other processes, the fluorescent technique was successful.

By the summer of 1956, the work showed so much promise that the Laboratory Branch applied for funds for a new research project that would investigate the application of the fluorescent antibody technique—FA as it came to be called—to communicable diseases of bacterial origin. In a handwritten note attached to the application, Hogan wrote: "This is one of the most promising approaches to laboratory identification of specific organisms to date. This program should be pushed even at the expense of other programs." His enthusiasm was echoed by his second in command in the Laboratory Branch, Dr. U. Pentti Kokko, who called it "an extremely important project which we should start as soon as possible."[31]

The fluorescent antibody technique was a Cold War activity that paid off in a notable peacetime advance. The process was quickly applied to streptococcal infections, then to staphylococcus, and eventually to rickettsia, viruses, and fungi. It permitted specific therapy to be instituted much more promptly. As CDC's assistant chief, Alan Donaldson, dramatically put it, "It was almost like putting a neon light on these organisms."[32] The technique was simple, specific, practical, and economical. And it was fast. The diagnostic time for bacteria could be reduced from five days to thirty minutes, of viruses from seven days to one day or less. The FA technique cut the cost of diagnosing poliomyelitis from $200 when a monkey was used to less than $10 with tissue culture, and reduced the time required from eight days to a few hours. Theoretically, it was possible to make a diagnosis by staining a single organism.

Reports of its successful application came in quick succession—for yellow fever, pertussis, malaria, syphilis, gonorrhea, streptococcus, and *Escherichia coli*. Dr. Wilbur Deacon used FA in diagnosing venereal disease. His work was particularly important because earlier tests for VD were either very difficult and therefore expensive, or they were not very sensitive. In CDC's Montgomery laboratories, Drs. Charles Shepard and Robert Goldwasser applied FA to rickettsial and viral diseases. In the first category were typhus and Rocky Mountain spotted fever, in the second, polio, encephalitis, and influenza. Also in Montgomery, Dr. Robert Kissling developed the FA test for rabies, first used in a field trial in 1959 with 100 percent accuracy. HEW Secretary Arthur Fleming was so enthusiastic he predicted that the ultraviolet diagnosis would open up an avenue "toward eventual eradication of rheumatic fever and rheumatic heart disease" and that it would bring almost immediate treatment of perhaps fifty communicable diseases. It was an indispensable tool for germ-warfare diseases. CDC's Technology Branch developed an air sampler that used FA to "read" the air for pathogens.[33]

It took four years of work and dozens of people to give a broadly applicable practical turn to Coons's theoretical study. Coons was very pleased with this "new way of looking at the world." The FA technique was popular with both scientists and the public. Important visitors to CDC were always taken to the laboratory to look through a microscope at the glowing disease organisms. The work made good copy for newspapers and magazines, and thus spread the word about CDC. More important, the FA technique made it possible for CDC to serve the states better.[34]

In the spring of 1958, CDC shifted its emphasis to staphylococcal infections. For several years, CDC had answered emergency calls from hospitals around the nation when staphylococcus infections broke out. The first call for help came in 1955 from Seattle, Washington, and in the next three years, there were twenty more requests. The outbreaks, while particularly severe among infants and nursing mothers, were not limited to the newborn and maternity units. They could show up anywhere in the hospital or even after the patient returned home. Epidemics brought under control broke out again.[35]

The "golden villain" in the hospital infections drama was the *Staphylococcus aureus,* so called because of its color. It is ubiquitous in nature, and when antibiotics were first introduced, it could be kept under control easily. But over the years the many strains of staphylococcus, fighting for their own survival, became resistant to antibiotics just as mosquitoes, flies, and other insects developed resistance to insecticides. With antibiotics seemingly offering a magic shield against the spread of infection, some hospitals abandoned the stringent aseptic measures that had kept staphylococcus at bay and kept the problem hidden for fear of censure by health departments.

CDC organized an institutional subcommittee on staphylococcal infections in June 1957. Epidemiology would answer the epidemic calls; Laboratory would teach the state laboratory personnel how to do phage-typing (the quickest, most accurate means of identifying staphylococcal strains); Technology would work on studies of airborne pathogens; and Training would make a film.[36]

Early in 1958, a major epidemic in Houston pushed staphylococcus to the top of CDC's agenda when sixteen infants died in a single hospital. Before the epidemic was brought under control, more than half the employees in the hospital's pediatrics department had been found to harbor the bacterial strain. CDC's laboratory had little time for anything but phage-typing. In May, the Laboratory Branch became the national staphylococcal phage-typing center.[37]

Staphylococcal infections became a national issue, and the American Hospital Association asked for a conference to discuss the issues involved. The surgeon general concurred and put CDC in charge. This conference, held in September 1958 at CDC, made several recommendations: all hospitals should organize infection-control committees and isolate infectious patients; home care for minor illnesses should be encouraged; and research should begin on hospital design, ventilation, housekeeping procedures, and sterilization techniques. Congress appropriated an additional $1.3 million for research on staphylococcus, a million dollars to go to the National Institute of Allergy and Infectious Diseases, the rest to CDC.[38]

The environmental aspects of staph infections seemed to be the most troublesome area, and in this fact, Sib Simmons saw an opportunity. Within a week after the national conference, he asked permission for the Technology Branch to do research on the effect of air-conditioning, heating equipment, and disinfectants on staph infections. It was one of those programs he just "eas[ed] into . . . before somebody thought about it. I knew the staph thing had not been worked on, but by the time [Epidemiology] waked up, I already had it. Epi got calls, and they sent people out, but the organization of the CDC program on hospital infections was started by us. We had a concrete program."[39] It was another building block for CDC.

Another of those blocks was tuberculosis control, for which CDC was given responsibility in 1960. Like the Venereal Disease Division, the Tuberculosis Division was proud, and its staff fiercely resisted the move to Atlanta. The unit had a number of black employees, who were worried about housing in a segregated city. One portion of the division successfully resisted the transfer. Tuberculosis research stayed in Washington, primarily because the deputy chief of that program, Shirley Ferabee, did not want to move. Her husband was chief of operations at the Bureau of the Budget, so her protests carried unusual weight.[40]

By 1960 tuberculosis was on the decline. Its incidence dropped by 75 percent between 1946 and 1956, and the length of time required for hospitalization was cut by two thirds—to only eight months. This was owing primarily to the use of antibiotics, particularly streptomycin, and the development of a research methodology based on statistics. In the late 1950s, research on tuberculosis control centered on a new drug, isoniazid, as a prophylactic. Eventually, isoniazid proved so effective it made tuberculosis hospitals unnecessary.[41]

As CDC broadened the scope of its programs at home, it extended its influence abroad. Numerous foreign visitors, many of whom held their nation's highest positions in public health, came to CDC to study for weeks at the time. In the late 1950s, these visitors stayed at private homes or boarding houses in Atlanta, a silent testimonial to the segregated nature of Atlanta in that decade. "We simply try to explain to the Negro and other dark-skinned visitors that there are certain customs and traditions in this country, just as they have at home," Joseph Borches, the training officer said. "They usually understand."[42]

At the same time, more and more of CDC's staff went overseas at the request of the International Cooperation Administration, the World Health Organization, and the Pan American Sanitary Bureau. This was not something new. A decade earlier, CDC had provided help with malaria control. Justin Andrews went to Iran, and Harry Pratt and F. Earle Lyman to South Vietnam. At that time Surgeon General Scheele described the latter effort as "a keystone of our effort to contain communism and win a permanent peace. Health may . . . play a crucial and constructive role in influencing human destiny."[43]

The same arguments were presented in 1958. President Eisenhower called for an international attack on disease in the strife-torn Middle East, where the most serious health problems were infectious diseases, CDC's specialty. Experts on mosquito control went to Iran, and many of CDC's foreign visitors came from the Middle East.

Many people at CDC thought internationally. When an epidemic of cholera and smallpox swept across Southeast Asia in the late 1950s, Langmuir proposed that CDC send a team of epidemiologists to help. The proposal went through the Department of State to the World Health Organization, and in the spring of 1958, to everyone's astonishment, the offer was accepted. It was the first time a CDC team had gone overseas.

The EIS spring conference, the biggest meeting of the year for the epidemiologists, was to begin in a day or so in Atlanta, but when the call came, Langmuir accepted at once and left the next day with Dr. Glenn Usher, CDC's representative in Washington, and an EIS officer, Dr. Fred Dunn. A Cold War urgency as well as the health emergency propelled them to instantaneous response. A Russian team and some Afghan vaccinators were headed for East Pakistan (now called Bangladesh), and Langmuir was determined to get there first. If the first principle of epidemiology could be coupled with the drama of the Cold War, so much the better.

Within a few days, four more EIS officers left for East Pakistan—Drs. Jim Mosley, Yates Trotter, Chandler Dawson, and Bruce Dull—and two more, Drs. Malcolm Page and Jacob Brody, followed shortly. They were committed to work in the area for three months, and by the time they were all assembled, a plan of action was worked out: accompanied by a Pakistani physician, they would go out into the country to verify the reporting of smallpox cases and deaths, reasonable roles for epidemiologists. Shortly after the Americans reached Pakistan, the six-member Russian team, who were primarily interested in cholera, arrived. They brought cholera bacteriophage with them, a method of cholera control abandoned in the West two decades earlier, and received so much unfavorable publicity they left after one month.

CDC rented a house in Dacca, from which the team fanned out into the countryside. They traveled mostly by train and jeep, but sometimes on bicycles, in tricycle rickshaws or primitive boats powered by coolies, or on foot. They found little validity to the case reports of smallpox but much validity to the death reports, so their surveillance came to be one of mortality. The Pakistani health department used the information to direct the efforts of the twenty thousand volunteers it recruited to battle the massive epidemics.

The epidemic could not be brought under control in a few months' time, even though twenty million people were vaccinated. But it did provide the CDC team with a chance to teach and demonstrate the principles of epidemiology. They got some valuable experience as well. They saw their first smallpox cases, tested dried smallpox vaccine and found it was potent, and learned how to work in the highly charged political atmosphere that surrounded the epidemic. (The government of East Pakistan fell while they were there.) It was valuable hands-on experience for an organization that in less than a decade would tackle the eradication of smallpox on a much wider scale.[44]

CHAPTER 7

1600 Clifton Road

CDC's credibility grew steadily during the 1950s, but the institution remained homeless. Five years after Emory University donated fifteen acres of land on Clifton Road for its headquarters, the site was still covered with woods. Plans were drawn for seven buildings, but no money was appropriated for construction and there was little hope for such a miracle. Not even the need for vigilance against biological warfare could shake loose money for a permanent home for CDC.

This quest for new buildings coincided with the presidency of Dwight David Eisenhower and a new era in the history of the Public Health Service. In 1953 the Federal Security Agency was elevated to cabinet status as the new Department of Health, Education and Welfare. Politics accordingly became increasingly important. Although the surgeon general was allowed to keep his authority over the PHS and its commissioned corps, he reported to the HEW secretary. More money than ever before was spent for public health during that decade, but the priorities changed. Ever more emphasis was on medical research. The liberally funded NIH boomed.[1]

This shift of emphasis probably accounted for CDC's difficulty in making a case for new buildings despite the force of its arguments. It occupied fifty-three buildings in Atlanta, Chamblee, and Montgomery, many of them makeshift shelters contrived from barracks, hospital wards, mess halls, and portable buildings. They were firetraps, expensive to maintain, and biologically unsafe. Cases of tuberculosis, diphtheria, brucellosis, and numerous undiagnosed respiratory and systemic infections occurred among the clerical and technical personnel, many of whom, after treatment at government expense, asked for a transfer.

CDC's laboratories did not have germ-proof walls, individual room air-conditioning, large-scale facilities for incubation, very low temperature refrigeration, or built-in hoods and inoculation chambers with exhausts and expelled-air incineration.

This desperate state was complicated by the withdrawal of Lawson Veterans Administration Hospital from Chamblee, where most of CDC's laboratories were located. Rumors abounded that the adjacent Naval Air Station would extend its runways directly through the site to accommodate jet planes. What would CDC do without even its makeshift facilities? From the Atlanta perspective, the argument for new buildings was compelling.

The view from Washington was quite different.[2] Surgeon General Scheele was not particularly interested in CDC's needs, and the Bureau of the Budget refused the request for $12,125,000 to fund construction. Despite repeated entreaties by Justin Andrews and Theodore Bauer, President Truman's order that no new buildings be erected except for defense purposes remained in effect long after he left office.

Help came from an unexpected source in the mid 1950s. Boisfeuillet Jones, vice president of Emory University and administrator of the university's health services, called Bauer for some information. Robert Woodruff, chairman of the board of the Coca-Cola Company and Emory's largest benefactor, wanted to know why no buildings had been erected on the site donated so many years ago by Emory, and indirectly by Woodruff himself. If the government did not want the property, he would take it back. Bauer explained the difficulty of getting any building request through the Bureau of the Budget, a conversation Jones in turn repeated to Woodruff, who was an old friend of the president's. (Eisenhower often went hunting on Woodruff's south Georgia plantation.)

Undeterred by the fine points of government bureaucracy and priorities, Woodruff telephoned the president, who was on a golfing vacation at the Cherry Hill Country Club in Denver.

"Ike, do you have a pencil and paper?" Woodruff asked the president. "I have a question to ask you. Why isn't the government building that CDC building in Atlanta?"

"Well, send me a note," Eisenhower replied, deflecting the inquiry.

"I'm not going to send you a note," Woodruff responded. "I asked if you had a pencil and paper."

Whether or not the president took notes on this conversation, he acted on it, because within a few days the White House got in touch with the surgeon general, who then asked Bauer why he had done nothing about the new building. He was ordered to get things started at once.[3]

By July 1955 the preliminaries were nearly complete. Both the House and the Senate approved an appropriation of $12,330,000, and the General Services Administration was authorized to let a contract. The buildings were to be erected under the Lease-Purchase Act, which provided that private interests would finance construction. The government, in turn, would pay for them over a period of years through a lease. But contractors showed little interest in the project, primarily because of the 4 percent ceiling on interest. Only a few bids were received, and they were all rejected.[4]

When Dr. Anderson became CDC's director in the fall of 1956, his charge was to get the building program under way. Plans drawn years before were out of date and had to be done over. The first step was to get money for planning, a process that began in the Bureau of State Services, and went, in turn, to the surgeon general, the budget office of the department, the secretary of HEW, the Bureau of Budget, and finally to Congress. Anderson was ultimately successful, only to be told by his own staff that they were short by half and he had to ask for more. Painful as it was to admit that he had underestimated by 50 percent, he swallowed his pride and repeated the whole tedious process.[5]

By the spring of 1957, ten years after Emory donated the land, construction was again put on hold when the president deferred all building projects. In Washington, Dr. Bauer, who by that time had become chief of the Bureau of State Services, did what he could to get an exception. Testifying before the House Subcommittee on Appropriations, chaired by Rep. John E. Fogarty of Rhode Island, he spoke forcefully of CDC's desperate need. Fogarty, a champion of public health, was easily convinced, but his influence alone was insufficient.[6]

Almost a year later Fogarty came to Atlanta to see for himself. He found an institution scattered in too many buildings to be efficient. He toured the facilities at Chamblee and was properly horrified. He wrote the president directly:

> When I say that conditions are deplorable I have in mind the dilapidated wood frame structures occupied at Chamblee. . . . originally constructed as temporary buildings for the old Lawson General Hospital. That Federal employees are required to work in such firetraps is, in my opinion inexcusable. I sincerely hope that the next time you are in Georgia you can find the time to visit this institution.[7]

Fogarty, a Democrat, accused the Republican administration of unnecessary delay, and predicted that the lease-purchase agreement—with payback in twenty-five years—would greatly increase the cost. This unusual method of financing public buildings kept the federal deficit down, but it was expensive. The government paid $20 million for buildings that cost only $13 million. The CDC structures were the only special-purpose buildings constructed under the Lease-Purchase Act. All the others were office buildings or post offices.[8]

In spite of the trouble CDC had getting money for its new headquarters, the decade before 1965 would in time be looked on nostalgically as the "good old days" insofar as getting money out of Washington was concerned. The process was always the same—through the hierarchy of the Public Health Service, into the maze of the Department of Health, Education and Welfare, then to the Bureau of the Budget, and finally to Capitol Hill. The hard part always came early in the process, and the amount CDC asked for was usually cut each step of the way through the Bureau of the Budget, watchdog of the Treasury. When the process reached Capitol Hill, it was necessary to touch base in only two places: Congressman Fogarty in the House and Senator Lister Hill, Democrat of Alabama, in the Senate. These two men headed the appropriations subcommittees that oversaw health matters. Authorization committees, which later came to play such an important part in the budget process, did not exist. The only authorization needed was the Public Health Service Act, which, as Anderson explained, directed that "the Surgeon General shall go forth and do good."

When the division chief (Anderson in the late 1950s) reached Congress, he was expected to justify exactly the amount approved by the Bureau of the Budget and no more. Because the administration was controlled by Republicans and the Congress by Democrats (some of whom were enthusiastic about public health), whoever testified was almost certain to be asked about the adequacy of funding. Often as not, Fogarty or Hill would lean across the table and inquire, "Are you sure, Doctor, you are asking for enough for these wonderful programs?" It was not unusual for Congress to increase health budgets sizably over administration requests.[9]

Anderson had especially good relations with Fogarty, whom he first met when he was head of the Tuberculosis Division. After Anderson moved to Atlanta, Fogarty let him know that he was especially interested in CDC. It was far from Washington, Fogarty said, and had no great lobby, and he wanted to help. While Anderson was director, even though he asked for big budgets for planning and construction, the CDC always got good increases for its epidemiology, laboratory, and training services. "We took advantage of every crisis," Anderson recalled. "When Asian flu came along, we were . . . at the door asking for more money for labs and EIS. When the staphylococcus infection scare [appeared], we asked for more money and got it."[10]

Congressman Fogarty was a colorful character, a man of great energy. He often wore bright green bow ties and sometimes did business over a few drinks. In the House he was known as "Mr. Public Health," a man who took great pride in what he was doing. Senator Hill was quite different, a distinguished-looking, courtly, old-fashioned southern gentleman who preferred to do business in his office. He put people at ease, listened, and made suggestions. His father had been a physician, and this may have been at the root of Hill's deep interest in public health, but whatever the reason, he was absolutely committed to it. He was always in control and always did his homework well.

The surgeon general, Fogarty, and Hill formed the base of CDC's support in Washington. Sometimes it was important to touch base also with Mrs. Mary Lasker, a well-to-do New York woman who made promotion of public health one of her main interests. Although she was primarily concerned with the National Institutes of Health, she sometimes supported CDC's projects. "It was axiomatic in those days," Bill Watson recalled, "if you wanted anything done, you touched four bases: the surgeon general, Senator Hill, Congressman Fogarty, and Mary Lasker."[11]

CDC, whose domain was service, was removed from the center of power both ideologically and geographically. It did not have a strong constituency—its budget was only a small fraction of that for NIH—and it was not easy to keep its presence felt in Washington. There were advantages to being out of Washington, however, and as the years passed, the Atlanta location was considered one of CDC's great pluses. It meant less involvement with the political intrigues of the Capitol, less contact with bureaucrats, more freedom of action, and best of all, many fewer meetings to attend. Distance was also conducive to the feeling of esprit so important to CDC's success. As one staff member put it, the Atlanta location was "salubrious." Atlanta benefited, too, and in the late 1950s began to take pride in the government health center being built in its midst.[12]

At that time Atlanta was a big country town with signs of racism everywhere. The CDC staff was as lily white as the leadership of its home city. There were no black persons in the Peachtree–Seventh Street headquarters, a fact symbolized in segregated Atlanta by something so simple as the existence of only two rest rooms there, one for men and one for women. In the years after the 1954 Supreme Court decision in *Brown v. Board of Education,* the South's determination to maintain a segregated society was demonstrated forcefully in many ways, including the existence of separate rest rooms, water fountains, and waiting rooms for blacks and whites. The matter of separate rest rooms bothered Anderson, who wondered what he would do when and if blacks were added to the staff. In planning the new facilities on Clifton Road, he handled the problem in the best southern fashion: there were two sets of rest rooms, one for blacks and one for whites. The building was barely open before both the law and the mood changed, and CDC found itself with twice as many rest rooms as it needed. There was never enough lab space, however, so the extras were gradually converted to better use. In a way this changed use of space symbolized an internal transition of CDC from a southern institution to a national and international one.

Racial problems affected the construction of the new CDC headquarters on Clifton Road, and it fell to Anderson to deal with these sticky issues. He had a run-in with the Georgia Power and Light Company over special lines to the construction site. The law required Georgia Power to post equal opportunity employer signs along the right of way, which it refused to do. HEW Secretary Arthur Fleming instructed Anderson and Mr. Lyle, the regional director of HEW at the time, to call on the president of Georgia Power, John J. McDonough, and educate him. The meeting began pleasantly and Anderson was thinking that the education process would go quickly when Lyle turned to him and asked, "Dr. Anderson, what was it we came here to talk about?"

There was nothing for Anderson to do but plunge in. "I understand that you won't put up the equal employment opportunity signs," he said. McDonough exploded out of his chair, protesting that the company had many black employees, especially in the home economics department. Perhaps the trauma of the visit made Anderson forget what happened next, because years later, he could not remember how the problem was resolved, but the power lines were put in and construction got under way.

Resolution of difficulties with the Atlanta Gas Light Company required negotiations in Atlanta and Washington. The company refused to sign the antidiscrimination clause in its contract to install large pipelines. Anderson reported this to Washington, only to be told by Secretary Fleming that he was to get the problem solved even if it meant running a pipeline from Savannah to Atlanta for the sole use of CDC. Anderson wondered how the Army's Fort McPherson and the Federal Penitentiary in Atlanta, both of which were served by the Atlanta Gas Light Company, got around the no-discrimination clause. A check with the Departments of Defense and Justice revealed that they did not even require it.

Secretary Fleming expressed disbelief at this startling disclosure, but when he double-checked with Defense and Justice, they acknowledged this was correct. The commission overseeing governmental construction contracts at first insisted that these other contracts could not exist, but finally decided that the problem could not be resolved on a case-by-case basis, and Atlanta Gas Light was allowed to proceed with the pipeline without signing the antidiscrimination clause.[13]

The electricity and gas crises threatened CDC's viability. Equally serious was the possibility that the Atlanta public schools would be closed. Bumper stickers emblazoned "Never!" appeared all over the South, and governors stood in schoolhouse doors proclaiming "Segregation forever." If Atlanta's schools closed, CDC's fate was surely sealed. Few scientists would move their families to a community without public schools, and science could not thrive in such a closed-minded atmosphere.

Racial problems complicated CDC's day-to-day business as well. Housing was always a problem for blacks on official visits until Anderson persuaded a small hotel close by the downtown headquarters to relax its racial policy. Office space was a problem, too. When even the new buildings could not house the rapidly growing institution, Anderson had to rent office space, but as an equal opportunity employer, CDC was barred from a suitable building in nearby Decatur. Anderson found one in Buckhead whose owner was amenable to having blacks work therein, and the immediate problem was solved. Another was certain to crop up. "Considering the climate in Atlanta," he recalled, "it is kind of amazing that we were able to do what we did."[14]

The first plan for Building 1 was for a large E-shaped structure with many windows. Marion Brooke thought this meant the laboratories would not be air-conditioned, and he was worried. His fears proved groundless, largely because construction was so long delayed. By the time it began, air-conditioning was no longer an exotic item.[15] The concerns of Brooke and others were probably instrumental in getting the plans changed to something quite different, two buildings in one: a central windowless part for the laboratories, surrounded by an outer shell with a large number of windows for offices. The laboratories, but not the offices, were to be air-conditioned. By the time construction was completed, however, air-conditioning had achieved wider use and the offices were cooled, too.

The laboratories were designed by a team that garnered ideas from around the country. Among the planners was Earl Arnold, who turned the modest facilities at Montgomery into a decent place to work. Arnold did not like the concept of windowless laboratories, but he was more concerned with safety than with esthetics. The problem of constructing laboratories where work with infectious materials could be done safely had never been resolved entirely, not even at NIH. But Arnold and the others did what they could to design proper equipment and air-filtration and air-incineration systems. There was no shakedown period. The concrete buildings were up, and the people fitted into them.

One of the new buildings was designed especially for the audiovisual unit, which turned out dozens of films and filmstrips a year. Its needs were quite specific. The four-story Building 3 contained two huge stages, each three stories high, numerous darkrooms, and an excellent sound department. It was everything Dr. James Lieberman, the movie maker, needed for producing and distributing films and other audiovisual aids.

Squabbling over space was probably inevitable. Epidemiology had more space than it could use immediately. Jim Steele, who headed the veterinary program, asked for twenty-six animal rooms in Building 7, even though he had only a few guinea pigs and two dogs at the time. Since Building 7 did not exist, no funds having been appropriated for it, a bit of wishful thinking did no harm. Dr. Donald Martin also eyed the nonexistent Building 7 for the Training Branch. He thought it should be like the new Center for Continuing Education at the University of Georgia, a gorgeous building with hotel space, pleasant dining facilities, an auditorium, and many meeting rooms. The Laboratory Branch had other ideas. It wanted Building 7 for the diagnostic reagents program and other work.[16]

When the new buildings in Atlanta were complete, the Montgomery lab was to close. This was a touchy situation, because Alabama was Senator Hill's home state. Anderson and Deputy Surgeon General Price called on the senator to break the news personally. Hill welcomed them cordially, but, as expected, he was not happy when he learned the nature of their mission. "Don't ever come to me with news that you are going to close something up in my state," he said. The tension was broken only when the senator laughed. He was mollified when the radiological health program laboratory was moved into buildings vacated by CDC.[17]

The Chamblee laboratories were to be closed, too. In fact, the miserable conditions at Chamblee, more than anything else, provided the raison d'être for the long campaign to get something better. Before the buildings at 1600 Clifton Road were complete, however, it was obvious that everything could not be squeezed in. Some programs would have to stay behind. Venereal disease lost out, and so did toxicology, which, much to Sib Simmons's dismay, was moved from Oatland Island into four buildings at Chamblee. Simmons thought this missed the whole point of moving—to be close to scientific, academic, and professional resources.

Moving days for those units assigned space in the new buildings were from May through June 1960. Murphy's Law was at work, however, and the final day set for moving turned out to be the first. Dr. Anderson was a casualty of the delay. He never occupied the large corner suite on the second floor of Building 1 reserved for him. Just as the move began, he was transferred to Washington. CDC's deputy chief, Dr. Clarence Smith, became the center's sixth director, and it was he who moved to the "Second Floor," CDC's version of the Oval Office.[18]

There is nothing ordinary about moving a laboratory. Postponement created the first problems. Mae Melvin packed up her parasitology lab in April, but it was a case of hurry up and wait. Her work slowed to a halt, so she unpacked bit by bit, and was about back to normal in late July when she was given just two days to get ready once more. The bacteriology laboratory moved then, too. William Ewing could never forget July 29, 1960. With the models of the laboratories drawn months before clearly in his mind, he ran up and down the corridor of his new lab all day directing the placement of refrigerators and boxes. Truck after truck came, and at day's end he was exhausted, but the bacteriology labs looked just like the models. It was a look that remained unchanged for many years.[19]

Moving the virus and rickettsia laboratory from Montgomery was more difficult. The staff, certain that their freedom would be inhibited, and that their productivity would suffer, did not want to move. They liked the lack of immediate oversight that being in Montgomery afforded, just as those in Atlanta relished their distance from Washington. The laboratory's director, Morris Schaeffer, decided not to move; he accepted a position in New York instead. The Montgomery group had a new leader, Dr. Telford Work.

Jim Paine worked out the moving-day logistics. In Montgomery, all reference specimens were kept at −70° F. The freezer manufacturer did not know how long these low temperatures could be maintained without power, so Paine's staff experimented for days before coming up with the sawdust solution: plastic bags filled with wet sawdust packed into every nook and cranny. The freezers were then taped shut and kept unopened for several days. One midnight they were loaded onto trucks, which arrived in Atlanta about 6 A.M. Their contents still frozen hard, the freezers were unloaded and plugged in again. Animals had to be moved, too. Dogs under long-term studies for rabies posed an especially difficult problem. A car "riding shotgun" followed the closed trucks carrying the dogs in their cages just in case a traffic accident should spill rabies-challenged dogs along the roadside.[20]

On September 8, 1960, the mostly windowless buildings on Clifton Road, which had the solid, serviceable look of a factory, were dedicated. A flatbed truck, draped with bunting, served as a platform. The sun bore down on the parking lot, the chairs were hard, and the program went on too long. It was nonetheless a momentous day for the center and, some said, for the health of the world. CDC employees wore Dedication Day ribbons as a reminder that people, more than buildings, made the center important. HEW Secretary Arthur Fleming and all of CDC's former chiefs came. Dr. Thomas Parran, who had trained so many of its leaders, was there, too. Surgeon General Leroy E. Burney presided. Neighboring Emory University shared the celebration. Scientists in both institutions looked forward to years of fruitful cooperation.

Congressman Fogarty was the speaker. In the warm, persuasive style for which he was well known, the congressman appealed to the American people to be vigilant in matters of health. The people, not physicians, he said, would determine how the "rich life saving gifts" that came from the center would be used. "Let the ingeniousness of the scientists employed here be matched by our own ingeniousness in adapting old ways, finding new ways, challenging tradition . . . to assure that when knowledge leaves the laboratory, it reaches promptly all the people, rich and poor, young and old, whose health it can protect."[21] Astute politican that he was, Fogarty knew that the political and social challenges would most likely be more difficult to resolve than the scientific ones.

CHAPTER 8

A Call to Arms

The first months in the new CDC headquarters coincided with a fortuitous shift in the national mood. President John F. Kennedy summoned the American people to duty and service on a "New Frontier." The sense of purpose emanating from 1600 Pennsylvania Avenue was reflected at 1600 Clifton Road. Proud of its expertise and anxious to work on a broader scale, CDC was ready to move forward.

Although most of the staff did not realize it at the time, they had a powerful new weapon in their arsenal. The announcement was made without fanfare at a meeting of the branch chiefs: "NOVS [National Office of Vital Statistics] was moved to CDC on September 30. We don't have any responsibility for publishing the morbidity report until January."[1] The laconic wording of the staff minutes correctly reflected the remarkable lack of enthusiasm for publishing the *Morbidity and Mortality Weekly Report*. Most of them could not see how this would benefit CDC, and they did not want the bother of a weekly publication. Since it increased the staff by only half a position and added but $16,000 to the budget, it hardly seemed worth the effort.

Alexander Langmuir did not see it that way. He used all the tricks he could muster to get *MMWR*, as it is universally known, transferred from Washington. Many at CDC looked upon it with disdain as a moribund journal that had served little use, but Langmuir saw great possibilities in it and argued persuasively that the agency charged with controlling and preventing disease should also collect and distribute morbidity and mortality data. *MMWR* could be used for epidemic reports, and it was perfect for relaying information to health officials. Still, the move was, as Langmuir observed, like "pulling teeth without anesthesia." Just as he had seen CDC as the "promised land" when others saw nothing but a bunch of technicians, he saw in *MMWR* the key to giving surveillance the power to make a difference. Establish a reputation for scrupulous accuracy, he maintained, and *MMWR* would add to CDC's stature.[2]

Publication began in January 1961, and *MMWR* quickly took on an Atlanta stamp. When published in Washington, it had contained mostly "non-vital" information, as one critic put it. Within a few months, it was transformed. Morbidity and mortality data, which came in every Friday from all the states and 123 major cities, were recorded in enormous ledgers by eye-shaded clerks perched on stools. The data were then carefully compiled for publication the following Friday. The printing press was in the basement, and it was a point of pride that *MMWR* never missed an issue. Even when snowstorms closed down the rest of CDC, the press deadline was met. In 1966, when CDC somewhat timidly entered the computer age, an effort was made to simplify and speed up data collection, but Langmuir had no use for computers and resisted vigorously. For years this was a losing battle.[3]

The very first issue of *MMWR* published under the aegis of CDC contained a report of a hepatitis epidemic in New Jersey. When *MMWR* was published at NOVS, the editor, Carl Dauer, sometimes included notices of epidemics, but his office had no way of doing an investigation. Since CDC did investigations all the time, reports of epidemics became routine. Quite early on, editorial comments were appended to articles, giving CDC a bit of leverage it had never had before. Dr. Michael Gregg, who became editor in 1967, explained: "We can present the science in the text and anyone can interpret it anyway he wants. But the editorial note is our opportunity. . . . to get the information out and make it work for us."[4]

Langmuir supervised the publication of *MMWR*. A stickler for linguistic precision, he expected the same from the editorial staff. Ida Sherman was his mainstay; the other staff were mostly EIS officers. (Among them was Dr. Lawrence Altman, who later became a medical reporter for the *New York Times*.) Quality data, investigated and explained, were the weekly's hallmark, and it quickly gained popularity. The circulation in 1961 was 6,000; two decades later it was more than 80,000. *MMWR* became a key factor in CDC's relations with the states and the press. Many countries and the World Health Organization imitated it.[5]

The buildings on Clifton Road were testimony in brick and mortar to

CDC's stability, but they were not perfect. Their design was flawed, and mechanical problems bothered everybody. Since the lot was so small, plans for expansion began at once. Space out of town for breeding experimental animals was urgently needed. Amazingly, when measured against the glacial pace of financing CDC's building program in the 1950s, money for these additions was appropriated speedily and with little trouble. The House Appropriations Committee, doubtless at the behest of Congressman Fogarty, readily approved $12 million for constructing a larger auditorium, an animal-breeding farm, and more laboratories. The committee criticized the existing center as built on "badly out of date plans under the ill-fated lease purchase scheme." Again everybody hoped to close the Chamblee labs, and room had to be made to relocate the Chapel Hill venereal disease experimental laboratory, the Southeastern Rabies Field Station (from Montgomery), and the rest of the Tuberculosis program, which was still in Washington. All these moved to Atlanta. Meanwhile, rumblings came from Savannah that the laboratories at Oatland Island were inadequate and difficult to maintain. At least some of the staff wanted to move.[6]

A mostly new staff directed CDC's stepped-up war against disease. Dr. Clarence (Larry) Smith became CDC director just as the new buildings were occupied, and within a year there were major changes in his command. The long-time chief of the Laboratory Branch, Dr. Ralph Hogan, retired to become an epidemiologist for the state of Florida. (Langmuir could hardly believe it. Once in Florida, Hogan's relationship with the Epidemiology Branch underwent a complete reversal. His cooperation was, according to Langmuir himself, "total.") Succeeding Hogan as Laboratory director was Dr. U. Pentti Kokko, a graduate of the University of Helsinki and of Johns Hopkins University. He and Langmuir were cordial, and the simmering conflict between the Epidemiology and Laboratory branches cooled. Dr. Alan Donaldson, who had been at CDC since the MCWA days, stayed on as deputy director, and William Watson, whom everyone called Bill, was appointed chief executive officer in September 1961. He was the first of the public health advisors to move into a CDC command post, and for more than two decades he played an increasingly important role. He became, as one colleague put it, "the conscience of CDC."

Another newcomer to the administrative office was Dr. David Sencer, just beginning a seventeen-year stint at CDC, eleven of them as its director. Sencer came out of the Tuberculosis Division and worked briefly in Washington in the Bureau of State Services before his transfer to CDC as assistant director. He was given a free hand, and as an old-timer with the Tuberculosis Division, he eased the integration of that unit into its new organization. Blessed with an incredible memory and a gift for detail, Sencer learned how to make CDC work. For all the glamour of the laboratory and epidemiology, he knew that it was administrative support that made the wheels turn: making sure that people had the things they needed—the media, the glassware, the equipment, the travel arrangements. A sense of pride was important, too. Bill Watson told a story that spoke eloquently to the point. "Have you looked at the flag?" one of the telephone operators asked one day. "It's dirty. CDC should not have a dirty flag."[7]

A sense of institutional pride and a determination to make things work forced CDC to confront the racial issue in Atlanta squarely. Larry Smith decided that insofar as CDC was concerned, race did not exist. CDC was a national organization with work to do. Many blacks came there to do business, and that made CDC's role different. It was not social. It was business. He pretended that Atlanta was not a southern town.

Bill Watson went to him and said, "I don't believe you understand," but Smith just blithely proceeded. There were blacks coming to a meeting and Smith and Watson scouted around until they found a hotel, the Peachtree Manor, that would take them. "We did the same thing with the finest, newest restaurant in Atlanta, Yohannan's at Lenox Square," Watson said. "Larry said we will take our black African visitors to dinner. I protested that the restaurants were segregated. 'But this is business,' he said. So we made [a] reservation at Yohannan's. The African wore native dress. We walked in that restaurant and sat down and they served us. No questions."

An improvement in race relations in Atlanta was essential before CDC could be transformed from a southern institution into a national and international one. Watson was particularly sensitive to racial injustice. On a visit to the Savannah laboratories, he noticed that a distinction was made in the laboratory's paging system. Some were called Mr. and Dr. and some were John and Jane. "So I stopped it. I knew Smith would back me. Everyone had a title after that." In Atlanta, the policy was to hire blacks and develop an active, vigorous in-house training program. Watson called it "our own internal kind of desegregation." When CDC was small enough to have a Christmas party, there was integrated dancing, unheard of in Atlanta, and it created quite a furor.[8]

Progress towards equality and protection of human rights was not always smooth. William Darrow, a public health advisor from New York, came to Atlanta for training as an interviewer in the venereal disease program in 1961. Interviews were conducted in a room with a two-way mirror so that the PHAs could be observed and recorded for later critique, but the patients were not informed. In those days, the Venereal Disease Branch was reluctant to hire women and blacks as public health advisors on the premise that health departments would not accept them. But Darrow, who became a recruiter for CDC, with Bill Watson urging him along, pushed for the hiring of more blacks. There was one touchy incident in 1962 when a young black man from New York, son of a United Nations official, quit a venereal disease study course when he was refused service in a restaurant. Two white trainees also quit in protest. When Congressman Adam Clayton Powell of Harlem complained to HEW, Secretary Abraham Ribicoff assured him it would not happen again.[9]

Sensitivity to racism did not extend to the Tuskegee experiment, which continued into its fourth decade. A changed social climate and the passage of landmark civil rights legislation in 1964 and 1965 did not stop it. Darrow once went to Alabama with a physician to test old black men for cardiovascular problems. "He asked me if I knew about the study," Darrow recalled. "I said, 'Not much, we aren't allowed to.' He said 'I feel very uncomfortable doing this.' That is when I knew something was going to happen sooner or later. This was before it all hit the press." The Tuskegee study was a time bomb ticking away.

Watson described the Tuskegee experiment as "one of those instances in which the sins of the fathers were visited upon their descendants, but the descendants did not see what was happening in society and they did not act soon enough." Watson is uncritical of Vonderlehr and his associates, who began the experiment on untreated syphilis in black males in the 1930s. He called them liberals for their time. "They saw blacks afflicted with this dread plague, syphilis. There's a great deal of paternalism in this, and they thought they were doing the right thing. . . . People forget in the antibiotic age that the pre-antibiotic treatments [for syphilis] were risky in and of themselves. But it is impossible to defend the fact that Tuskegee was not terminated earlier."[10]

CDC had no more implacable foe than venereal disease. The fight against it occupied more than half the staff, and in 1961 it seemed as if the battle would be lost. Syphilis rose an alarming 200 percent in just two years, and other venereal diseases, particularly gonorrhea, increased too. Funds for control were dangerously low. In 1950 state and federal governments spent twenty cents per capita on venereal disease control; in 1960, only eleven cents. During that time, rapid urbanization and a changing lifestyle increased the opportunity for venereal disease to spread. Primary and secondary syphilis reached their lowest incidence in 1957: 6,251 cases, or 3.8 per 100,000 of population. Then the upward spiral began. In 1961 there were 18,781 new cases, a rate of 10.4 per 100,000. Major organizations long concerned with venereal disease control were alarmed. Three of them—the Association of State and Territorial Health Officers, the American Venereal Disease Association, and the American Social Health Association—asked the government to double appropriations for the fight against VD. Surgeon General Luther Terry responded with a proposal to *eradicate* syphilis. He appointed a task force to tell him how to do it and set a timetable. Headed by Dr. Leona Baumgartner, commissioner of health for New York City, the task force worked through the autumn of 1961. Its plan was full of hope and loaded with "ifs": "If personnel can be secured and developed to the required level by 1963, and if a comprehensive, dynamic, promotional education program is developed, the epidemic spread of syphilis in this country can be stopped within ten years."[11]

This special call to arms required a major shift of emphasis: the National Venereal Disease Control Program became the National Syphilis Eradication Program. In the "can do" atmosphere of the early 1960s, anything seemed possible. The campaign's major weapon was epidemiology. The number of field staff personnel in the VD branch jumped from 300 to 480 in 1962. They worked in forty-three states, the District of Columbia, the Virgin Islands, and Puerto Rico.[12]

What they learned was discouraging. The number of cases of primary and secondary syphilis increased dramatically to more than 20,000 in 1963, but that was less than half the story. Epidemiologic follow-up showed an additional 124 cases for every 100 infectious patients interviewed. Syphilis could be wiped out *if* there was more money for follow-up, *if* there was better reporting by doctors, and *if* the public could be educated. But syphilis was not included in the curricula of most secondary schools and received short shrift in medical schools. Only a few physicians had had as much as two hours' training in syphilology, and fewer still had ever seen a clinical case. When public apathy was added to the medical profession's low index of suspicion, the magnitude of the problem facing public health officials was tremendous.[13]

In spite of this, progress was made. "Operation Pursuit" considered every index case as the beginning of an epidemic, quickly followed up all disease contacts, and treated them whether or not they showed symptoms. By 1966 the number of cases of infectious syphilis in the United States began to level off. Yet William Brown, who directed the work, was ever mindful of Brown's Law: "As the point of eradication is approached, it is more often the program that is eradicated than the disease."[14]

In the laboratory, the diagnosis of syphilis was steadily improved. The rapid plasma reagin test gave results in a few hours and was especially useful along the Mexican border, where all migrant workers were screened and treated. Fluorescent antibody tests speeded up diagnosis still more. By 1967 a completely automatic serologic test for syphilis was practicable. There was hope, too, that a vaccine for syphilis could be developed, the only certain way to stop the disease.

The task force had recommended an intensive educational program for both professionals and the public. The Venereal Disease Branch set up a behavioral science unit in July 1963 to find out what worked best. Physicians had to be persuaded to report more than one of every nine cases of syphilis, and adolescents and young adults, whose patterns of sexual behavior were changing rapidly, needed to know how syphilis was spread. To educate physicians, CDC prepared a "Professional Education Package" containing printed materials, slides, and a film. Educating the public was more difficult. Public controversy over the school curriculum threatened the essential educational process.[15]

Two books on venereal disease written by William F. Schwartz, an educational consultant at CDC, attempted to separate venereal disease from sin. Schwartz intended "to take venereal disease out of its moral context and . . . [make] it a disease." He did very well until the national Columbus Day Committee discovered that he had "slurred" the honor of the Admiral of the Ocean Sea. Schwartz wrote that Christopher Columbus had died in jail, paralyzed and quite mad from syphilis. The chairman of the national Columbus Day observance kicked up so much fuss that the HEW secretary asked the National Library of Medicine for a thorough review. When the search showed differences of opinion about the cause of Columbus's madness, the secretary asked Schwartz to delete all mention of Columbus in future editions. The author reluctantly agreed. Even with Schwartz's pledge not to slur America's discoverer again, the issue would not die. The Knights of Columbus appealed to President Lyndon Johnson's special assistant Jack Valenti to do something. The "something" turned out to be the physical excision of all references to Christopher Columbus from the 52,000 existing copies of the book. Fortunately, the snipped-out page began and ended with a paragraph.[16]

CDC undertook the eradication of syphilis with some enthusiasm, but not another eradication program that came its way about the same time. Hardly anyone saw the eradication of the *Aedes aegypti* mosquito, vector for yellow fever and dengue, as a pressing health concern. Dengue was a problem in Puerto Rico, and it cropped up occasionally in the states, but there had not been a case of yellow fever in the United States since 1905. Better use could be made of the public health dollar than to wage an expensive campaign against this "city slicker" mosquito that liked to breed in old tires, bottles, tin cans, and water barrels.

The decision to eradicate *Aedes aegypti* in the United States was a political one, a matter of foreign policy. Latin American nations wanted it. Two decades earlier, Dr. Fred L. Soper of the Pan American Sanitary Organization had developed a program that successfully eradicated the yellow fever mosquito from Brazil, but there was danger of reinfestation so long as the carrier existed anywhere in the hemisphere from Oklahoma to Argentina. An eradication program was again proposed in 1942 but because of the war, no action was taken. Not until 1947 was an eradication plan approved. Countries in South and Central America got started at once and claimed much success, but the United States did nothing. Soper, who became a consultant to the Public Health Service, actively lobbied for the program, to which the United States had made a formal commitment. In 1961 the Pan American Health Organization (PAHO) approved a resolution calling for eradication of *Aedes aegypti* and the United States signed on, but again did nothing. The next year Mexico's minister of health pointedly presented Surgeon General Luther L. Terry with "the last two *Aedes aegypti* mosquitoes in Mexico," neatly embedded in plastic.[17]

The point struck home. CDC fought the program "tooth and nail" because public health funds could be better used elsewhere, but the political pressure was too great. In the spring of 1963, the House Appropriations Committee turned down a request for $5 million for the program, but six months later, yielding to political inevitability, approved $3 million. As Congressman Fogarty said, "It is not very often that we have a foreign aid program where the money can be spent in the United States."[18]

CDC accepted the order and the timetable to get rid of the *Aedes aegypti,* a more formidable and expensive task than eradicating a disease. The *Aedes aegypti* Eradication Branch was created, with Donald Schliessmann, a sanitary engineer who had been at CDC since its MCWA days, as its chief. The mosquito was found in nine southern states, from Texas to Florida, in Puerto Rico, and in the Virgin Islands, and its elimination required separate, closely supervised programs for each place. A pilot study done by the Technology Branch in Pensacola, Florida, from 1957 to 1961 provided a model. Power sprayers mounted on trucks were used routinely, but sometimes teams of men armed with hand sprayers checked around private homes several times each mosquito season. "We . . . will use the most democratic methods we possibly can," Schliessmann explained, but clearly cooperation and goodwill were as vital as insecticide to successful completion of the task.

The program began in the spring of 1964 in those places where the infestation was heaviest—Texas, southern Florida, Puerto Rico, and the Virgin Islands. It would have been better and cheaper to start everywhere at once, but this was impossible for reasons of both budget and biology. Old-timers at CDC must have had a sense of déjà vu. They were back in the transportation business. CDC leased hundreds of trucks, launched intensive recruitment efforts, and stockpiled supplies. "I'm about to buy five miles of muslin," the procurement officer, John Barron, told David Sencer one day. "The *Aedes aegypti* program will buy five miles of muslin so that they can tear it into little squares, tie stones in the corners, and put it over the water barrels in the Virgin Islands where people collect their drinking water so that mosquitoes won't lay their eggs."[19]

The program was the most expensive insect-eradication program ever launched by the PHS. Although progress was made, it was obvious the *Aedes aegypti* would not be eradicated in five years. There were delays and controversy. Entomologists were irate when they thought that "eradication" would apply to their research colonies. They considered their work vital to the success of the program. There was much to learn about the vector of yellow fever and dengue, like the fact that it was not so domestic after all. It often bred a half mile from human habitation in tree holes and palm fronds. Sib Simmons's Technology Branch called for more research on alternate methods of eradication. Insecticides alone would not accomplish the goal.[20] Two years later, Sencer outlined a new approach. Instead of trying to eradicate *Aedes aegypti*—an enormous, if not hopeless, task—he wanted to pay more attention to basic and operational yellow fever research, surveillance, and prompt epidemic assistance. Much more needed to be known about the natural history of the dengue viruses, too, so that control could be achieved with or without the eradication of the vector.[21]

In the summer of 1968, just as research that might have made the program work was maturing, the *Aedes aegypti* program was transferred from CDC to the Consumer Protection and Environmental Health Service. A year later, the entire program was abandoned. The government had spent $53 million on it, and the budget-conscious newly elected Republican administration cried enough. David Sencer was among those dispatched to the meeting of the Pan American Sanitary Bureau in El Paso to allay the fears of Latin America that swarms of North American mosquitoes would swoop across the border bringing death in their wake. The cost of the program, the legal difficulties involved (many Americans objected to the intrusion on private property of men in search of mosquitoes), and the rising tide of opposition to massive use of DDT all dictated that the program end.[22]

Sencer had always objected to the program, but he would not say the money had been wasted. The program produced an extremely effective insecticide that could be sprayed from an airplane at low altitude. CDC used it to fight encephalitis in Texas and malaria in El Salvador. Many American communities looked better, too, because much debris where mosquitoes bred was cleaned up. Few, if any, Americans fretted about the return of yellow fever. Devotees of surveillance knew that a good vaccine and a careful watch offered defense enough.[23]

These two eradication programs—one against an ancient disease, the other against an insect—did not originate in Atlanta, but CDC accepted responsibility for them. Few at CDC believed that syphilis could be eradicated, but they hoped that a massive dragnet would reduce it to a low level. The search-out-and-treat system worked well, but interest lagged, federal money dried up, and the job of control was more and more turned over to the states. Brown's Law went into effect. CDC was never enthusiastic about the *Aedes aegypti* program and gave it up without regret. These two programs were to CDC what the Vietnam War was to the nation. By the time they ended, attention was turned to other projects where the chances of success were much better.

CHAPTER 9

The Candidate for Surgeon General

For career officers in the Public Health Service, an administrative post at CDC was usually preparation for a higher position in Washington. When he learned the surgeon general wanted to see him, Larry Smith knew instinctively that he would be moving. He did not want to leave Atlanta; he felt a loyalty to CDC, perhaps the first director really to care about the institution since the old MCWA days. Sentiment, however, had no place in PHS appointments. Smith became deputy director of the Bureau of State Services, CDC's parent organization in the Public Health Service, and Dr. James Goddard took over as CDC chief in September 1962.

Goddard was as reluctant to go to CDC as Smith was to leave it, even though the promotion put a star on his uniform. Goddard's goal was to become surgeon general, but he hoped for some other road to the top. When Assistant Surgeon General Arnold Kurlander asked him why he deserved a star, Goddard replied that he had noticed the recent recipients of stars, and "I just happen to think I'm about as good as any of those are."

There were but three possibilities for a star appointment—head of the Indian Health Service, chief of the Hospital Division, or CDC chief. Goddard was to think it over. The post at CDC was his third choice. "I do not know anything about communicable disease other than what you get taught in medical school," he told Kurlander. "And you know, it's not my bag, Arnie."

"Congratulations, you're the new chief of the Communicable Disease Center," Kurlander replied.

"You bastard!" was all Goddard could say.

Kurlander and Surgeon General Terry had made the decision. In answer to Goddard's inevitable "Why?" Kurlander said, "Well, Jim, we think you still got a little growing to do, and we think that's a good place for you to do your growing. So you go down to Atlanta September 1."[1]

Goddard was, by his own admission, "young and brash" in 1962. At thirty-nine, he was the youngest man ever appointed chief of CDC. After graduating from George Washington University Medical School, he interned in the Public Health Service—again his last choice—and entered private practice in Kalida, Ohio. He became a PHS officer in 1952 in response to a collect telegram offering him a commission in the regular corps. He accepted because he wanted his life to make a difference, and he thought public health provided a better opportunity than private practice.

He had assignments in Colorado, North Carolina, and New York before he was loaned to the Federal Aviation Agency in 1959, where he raised an immediate stir. When he discovered there were no standards for balloon pilots, he applied for and got a license. FAA established qualifications at once. Goddard clashed with FAA's director, Najeeb Hallaby, however, and asked to be returned to the PHS. He was in charge of accident prevention when the summons came to go to Atlanta. Though he did not want the CDC job, he insisted on a very public signal that he was in charge. His personal star flag, to which his recent promotion entitled him, flew on CDC's pole—white when he was on board, yellow when he was away.[2]

A contemporary likened Goddard to "a guy who gets a new watch, takes it apart to examine all the pieces, then puts it back together. Except Goddard would try to improve on it." He began his new job by visiting all the field stations. The yellow flag flew at CDC while Goddard "took the watch apart."[3]

Goddard found work under way on vector-borne diseases at three stations: encephalitis in Greeley, plague in San Francisco, and schistosomiasis in San Juan, Puerto Rico. Work at the Phoenix field station had expanded to include hepatitis; virologists joined bacteriologists and epidemiologists who had studied diarrheal disease for more than a decade. At the Kansas City Station, Dr. Michael Furcolow studied histoplasmosis. By the time of Goddard's visit, Furcolow knew that this was not a rare disorder but a common ailment, especially in the Midwest. As many as thirty million Americans had been exposed. Assistant chief at Kansas City was thirty-two-year-old Dr. T. D. Y. ("Too Damn Young") Chin, the resident expert on ECHO viruses. The work in both Kansas City and Phoenix was indicative of CDC's expanding interests.

The physical facilities of the field stations mirrored those in Atlanta and Chamblee, ranging from very good to barely passable. The Kansas City Station was by far the best. After fifteen years in a quonset hut, it moved into a half million dollar structure at the University of Kansas Medical Center paid for by the Kansas Endowment Association. The Greeley station occupied a pre–World War I clapboard building, and the staff was anxious to move, preferably to Boulder or Fort Collins, where, like their colleagues in Kansas City, they would have a university connection. At the Phoenix Laboratory, Dr. Melvin Goodwin had won approval for a new building while Anderson was CDC's director, but nothing had been done. He told Goddard the need was urgent. The city of Phoenix was about to widen Seventh Street and take away half the laboratory.

Goddard's preparation for his job in Atlanta included a warning to look out for Alexander Langmuir, a troublemaker. While the Epidemiology chief insists he never sought out controversy—rather controversy sought him out—"Langmuirian thunder" was the stuff of legend. "See that little vent pipe there in the roof?" a secretary in his office asked a reporter one day. "When we see that smoking we hardly move because we know he's blowing off steam."[4] Langmuir was irascible and unpredictable, droll and witty, and shrewd about getting what he wanted.

Goddard arrived in Atlanta resplendent in his uniform, his reputation as an autocrat established. The two might well have clashed. Instead they got along well. Goddard liked Langmuir. When he got the impression at a budget meeting that Langmuir was not presenting the budget he wanted, he asked if this was really enough money. Langmuir said he could use more EIS officers. "How many?" "Sixty," Langmuir replied. "Fine," Goddard responded. The result was the largest EIS class ever.[5]

By the 1960s, Langmuir's reputation as the "hard-nosed epidemiologist" was well established. He liked the description and took much satisfaction in the ability of the EIS to handle any emergency. The group amassed a number of names—shoe-leather epidemiologists, disease detectives, fire fighters. Their hallmark was instant availability. Personal plans never took precedence over a call for help. Occasionally, they left without luggage. Sometimes an officer would return from one call only to be met at the airport with orders to catch the next plane for an emergency in another city. Such speed called for flexibility in financing travel, so the EIS operated on a "travel now, pay later" plan. Every officer had a booklet of blank tickets called TRs. If there was no time to go through channels, he just filled out a TR with a cost accounting number. Irregularities were commonplace and the despair of Helen Richardson, travel clerk in the EIS office, who had to justify everything, even a trip by dogsled to a remote corner of Alaska.[6]

Outbreaks of hepatitis kept the EIS especially busy. The problem surfaced in 1960, when there were sixty-five thousand cases and eleven epidemic calls. That year the concern was serum hepatitis. In 1961, there was a new worry, infectious hepatitis, traced to consumption of raw oysters and clams contaminated by sewage pollution. An epidemic in New Jersey was traced to a New Year's Eve Party where raw clams from Raritan Bay were served. In Mississippi, outbreaks were traced to raw oysters pronged in the mouth of the Pascagoula River. Dr. D. A. Henderson, the EIS chief who led the New Jersey investigation, called eating raw shellfish "Russian roulette on the half shell."

Control depended on surveillance and research. Dr. James W. Mosley was given a lab and named chief of the hepatitis investigations unit. It was his job to establish a base so that new control procedures could be quickly applied. "In the K[arl] F. Meyer tradition," Langmuir explained to CDC's chief, "field problems must be referred to the laboratory and rapidly back to the field if effective progress is to be made." Mosley worked in Atlanta, but when the new laboratory was built in Phoenix, Goodwin saw an opportunity to expand that laboratory's work in hepatitis. The National Aeronautics and Space Administration needed a place to house its chimpanzees, and Goodwin agreed to take them in if they could also be used for medical studies. That decision put CDC's Phoenix laboratory in the forefront of hepatitis research.[7]

After a decade of relatively little progress, 1961 was a "breakthrough" year in hepatitis. The discovery of shellfish as a source of infection, the question of carriers, and the use of gamma globulin as prophylaxis all pushed research along. The popular press dubbed hepatitis the "mystery disease," although there was nothing new about what once was called jaundice. Goddard compared hepatitis to Jack the Ripper. "It leaves its mark and we know it has struck, [but] . . . we have not isolated the virus, and therefore we have no vaccine."[8] Langmuir saw all the fieldwork in hepatitis as preparation. "We should be so knowledgeable about what's going on in this country that when the virus is isolated, when there is a tool to work with in hepatitis, we are there first with the most. This is going to break somewhere in the world. . . . Let's be ready!"[9]

Goddard was especially interested in the rapid increase of salmonella outbreaks, and nothing he learned at CDC better prepared him for his next job as commissioner of the Food and Drug Administration. The increasing complexity of the food chain turned what had been a medical curiosity into a major national problem. CDC began surveillance of salmonellosis in 1963 after dozens of cases attributable to *Salmonella derby* appeared in hospitals in the Northeast. Those outbreaks were traced first to contaminated eggs, then to powdered milk, frozen turkey, smoked fish, ground beef, dog food, and peppermint sticks. The ubiquitous salmonellas are hardy and, with the nation's food-distribution system undergoing radical change, they found their way into packaged foods such as cake mixes and assembly-line items like frozen foods. One plant could spread infection throughout the country. James Steele said the spread of salmonellosis was a "national disgrace," and Goddard urged physicians to be much more careful in reporting cases. One source of infection was animal feed, particularly fish meal, which is hard to keep sterile.[10]

The biggest outbreak of salmonellosis occurred in Riverside, California, in 1965, when 15,000 people were affected with varying degrees of diarrhea, nausea, and fever. The call for help came to CDC at 3 P.M. on Friday, and by midnight seven people from Atlanta were in Riverside. They first suspected powdered milk, then dried eggs, cake mixes, or a hotel banquet, but the pieces of the puzzle did not fit. Patients were scattered over the city, and they had bought their food in many markets. The only common denominator was residence in Riverside. Thousands of laboratory tests had to be made, so the laboratory went to the epidemic. John Boring, who led the lab team, zeroed in on the water supply, even though it came from a supposedly safe deep well. His suspicions proved correct and within a few days *Salmonella typhymurium*, which ordinarily does not live in water, was isolated as the cause. No epidemic this size had been produced by contaminated municipal water in modern times, and it was an ominous warning. Danger lurked everywhere.[11]

The year of the Riverside epidemic, EIS officers were called to Washington, D.C., to investigate a mysterious respiratory ailment that struck patients at St. Elizabeths Hospital. All the victims were in the hospital's west wing, but the search came up empty. Having grown accustomed to success, the EIS officers found the St. Elizabeths problem frustrating. All they could do was bring their specimens back to Atlanta and put them in the freezer. They waited eleven years for an answer. (See chapter 18.)

Tall, rangy Jim Steele, whose job it was to watch out for zoonoses, thought these would prove increasingly important. In the jet age, they could come from anywhere. (A soldier, returning from Vietnam in 1964, brought the first imported case of plague in forty-two years.) Steele was especially concerned about rabies and encephalitis. Intensive campaigns to inoculate dogs against rabies proved very effective, but when the disease spread to wild animals, hope of eliminating it vanished. Rabid foxes, skunks, raccoons, and other wild animals posed more of a threat to human health than rabid dogs. By 1961, work that Denny Constantine did in the bat caves of the Southwest proved what CDC had feared since 1956—that in confined areas like a bat cave, rabies is an aerosol. In the National Rabies Laboratory at Chamblee, work progressed on developing a less toxic pre-exposure rabies vaccine for humans and a gamma globulin serum loaded with anti-rabies antibodies to use on those who had been severely bitten on the head and neck. Blood donations came from veterinarians across America who had received anti-rabies shots.

CDC used chickens as an early warning system against encephalitis. Like wild birds, they are hosts to the virus, and build up antibodies against it. Sixty-five flocks of guardian chickens were scattered about the country in 1963, and there was no encephalitis outbreak that year, but in 1964 when these sentinels were not used, encephalitis struck hard in Houston, Texas. A crash program of mosquito control was initiated, and CDC sent a fourteen-man team to help. They could offer very precise aid because two years earlier Dr. Roy W. Chamberlain, CDC's mosquito specialist, had isolated the St. Louis encephalitis virus. The principal avian host for the Houston epidemic was the common house sparrow, but almost a quarter of Houston's wild and domestic birds had St. Louis encephalitis antibodies.[12]

The activism of the 1960s expressed itself in the vigor of the attack on tuberculosis. When the Tuberculosis Division moved to Atlanta in 1960, the national case rate for the disease was 31 per 100,000, but with new drugs and surveillance, the division hoped to cut it to 10 per 100,000 by 1970. Streptomycin and isoniazid (INH) reduced the number of deaths from tuberculosis, and by 1960 it was known that drugs, if given long enough, would actually cure the patient. In the short run, this meant that incidence of the disease could be reduced sharply. In the long run, it meant the end of tuberculosis sanitariums.

In 1962 Congress authorized grants for treating tuberculosis patients outside hospitals. Two years later, Surgeon General Terry appointed a national task force on tuberculosis, which met at CDC and outlined a ten-year course of action. Project grants would provide outpatient treatment, identify contacts, and begin long-term service for persons at risk—migrant farm workers, blacks, and the poor wherever they were found.

The most used drugs to fight tuberculosis were the inexpensive INH and para-aminosalicylic acid (PAS), which were effective in curing 95 percent of the cases. INH had the additional benefit of keeping persons exposed to tuberculosis from contracting the disease. Dr. Alfonso Holguin, chief of the TB program, took pride in the progress made since the days when strict isolation or mutilating surgery was the only recourse. There was timely aid from the laboratory. The fluorescent antibody technique was used to type the tuberculosis organism, making speedier treatment possible.[13]

At CDC, Goddard found more "true pros" than he had ever encountered, and every Friday he toured the labyrinthine halls to speak to as many as he could. At the top of his list was Dr. Charles Shepard, one of CDC's most distinguished scientists, who for thirty years was chief of the leprosy section. A quiet, retiring man totally dedicated to excellence, Shepard was the center's best read, most knowledgeable person in infectious disease research. He had accomplished much himself, and he expected the best from those who worked with him. "He did not suffer fools," one colleague remembered, "but once young people . . . showed their colors, then you saw this magical relationship." Shepard found time to chat with those people in the halls, a mark of his approval and, consequently, of their "arrival" at CDC.

In a career in the PHS that spanned forty years, this Nebraska native worked first at NIH, where he pioneered the techniques that allowed serologic differentiation in murine and epidemic typhus. At the Rocky Mountain laboratory, he concentrated on Rocky Mountain spotted fever and Q fever. At CDC, first in Montgomery and then in Atlanta, Shepard worked on leprosy. While in Montgomery, Shepard accomplished what had been deemed impossible: he cultivated the causative agent of leprosy, *Mycobacterium leprae,* in the foot-pad of a mouse. The work changed the course of leprosy forever. It shortened the time for antibiotic sensitivity-testing from several years to several months and paved the way for vaccine studies.[14] No disease was more feared or mysterious than leprosy, and until Shepard's study, humans whose only reward was the faint hope that others would profit were the experimental animals.

Shepard did a prodigious amount of work and set exacting standards for himself. Report followed report. On the cutting edge of his discipline, he always used the latest techniques, including the early computers. He loved science and told his staff, "Your only job is to be the best scientist you can." He often posted a calculation on a small chalkboard outside his office door to stimulate them. On the same board, he listed the places he had visited the year before. The list was long, for Shepard was in demand all over the world. He had no personal ambition to rise in the ranks of public health administration, and in this regard he and Goddard could not have been more different. Shepard loved science for science's sake, and that was reward enough. One of his favored young people, Joseph McDade, remembered him as proud, dignified, and humble, and quoted the dictum that shaped his life:

> "If you really know and understand science you realize that any contribution you make is very small compared to the total amount of information that needs to be added." So he was humble when he measured his successes against nature and the universe, and he was proud of his accomplishments, because he realized that a lot of them came from good hard work, and not necessarily from native spontaneity and genius. So he was both humble and proud . . . and disdainful of people who did not put in that same kind of devoted effort.

In his laboratory, Shepard gave directions to the technical people, but he left the professionals alone to pursue science in their own way. Whenever they did not measure up to his standards, he let it be known, and after a while, they did not work there any more. Shepard himself worked long hours, often into the night and on weekends, but he had broad interests. He walked to work to enjoy the air. He read widely, dabbled a bit in painting, and never missed a symphony performance.[15]

There was always respect and sometimes levity in Shepard's lab. After he successfully cultivated the leprous bacilli in the mouse's footpad, he looked for other animal models. Success with the mouse footpad pointed to animals with naturally cool temperatures, so Shepard and a colleague, Fred Clark, decided to try reptiles, amphibians, opossums, and finally alligators.

The alligator *Mississippiensis* was an endangered species and could be used for research only with permission from the Fish and Wildlife Service. Clark was dispatched to pick up the ten alligators promised for

the project from the Blackbeard Island refuge where they were deci-
mating waterfowl.

> I followed directions one steamy summer morning through endless man-
> grove swamps to the end of the road at what was clearly an alligator poach-
> er's camp. There I was confronted by a few of the seamiest most disreputable
> looking characters I have ever seen. I told them I was there from the gov-
> ernment to get my ten alligators. The spokesman of the group did not speak
> to me, but simply grunted and kicked a burlap sack on the ground. I did not
> stop to examine the contents. I grabbed the sack and got out of there.
>   There were only seven alligators and only one large one, a four footer. He
> was very gentle at first. I kept him in my laboratory sink. He emerged each
> night and wandered about the laboratory. First thing every morning I lo-
> cated him and placed him in the sink. Suddenly one morning he . . . attacked
> me, [so] I bought a 200 gallon cattle watering tank and placed it in a useless
> walk-in autoclave some bumbling bureaucrat had constructed in Shep's bai-
> liwick. Come mating season the following spring we learned that our friend
> really was a male. The magnificence of his bellowing reverberations first in
> the water tank and then in the giant relic autoclave was beyond imagination.
> Tchaikowsky would have incorporated it in the 1812 overture.[16]

Discovery of the armadillo as the ideal laboratory animal for the
study of leprosy was a bit of luck, in which Shepard played an important part. On a visit to a Baton Rouge chemist whose wife raised
armadillos for her genetics research, it occurred to Shepard that armadillos might be useful for leprosy research since they had a body temperature of only 30° C. "So I called Wally Kirscheimer over at Carville
and told him about this," Shepard informed David Sencer when news of
the successful experiment was about to be published. "He went over
and got some of these and sure enough he could grow [the leprosy
bacilli]." It was "typical of Shep," Sencer said, that although the idea
was his, he sought no credit for it.[17]

Goddard always took CDC's visitors to see the laboratories' dish-
washing facilities. Eight million pieces of glassware a year were washed
there, and Goddard told the visitors, "This is the heart of CDC. If this
shuts down, we are out of business." The work of the laboratory was
central to CDC's operations. The newest laboratory tools were tested
for better, faster means of identifying disease organisms. A serum bank
was established where suitable specimens collected by any unit in the
center were carefully stored for research purposes. The bank tied CDC
into a national and international network of sera exchange. The laboratory's tissue-culture unit produced high-purity antigens, antisera, cultures, and reagents for use in nonprofit medical labs. By 1964 the unit
was so efficient—it reduced the cost of a culture from twenty cents to

nine cents—it won a presidential citation for saving the government money. Key to economy in production of viral reagents was the use of large animals like horses and goats as the source of antisera. They not only produced much larger quantities of uniform sera per animal but were easier to handle than small animals.[18]

A problem that had long been a concern of CDC—the quality of work done in the nation's private laboratories—came to a head in 1961. Dr. Morris Schaeffer, who had taken a job as New York City's health officer, launched an investigation of private laboratories and found the situation "deplorable and shocking." They operated without inspection and with untested personnel, and some were so bad they were closed down. The national press covered the story, and the following year a national laboratory improvement program was established at CDC, which provided training, consultation, and standardized reagents to the nation's labs so that they could function better.[19]

If Goddard went to Building 3 on his Friday tour, he found himself beyond the confines of CDC. The audiovisual unit, once part of the Training Branch, still occupied the building, but was by then a separate unit of PHS. In the early 1950s, when the Clifton Road facility was still on the drawing board, Dr. Bauer thought that the audiovisual unit would have to produce a million dollars worth of films annually if it was to merit so grand a space. Under the energetic direction of Dr. James Lieberman, it took giant strides towards that goal in a remarkably short time. Lieberman hired writers and directors from Hollywood, learned to do the seemingly impossible (make cockroaches stand still for the camera), and made many films on how diseases were spread. He was so successful, his unit was separated from Training Branch in 1961 and took a sizable portion of the budget with it. In February 1962, it got a new name, the National Medical Audiovisual Facility.[20]

The ambitious Lieberman, a veterinarian by training, used the creation of NMAV to promote himself and settle a score with Jim Steele, with whom he often clashed. Bypassing the Atlanta chain of command, he interceded with the assistant secretary for health at HEW to get star rank. He would have been the first veterinarian in the service to achieve that goal had not CDC intervened to get Steele promoted at the same time. Lieberman had a flagpole erected on Building 3 just outside Steele's window and hoisted his own star on it. He also ordered flagstaffs for the NMAV annex and for his car, and posted signs around town pointing the way to NMAV. CDC countered with its own signs to direct visitors; Lieberman put up still larger signs. "There were many childish squabbles," Sencer remembers.

If success were measured in budgets, then NMAV was a triumph. Its budget increased dramatically, going up each year. In 1963 it was $475,000; in 1967, it was $2,140,000, and President Johnson plumped the program to Congress as the way "to turn otherwise hollow laboratory triumphs into health victories." But budgets are not everything, and in 1967 Lieberman's hopes of personal glory began to fade. Over his vigorous objections, NMAV was transferred to the National Library of Medicine, which ordered him to take down his flagpoles. Eventually, the unit was physically as well as organizationally moved out of Atlanta. In time it was discontinued altogether.[21]

The public health policy of the United States underwent a radical change in the early 1960s. Landmark legislation put the federal government in the business of providing patient care as well as protecting the health of the populace. Passage of the Vaccination Assistance Act during the Kennedy administration was in the tradition of preventive medicine. Passage of the Medicare-Medicaid legislation of 1965 as part of President Johnson's Great Society program made government the health provider for millions of Americans. Goddard believed this legislation narrowed the artificial separation between public health and private medicine, but others at CDC complained that it complicated the budget process. So much money went for Medicare-Medicaid that funds for prevention seemed harder to get. Old-timers looked back nostalgically on the days when they had only to check in with Hill and Fogarty.

By the 1960s, the Epidemiology Branch at CDC had expanded its interests to include chronic disease. When clusters of leukemia cases first appeared in Niles, Illinois, in 1961 and later in other parts of the country, Clark Heath started a surveillance program, paid for by the National Cancer Institute. Heath's work illustrated perfectly Langmuir's philosophy on research: "We give the maximum to service," he said, and "we find all sorts of wonderful things that nobody else knows about and we convert these into our research activities." Heath discovered a connection between leukemia and certain birth defects; this set in motion a project that in time evolved into the world's best data base on birth defects.[22]

A few years later, another EIS officer, Nicholas Wright, was unhappy in his assignment in a New England health department. Langmuir, remembering the speech Margaret Sanger had made at Harvard, decided to assign him instead to Emory University's family-planning program at Grady Hospital. He looked for approval to Goddard, who assured him that nobody in Washington would know about it. The word leaked out, however, and some months later a communiqué demanded to know what CDC was doing in family planning. Goddard and Langmuir replied truthfully that one person was so engaged and got their knuckles rapped for spending communicable-disease money in this fashion. Those higher up in PHS, however, reflecting the broadening scope of public health, approved the program, and CDC was soon heaped with praise for having the nation's only public health service officer engaged in family planning. Within a year, the program expanded. Carl Tyler and Bob Hatcher were recruited specifically for it. Family planning rapidly became one of CDC's major interests.[23]

Langmuir later called this dispersion the "EIS Diaspora." Besides staffing units in family planning, leukemia, and birth defects, Langmuir peeled off one officer after another to take on major projects. D. A. Henderson and Don Millar went to the smallpox eradication program, Bob Kaiser to the international malaria program, and John Witte to the immunization program. Tom Chin was set up independently as head of ecological investigations, a program that tied all the western field stations together. They were to apply the best principles of epidemiology and surveillance to new fields of endeavor.[24]

In time, Goddard came to like his job as CDC chief. He cherished Atlanta's distance from Washington and the independence that it lent to the organization he headed. Once a week he flew to Washington for a staff meeting of the Bureau of State Services, until it seemed prudent to stay away. Dr. Aaron Christensen, a conservative midwesterner who did not like commotion and argument, was head of the bureau, and it was inevitable that he and the outspoken Goddard would clash. For everybody's benefit, Goddard persuaded Christensen that it would be better if he "attended" the meetings by speaker telephone. The taxpayers would save the cost of an airline ticket, and Goddard would save time. During that hour every Thursday morning, he and Dave Sencer went through the mail, and sotto voce handled other matters. Every once in a while, Christensen would say, "Do you hear that, Jim?" and Goddard would reply, "Oh, yes, I'm with you," and go on with his work.[25]

CDC's relative independence from the bureaucracy is illustrated by its victory in controlling its publications. An edict from Washington dictated that all material not printed in CDC's own shop had to be cleared by the bureau's public affairs office. A giant bottleneck resulted. For example, there was the case of a comic book the Venereal Disease Branch wanted to publish as part of its education effort, which sat on a Washington desk for two and a half months. The man charged with approving publications refused to approve it because it showed some young people in a drugstore booth smiling and talking about VD. He did not think it appropriate for people to smile when they talked about VD. Goddard, "fed up to the gills," determined to do something about it.[26]

To illustrate the magnitude of the problem, he asked his executive officer, George Tremmell, to gather together all the training manuals, comic books, film cans, and technical papers produced by CDC, put them on one long table, take a color photograph, and make a giant print. Goddard took it to the next staff meeting in Washington. At the end of the meeting, when Christensen asked for new business, Goddard said that he wanted to talk about the matter of clearance. "Yes, George has to clear everything up here," Christensen replied. Out came the giant color photograph of CDC's production for one year. "What do you want us to do?" Goddard asked. "I want to adjourn the meeting," Christensen replied. Later he spoke to Goddard privately, in effect conceding defeat. "Jim, just run CDC." What about clearance? "Just run CDC," he replied.[27]

So Goddard ran CDC. He wore his uniform to work, a custom that set him apart from the other chiefs. At awards ceremonies, he required all commissioned officers to wear uniforms, brought in the Army band from Fort McPherson, and ordered flowers for the stage. He never missed an opportunity to show off CDC in the best light. When Lady Bird Johnson planned a one-day visit to Atlanta in the spring of 1964, Boisfeuillet Jones, an Emory University official then serving as special assistant to the HEW secretary, asked Goddard to help. He arranged a ground-breaking ceremony for a $12 million addition to CDC, money for which had been authorized but not appropriated, and ordered two silver shovels for the ceremony, one for Mrs. Johnson, and one for himself. Before the day arrived, staff members with less flair for the dramatic switched to more modest implements. The First Lady toured the center, saw how eggs were infected with the influenza virus, and bent over a microscope so she could see the "little green cells" revealed by the fluorescent antibody technique. The ground-breaking ceremony followed, with Goddard, dressed in his white PHS uniform, presiding. Top officers of the three military services were there, and Mrs. Johnson made a speech. Then she took the shovel, not silver but still ceremonial, to lift the first spade of dirt. The ground was so hard, however, that she was unable to dig into it. Columnist Hugh Park of the *Atlanta Journal* explained why:

With professional thoroughness [Bob Shackleford had] a parcel of ground . . . spaded up, refilled with light peat moss, and then everything [was] smoothed over so not a trace would show.

It was too good a job of camouflage.

To the consternation of officials, neither they nor Mrs. Johnson could find the prepared hole. Finally, with the help of DeKalb Commission Chairman, C. O. Emerich, she stuck her spade in the right place which offered such a contrast to her previous strenuous efforts that she lurched and almost fell in.[28]

Mrs. Johnson broke ground for a new auditorium at CDC's Clifton Road facility. Other new buildings for CDC were completed while Goddard was director, all of them out of town. Besides the long-awaited building at Phoenix and a new laboratory on the campus of Colorado State University at Fort Collins, there was the large facility at Lawrenceville, about twenty-five miles from Atlanta, for breeding experimental animals. Planned before the women's movement of the 1960s was visible to any but the most sensitive, the Lawrenceville buildings included no women's rest rooms. "We just weren't thinking about women doing those jobs." Goddard remarked later. "We had stereotyped ideas."[29]

While running CDC, Goddard never lost sight of his personal goal, appointment as surgeon general. In January 1965, at the beginning of a new administration, he called on Surgeon General Terry to tell him that he wanted his job. When Terry was reappointed, Goddard began to campaign actively for the post whenever it became vacant. He sought support from the American Medical Association and the American College of Surgeons, and he went to Capitol Hill to call on Congressman Fogarty and Senator Hill. He outlined his plans for reorganizing the Public Health Service. They listened but would not support him. He did not ask Mary Lasker, head of the Albert and Mary Lasker Foundation, the third most influential person in America in getting appropriations for medical research. Only Hill and Fogarty had more power. "I was not about to be another one of Mary's little lambs," Goddard said. The word got back to her, and she actively opposed his selection. Goddard never became surgeon general. After Terry resigned, Goddard was briefly hopeful, but Dr. William Stewart, a member of the first EIS class, was chosen instead.[30]

The decision was made by the new secretary of Health, Education and Welfare, Dr. John Gardner, an intellectual who took over the post in July 1965. He saw HEW as comparable to a university, where many subjects are studied and many departments struggle among themselves for recognition. He had about ten decisive appointments to make, among them the surgeon general and the commissioner of the Food and Drug Administration (FDA). It was not long before Secretary Gardner invited Goddard to stop by for a chat the next time he was in Washington. He offered him the post at FDA. Again, it was not a job Goddard wanted, but he took it and found the work exciting. It was a "remarkable change" to go to a regulatory agency from CDC, where the emphasis was on training, helping people, and solving problems.

Throughout much of his term as CDC director, Goddard left the hands-on operations of CDC to his deputy director, David Sencer, and to Bill Watson. Goddard—handsome, articulate, and dynamic—was good at promoting CDC's interests outside the bounds of Atlanta, and in both Sencer and Watson he had aides who were skilled managers who could take care of things at headquarters. Sencer loved being left in charge. In fact, he wanted Goddard's job so much he could taste it. Goddard had been in Atlanta but six months when he told Sencer, "This is the wrong place for me. I need to be in a small place and make it grow, or a place that is in trouble and shake it up and this is neither." So, as Sencer remembered it, Goddard just "did his own thing." Goddard was aware that Sencer wanted his job, and he knew it was probably difficult for Sencer to serve as deputy when he wanted so much to be chief.

Although he was well known in the commissioned corps, and Goddard promoted his candidacy, Sencer does not know how he got the top job at CDC. It may have been because he was just "there," summoned to help reorganize the Public Health Service by Surgeon General Stewart. It was a serendipitous appointment. It put Sencer, an extraordinary administrator, in a job he loved at a time when PHS launched new ventures.[31]

CHAPTER 10

Immunization:
The First Crusade

The job of controlling polio in the United States became CDC's responsibility in the summer of 1961. This important assignment was a mark of the surgeon general's willingness to make a politically sensitive decision. The staff, noting the transfer of the activity "down here," pledged "to keep everyone 'over-informed' and be sure that we have an on-going program that is adequate."[1]

Control of polio was an emotionally charged issue, and many interest groups inside and outside government were involved. Public policy dictated that the oral vaccine be administered without regard to previous Salk immunization in the hope that "community immunization" would eliminate the circulating wild virus. To secure the essential cooperation of the public, polio immunization was tied to existing programs of protection against diphtheria, whooping cough, and tetanus; the public was more likely to accept a campaign against multiple diseases than against one.

David Sencer, CDC's number three man in the early 1960s, who for a time directed the program, was among the most enthusiastic boosters of a multi-disease approach to immunization. He suggested that a "circulating stockpile" of antibodies against disease in 180,000,000 Americans could be interpreted as a civil defense measure, one that would have "many [other] benefits to the individual and the community."[2]

Polio was still a problem a half dozen years after the Salk vaccine was introduced, because too few people had been immunized. CDC was introduced to the difficulties of mass immunization in its "Babies and

Breadwinners" campaign. Those most in need of immunization were the hardest to reach; hoopla and gimmicks did not work. The most positive result of the "Babies and Breadwinners" effort was the use for the first time of public health advisors for something other than venereal disease control. They did such good work, they made themselves indispensable to future immunization efforts. Windell Bradford, a PHA who became one of CDC's managers, explained why: the PHAs, young college graduates who were nearly all liberal arts majors, were interested in society and its concerns. Like the Peace Corps, they were committed to service and gave themselves without stint to jobs with the potential to make life better. Immunization campaigns were tailor-made to their idealism. When broad-scale immunization programs were funded for the states, public health advisors were in great demand to run them.[3]

The Sabin oral polio vaccine (OPV) was the key to success of the extensive campaign against polio. It was easier to administer than the Salk vaccine, and possibly more effective. President Kennedy was enthusiastic about it, and within months of his inauguration asked Congress for $1 million to purchase oral polio vaccine for use in emergencies. The fund was first suggested by Alexander Langmuir. Like others in the PHS, he was frustrated by the opposition of the American Medical Association to the proposed medicare program. When efforts to do something for the elderly were stymied, the PHS shifted its emphasis to children. Langmuir was at a meeting in the early 1960s with a "clutch" of assistant surgeons general trying to think of something to do. As an extreme shot, he suggested the setting up of a special "epidemic aid fund" to buy polio vaccine for emergencies. "When asked how much money, I said off the top of my head, 'A million dollars should suffice.' Within two weeks, incredibly, a special emergency appropriation had passed Congress. When asked to define epidemic I said, 'Two cases of paralytic polio either of which [has] been typed.'"[4]

The production of OPV was beset with difficulties. The live polio vaccine was grown in monkey kidney tissues and could not be marketed until it was rid of simian viruses. These contaminated the vaccine produced by two of the five pharmaceutical houses manufacturing it.[5] Rigid government safety standards, purposely set very high in an effort to prevent another Cutter incident, also slowed production. The National Foundation, which had financed the research and field trials for the Salk vaccine, was adamantly opposed to the oral vaccine. Basil O'Connor dug in his heels and ordered nine million doses of the Salk vaccine while field trials for the Sabin vaccine were under way.[6]

The contest between Drs. Sabin and Salk posed a real dilemma for public health, and especially for CDC. The American Medical Association endorsed the Sabin vaccine in preference to Salk's killed-virus vaccine (IPV), and pharmaceutical manufacturers slowed or eliminated production of the Salk product. The government rejected all oral vaccines except the Sabin strains, and it was slow to license these. Vaccines for Types I and II polio were licensed in the summer of 1961, but the vaccine for Type III was not approved until March 1962. For a time, supplies of both Salk and Sabin vaccines were in short supply.[7]

The thesis that communitywide use of oral polio vaccine would eliminate the wild virus had to be tested. In May 1961, Dr. Henry Gelfand began the work in two Atlanta housing projects. He gave Type I OPV to 5,000 people and collected stool specimens from nearly 600 children aged eighteen months to three years. By the end of the month, in a year when polio viruses were unusually scarce, there were two cases of paralytic polio in the group, and Gelfand's samples showed a high prevalence of wild Type III virus. This could portend an epidemic. This was the first time a potential polio epidemic was predicted on the basis of routine laboratory evidence. Plans to feed OPV for Types II and III in mid June had to be looked at carefully, if not abandoned entirely. As Chief Smith explained to the surgeon general, "if attenuated Type III were fed and cases of paralytic polio occurred, there could be great confusion and misunderstanding, possibly liability actions." The community might think the epidemic was caused by the vaccine. "Scientifically this will not occur," Smith wrote, "but emotionally it might." On the other hand, the possibility of an epidemic in Atlanta presented an opportunity to test the hypothesis of epidemic control through feeding live-virus vaccine.

A conference at the surgeon general's office determined that the threat of an epidemic in Atlanta required an all-out attack. The state health department recommended three Salk shots for everyone under forty, and Sabin offered his entire supply of the not yet licensed Type III vaccine so that all Atlanta children under fifteen could be vaccinated promptly. The first shipment of 300,000 doses, 86 percent of the nation's supply, arrived by air and within a few days was distributed through schools and health centers.[8]

The second test came in August, when there were eighteen paralytic cases of Type I polio in three New York counties. Health authorities requested 350,000 doses of OPV from CDC's vaccine bank. Before the scare was over, twice that many doses were shipped. George Stenhouse,

CDC's public information officer, went to New York to help. He took films from the Atlanta epidemic and warned health officials to expect huge crowds on opening day, but no one was prepared for the ensuing crush. Some distribution centers ran out after fifteen minutes; such bedlam ensued that the sheriff and the police department were required to restore order. The New York experience provided many object lessons for the future distribution of the Sabin vaccine: a definite responsible coordinator had to be appointed, a prescribed method of administering the vaccine determined (not the eight different ways used in New York), and areas of coverage strictly circumscribed.[9]

Ideas for the Vaccination Assistance Act of 1962 crystallized over a period of months. J. Stewart Hunter, assistant to Surgeon General Terry, suggested buying oral polio vaccine and distributing it to the states, just as the PHS had provided Salk polio vaccine to the states from 1955 to 1957. The states had received no funds to distribute the Salk vaccine, however, so they distributed it in the easiest possible manner—through school systems. This left preschool children unprotected, and no arrangements were made for immunizing infants in the future. During the last months of 1961 and early 1962, plans for a different kind of vaccination program began to take shape.

CDC proposed an immunization campaign that would concentrate on children under five and would provide not only vaccine but money for personnel. The plan, approved by the Public Health Service and the American Medical Association, called for communitywide efforts to distribute the vaccine at appropriate intervals. Everyone hoped that enthusiasm for the new oral polio vaccine would increase protection against other childhood diseases. President Kennedy expressed that hope in February 1962 when he asked Congress to fund a wide-ranging health program: "There is no longer any reason why American children should suffer from polio, diphtheria, whooping cough, or tetanus—diseases which can cause death or serious consequences throughout a lifetime, which can be prevented but which will prevail in too many cases."[10]

CDC's Director Smith went to Washington for the congressional hearings. His only opportunity to brief Secretary Ribicoff on the details was during the short ride from HEW to the House Office Building, but it was time enough. The hearings went smoothly. The House approved the Vaccination Assistance Act in June, the Senate in early October. President Kennedy signed it into law on October 23, 1962, the day after he addressed the nation on the Cuban missile crisis. That news far overshadowed the signing into law of the relatively modest Vaccination Assistance Act. It called for $14 million for the first year and smaller amounts for the next two, but funds were not actually appropriated for another seven months. The Vaccination Assistance Act funded an enormously successful program, "as near to perfection as we can get," according to Jim Goddard. The bill provided not only for the immediate vaccination of children under five against four diseases, but for similar attacks on other infectious diseases when vaccines were developed. Translated, that meant an attack on measles. "We'll get a measles vaccine this year," said J. Stewart Hunter who had first suggested the program. "It's pretty imminent."[11]

The immunization program was an immediate success. David Sencer, its acting director, put together a small staff in the summer of 1963. Harold Mauldin, a public health advisor, handled field operations, and Jim Bloom, recruited from the Bureau of State Services in Washington, oversaw the budget. Later Dr. Robert F. Freckleton came from Washington to take Sencer's place. During the first year, CDC made sixty-one grants for vaccination assistance—thirty-four to states and twenty-seven to local health departments. The funds provided vaccine for children under five, the most susceptible group, and covered some administrative costs. Public health advisors were in great demand.

The campaign had three goals: to reach the five million previously unimmunized young children, to give booster shots to nine million others with partial immunization, and to develop early immunization programs in communities across the nation. Pockets of susceptibles often left immunization levels dangerously low. Unimmunized children most likely were in city slums, migratory and marginal farm families, and minority ethnic groups, few of whom ever saw a doctor. Nothing on the scale of this immunization program had been attempted before, and no one knew how or whether parents would respond. As Goddard said, "The art of persuasion, not the art of medicine, is now on trial."[12]

The immunization program would succeed only if the medical profession was supportive, the state health departments were persuasive, the volunteers competent and willing to give their time, and the public cooperative. How well all these groups worked together was demonstrated in the successful "Sabin Sundays," when millions lined up to get their lump of sugar spiked with OPV. Despite the outward appearance of success, public apathy still posed a threat.

A problem with any immunization program is that no vaccine is 100 percent safe. That oral polio vaccine was no exception became evident in 1962, only a year after the vaccine was licensed. A special advisory committee, appointed by the surgeon general to investigate, concluded that 18 cases of paralytic poliomyelitis were "compatible with the possibility of having been induced by the vaccine." The risk was about one per million overall, but it was somewhat greater for those over thirty. By the end of June 1964, when about one hundred million doses of each of the three types of vaccine had been distributed, CDC's polio surveillance unit found 123 cases of paralytic poliomyelitis in persons who had received the vaccine less than thirty days before. Of these, 36 were in epidemic areas and occurred in conjunction with emergency vaccine feeding programs. However, 87 were widely scattered throughout the country in nonepidemic areas and 57 of these were compatible with vaccine-induced disease.[13] In a carefully worded report, the advisory committee concluded

> that it is not possible to prove that any individual case was caused by the vaccines and that no laboratory tests available can provide a definitive answer. Nevertheless, considering the epidemiologic evidence developed with respect to the total group of compatible cases, the Committee believes that at least some of these cases were caused by the vaccine.[14]

The risk was greatest for Type III polio, about two and a half times greater than for Type I, and negligible for Type II. The committee recommended that the order of distribution of OPV be changed so that Type II was given first and that teenagers and adults be given the vaccine only when there was special risk of exposure.[15]

The discovery of vaccine-related cases of poliomyelitis put CDC squarely in the middle of the ongoing Sabin-Salk fight, and, as Langmuir observed, "When you tangle with Albert Sabin, you have a tiger by the tail." Sabin objected to changing the order in which the vaccines were given, and he objected to excluding individuals over fifteen. He regretted that so much emphasis was put on immunizing infants under one year without specifying the oral vaccine as opposed to the killed virus vaccine. He complained in a letter to Goddard:

> Although OPV is gradually being used more and more in routine pediatric immunization by private physicians and health departments, IPV is still being used on a large scale for such purposes—to the *detriment* [emphasis added] of achieving the optimum immunization of both the individual and

the community. With this the "attorney for the defense" concludes his case.[16]

If Sabin thought the report was too strong, others on the committee thought it was too weak. Dr. Gordon C. Brown, of the School of Public Health at the University of Michigan, said the risk following administration of this vaccine had been played down. A large proportion of the adult population were already immune to polio so "the few cases that have occurred are all the more significant. . . . We should be honest about these facts and not be browbeaten like timid children by the eloquent argument of one person who would like to alibi and explain away every single case that has occurred." He objected particularly to Sabin's use of the word *detriment*. "He apparently would like to write off completely the record of IPV in reducing poliomyelitis in this country to such a low level that we are now able to detect the cases caused by OPV."[17]

Dr. Archie L. Gray, of the Mississippi State Board of Health, also objected to the mild tone of the committee's report. The reference to a very minor hazard "demonstrates fear on somebody's part to stand for the facts being given out." He particularly objected to the "womb to tomb" aspects of the immunization effort, calling it "mass madness. . . . [I]t is simply misleading the public to believe there is a great hazard of polio in the adult population." The crucial sentence in the report was "the Committee believes that at least some of these cases were caused by the vaccine." It expressed a compromise position achieved with difficulty. The word *believes* was originally *concluded*. One committee member wanted the word *probably* inserted before "caused"; another wanted *presumably* as the modifier. Langmuir acted as moderator for the linguistic debate. "Albert will probably want the whole sentence deleted," he wrote William McD. Hammon. All those modifiers offended Langmuir. "I personally feel that the use of the word 'concluded' with the later qualification of 'probably' is just poor use of the English language." He liked the suggestion of David Bodian of Johns Hopkins University that the need for mass immunization programs in the United States had passed: "The precipitous drop in the incidence of polio and the disappearance of significant outbreaks signals the end of an era of achievement. At this time, the most urgent need is for continuing immunization programs focused upon infants and preschool children, among whom most of the future cases will occur." Langmuir agreed totally with this "beautifully worded paragraph," but he knew that the majority of the committee would not go along. Hammon did not want to rock the boat that much, and Goddard was unwilling to take such a radical proposal to the surgeon general.[18]

The controversy over the safety of the Sabin vaccine led the surgeon general to appoint a permanent Advisory Committee on Immunization Practices (ACIP) in May 1964. HEW Secretary Anthony Celebreze had approved the concept of the committee in 1962 when it became obvious that vaccines were becoming a more structured part of preventive medicine, but the committee did not meet until two years later. The ACIP, composed of seven health experts from outside the Public Health Service and members of the CDC staff, took the place of numerous ad hoc committees the surgeon general had appointed from time to time. Like the Armed Forces Epidemiological Board or the Red Book Committee of the American Academy of Pediatrics, ACIP was organized to make recommendations. A new vaccine for measles, the possibility of one for rubella, and the ongoing controversy over who should receive influenza shots gave the new committee much to do.

Dr. Goddard chaired the first meeting, and Dr. D. A. Henderson was the secretary. On the agenda were simplifying vaccination for diphtheria, pertussis, and tetanus; the severe outbreak of rubella then sweeping across the nation; and the two new vaccines for measles. When the committee met again two months later, the focus was narrower. The discussion centered entirely on vaccine-related polio cases.[19]

The early meetings of ACIP were notable for the debates between Langmuir and Dr. U. Pentti Kokko, chief of CDC's Laboratory Branch. Langmuir initiated them with a broad statement, which Kokko might challenge, and then the committee would participate. Bruce Dull, who succeeded Henderson as secretary, remembered them as a performance. "Both are charismatic [with] strongly held opinions. . . . [They] had a way in their debates . . . of pointing out issues that the advisory committee needed to resolve."[20]

The Vaccination Assistance Act of 1962 was limited to control of just four common childhood diseases, but CDC anticipated a campaign against measles, which struck four million American children every year, left some with complications like encephalitis and feeblemindedness, and caused five hundred deaths annually. When the Vaccination Assistance Act was renewed in 1965, it included millions of dollars for the national attack on measles that would be the centerpiece of CDC's second immunization crusade (see chapter 12). Meanwhile, a team from the surveillance section accompanied Henry Meyer of the Division of Biologic Standards to the Congo to study the feasibility of conducting a national measles-vaccination program in a country where measles posed a more serious threat to the lives of children than smallpox.[21]

While the effectiveness of polio and measles vaccines was quickly established, the usefulness of influenza vaccines was a subject of hot debate. In an address to the American Public Health Association in November 1963, Langmuir entered the fray on the side of caution: "There is little evidence that recent [polyvalent] vaccines have significantly prevented clinical illness and similarly little evidence in either direction to evaluate the effect of the vaccine on mortality of older persons and the chronically ill," he said. "It is, therefore, problematic how long such a program should be continued without better scientific evidence to justify the major costs to the general public that are entailed."[22]

Langmuir based his conclusions on surveillance of influenza. The figures on excess mortality—the most important consequence of epidemic influenza—indicated that influenza shots were no more than 20 to 25 percent effective. In spite of this poor performance, however, he called for continued use of the vaccine in high-risk groups, a policy CDC had recommended since 1960. Dr. Fred Davenport, professor of epidemiology at the University of Michigan, took exception to Langmuir's paper, calling the evidence "flimsy" and the recommendations confusing. The debate grew out of the elusive, ever-changing nature of the influenza virus and moved quickly from the scientific level to the popular press. Dr. Kokko compared the influenza virus and the vaccine to a lock and key: each flu vaccine was a key that fit only one specific flu virus, and there were thousands of them. Langmuir said that "it would be wrong to give the public the false hope of certain protection in the next epidemic" because existing vaccines could not work on a new strain of the virus. Goddard, "usually a glowing optimist," admitted that he saw no solution for the immediate future. The nation was lucky in 1957, Langmuir told a reporter. The outbreak came in April in the Southern Hemisphere, and there was time to get ready for its impact in the Northern Hemisphere about six months later. "Purely fortuitous, pure chance, that was."[23]

In the spring of 1965, just two years after the first grants were made to the states under the Vaccination Assistance Act, a national immunization conference was held in New Orleans. The major problem that came up at the session—the fact that 30 to 40 percent of children under the age of one still had not been immunized—had nothing to do with medicine and much to do with human nature. Reaching these children, whose parents had different priorities, would not be easy, but it was necessary. A different approach to enhancing the nation's health was also bandied about in New Orleans: take the attack on infectious diseases overseas. Immunizing the hard-to-reach at home and abroad would challenge CDC's ingenuity for years to come.[24]

CHAPTER II

The Lengthened Shadow of a Man (2)

A half dozen years after coming to Atlanta, Dr. David Sencer was at last in the job he wanted more than anything in the world. "It is a great honor," said the new chief of the Communicable Disease Center, "and in my opinion, it is the best job in the Public Health Service."[1]

The time was right for CDC to make a major thrust. Just entering its third decade, it was firmly established and had a reputation for solid accomplishment. There was an intense national interest in science. Despite the violence that dampened the decade's earlier exuberant expectations, the social climate of the 1960s fostered a belief in progress. Prodded by President Johnson, Congress passed major legislation to make war on poverty, protect civil rights, and improve higher education, health, and mass transit. Rioting in America's cities in the summer of 1965 made the need for improvement in the lives of the disadvantaged compelling. For a man of Sencer's energy, drive, and commitment, the job as chief of an agency whose stated mission was to control disease and to serve offered exciting opportunities. When he moved to the big corner office on the second floor of 1600 Clifton Road, the man and the institution were fortuitously matched at a time when it was possible to get something done.

Like many others, Sencer was introduced to the Public Health Service as a result of the doctor draft during the Korean War. His eighteen months' service as an enlisted man in World War II was not enough to exempt him from service in the 1950s, although for a time he was classified 4-F because he had tuberculosis. He was doing his residency at University Hospital in Ann Arbor when the chief of medicine told him that his 4-F status no longer applied and the military was looking for him. Turned down by the Navy as a volunteer, he took the suggestion of a colleague and joined the Public Health Service, where he could continue his tuberculosis work. The PHS assigned him to Idaho where, almost single-handedly, he developed ways to mitigate the hopeless health conditions of migrant farm workers. At the same time, he discovered the pleasure of getting things done involving many people.[2]

From Idaho, Sencer went to Muscogee County, Georgia, as head of the Tuberculosis Field Research Facility, where he worked in epidemiology and, aided by his own experience with the disease, laid the foundation for the modern outpatient approach to tuberculosis control. Having determined to make public health his career, hs went to Harvard for a Master of Public Health degree, and was back on the job in Georgia when a chance encounter changed his life. As he was returning from a business trip to Mississippi, his plane stopped in Montgomery, Alabama, where Dr. Robert Anderson, then director of CDC, and Dr. David Price, deputy surgeon general, got on board. Sencer knew Anderson, but he had never met Price. On the short hop from Montgomery to Columbus, the three men chatted. Price was so impressed with Sencer that he had him transferred to Washington as program officer in the Bureau of State Services. For Sencer the next two years were as miserable as they were valuable. He hated the job, but gained an encyclopedic knowledge of the bureau's many programs and their interrelationships, which later served him well. He came to Atlanta in 1960 to ease the transition of the tuberculosis program into CDC.[3]

In 1966 CDC was a bustling place. It was just launching one of its most ambitious—and ultimately triumphant—projects, the eradication of smallpox in West Africa (see chapter 14). Immunization was entering its second phase with measles as the target (see chapter 12); the time seemed ripe to eradicate malaria from the world (see chapter 13); and two more PHS units, pesticides and foreign quarantine, were waiting for imminent transfer to Atlanta. It was a lot to juggle at once, but Sencer believed that CDC could do anything, and he set out to make it work. He liked the description a Georgia State University management expert applied to CDC: "You run this place like a country store and it works." Sencer made CDC his "country store." He was the one person in charge; he knew everybody, what they were doing at work, and how their lives were going at home. He assumed complete responsibility for the necessary business with Washington so that no one else would be bothered. He reveled in handling details. If he wanted someone to be elsewhere in a hurry, he got the airline tickets and passports himself.

"What are you doing this morning?" he asked Dr. Lyle Conrad in a telephone call to the epidemiologist's home about nine o'clock one Saturday. Informed that Conrad and his family were on the way to the mountains, Sencer replied, "Terrific. I'm glad that you are all packed up. Just tell Connie and the kids that you will be a little delayed. I need you to take an airplane out to South Africa this afternoon." Protests from Conrad that he had no ticket, no passport, and was scheduled to speak to the immunization conference the next week were brushed away with "I'll take care of it." A few hours later, Conrad was on a plane with $50, an American Express Card, and a passport without a visa. When his plane landed in New York he got the necessary visa from two distinguished gentlemen, who greeted him and asked him to "step this way." Sencer had indeed taken care of everything.[4]

Sencer liked to walk around CDC. A friendly man, he took a direct interest in what his staff was doing, not just in what they were supposed to do or in their major goals. Dr. Michael Gregg, editor of *MMWR*, remembers that Sencer would drift into the office, read a draft of an article, comment on it, and be on his way. He read very fast and remembered everything and everybody. He could pick up a conversation several weeks after the initial encounter at the exact point where it had broken off. He reveled in knowing important, personal details. "I hear that your secretary is having a baby," he said to Conrad one day, thus breaking the news.

The CDC of the Sencer years was a "people place," still small enough to know everybody, small enough for all the staff to have a "feel" for the institution's direction. Many of them had been around since the MCWA days and felt an extraordinary loyalty to CDC. They believed passionately that they were doing important work, and Sencer was determined to make it possible for them to work with the least possible interference.[5]

Sencer took over CDC at a time when major changes were made in the PHS, which had been criticized for not being sufficiently responsive to the nation's rapidly changing health needs. HEW Secretary John Gardner, determined to address these criticisms, issued a secretarial directive in April 1966 that transferred authority from the surgeon general to the secretary. Gardner wanted to reduce the dominance of the commissioned corps and the surgeon general in the PHS and increase the number of civil service employees. Before the year was over,

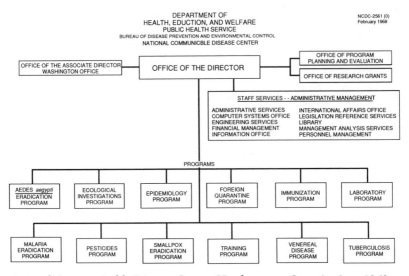

National Communicable Disease Center, Headquarters Organization, 1968

the new structure, designed by Surgeon General Stewart and his staff, including Sencer, was in place. It was streamlined for efficiency and reflected the radically changed role of the federal government from mere protector of public health to provider of health care for all who needed it. For the time being, the surgeon general was still in control of the five divisions embraced in the greatly altered PHS. One of these was the Bureau of Disease Prevention and Environmental Control, which included CDC.[6] Dr. Richard Prindle, a former EIS officer and a veteran of the PHS commissioned corps, was named bureau director.

The initial restructuring lasted fifteen months; in the next dozen years, there were eight major reorganizations of PHS as the government struggled to find the best means of fulfilling its vastly increased responsibilities for health care. The most drastic of these came in 1968, when the surgeon general lost line responsibility for public health programs to the assistant secretary for health and scientific affairs. Surgeon General Stewart thus became the deputy to Dr. Philip Lee, the first person outside the commissioned corps ever to provide leadership for the PHS. From the viewpoint of Washington, the move made sense. Lee's clinical background (he was a practicing internist) was important to implementing Medicare. From Atlanta, a stronghold of the traditional belief in public health practice, the move was alarming. It stripped the PHS of its power and independence. Sencer graphically stated his own sense of loss: "[Stewart and Lee] gave away the family jewels—the budget program, everything. They wanted to run a tight little office and it did end up that way: neat, tight, and little." He said that Jim Kelly, comptroller of HEW, stripped the PHS of all its staff, until they had just themselves and two secretaries. In time, like Samson shorn, the surgeon general, whose word had once been law, lost much of his power to the politically appointed assistant secretary for health.[7]

The various shake-ups in Washington inevitably affected CDC, including a change of name. Its initials had a much prized cachet, but CDC lost them in 1967 when it became the National Communicable Disease Center (NCDC). This was Dr. Prindle's idea, but it was so disliked in Atlanta the change was given only minimal attention. The first reference to the institution in any document was always to NCDC, but after this bow to orders, the familiar CDC was used.[8] The reorganization of PHS in 1966 moved CDC from division to bureau status within in the Public Health Service, which was itself an agency in the Department of Health, Education and Welfare. Sencer, whose title was changed from chief to director, liked to emphasize the institution's unity in spite of rapid organizational changes. He devised an organizational chart of CDC as a gear. "One tooth was Epi, one was Lab, one was Training, and they all fit," Sencer explained.[9]

Sencer prided himself on being more responsive to "downtown Washington" than NIH was. He flew up once or twice a week "principally to keep Washington off the back of the rest of the staff." He may have disliked some of the changes in the national office, but he made certain that CDC changed with the times. It was ready to apply the principles of communicable-disease control to a host of different problems and to become a full partner in international health agencies.

Expansion into new areas took more than scientists and physicians, important as these were. A cadre of carefully trained administrators was needed, too, "the Bill Watsons and the Windell Bradfords and the people who come along behind the doctors to make sure that something happens more than just studies." In short, CDC needed its public health advisors—the 685s in government lingo—and these were recruited by the hundreds. They always trained in the venereal disease program, but they moved into immunization, tuberculosis, or smallpox eradication whenever they were needed.

Sencer cites CDC's handling of an outbreak of plague in Indonesia as an example of its efficiency. He was at home in Atlanta one Tuesday when a call came from the State Department asking for help in controlling an epidemic of plague in the mountains of central Java. Authorities there asked for "cyanide, gas masks, and things for killing rats on ships." Sencer, doubting that infested rats from central Java would be getting on ships, cabled back, "Don't you need some epidemiologists, plague vaccine, vector control, a mobile lab?" Assuming the answer would be yes, everything was ready the next day, and on Friday, the formal request came through. By Saturday, a staff of five and all the supplies but the cyanide were at the airport in San Francisco ready to go. The cyanide went on a military plane from the Philippines. "If we had been in Washington we could not have done that," Sencer said.[10]

The hallmark of the Sencer years at CDC was growth, some of which was accomplished by tacking new programs on existing ones. In 1966 the $6 million Office of Pesticides moved to Atlanta from Washington. It had been created in 1964 in the wake of widespread public reaction to the publication of Rachel Carson's *Silent Spring*, which detailed the threat that pesticides, particularly DDT, posed to the environment. The Office of Pesticides coordinated the activities of three departments— Agriculture, Interior, and HEW—in registering pesticides. For the most part, it was run by people who knew little about them. The move to CDC, where it was merged with Dr. Wayland Hayes's ongoing toxicology program, put experts in charge. The renamed pesticides program, with Dr. S. W. Simmons, formerly of the Technology Branch as its head, included a laboratory in Perrine, Florida, a staff of 130, and grant programs in a dozen states. Its job was to get hard data on the long-term effects of exposure to pesticides and, whenever necessary, to issue warnings. The program had been in Atlanta only a few months when Hayes, addressing the Royal Society in London, warned against shipping food and pesticides together. Simmons had long been interested in biological and genetic control of disease vectors, but the pesticides program was concerned only with the toxicity of pesticides, a narrowing of interests Simmons considered inefficient.[11]

Only two years after the pesticides program came to CDC, it was transferred to the Consumer Protection and Environmental Health Service, a division of the Food and Drug Administration. From there it was moved a year or so later to the Environmental Protection Agency. The transfer from Atlanta cost the program much of its effectiveness and many of its best people, who claimed that away from CDC's careful tutelage, it was "shot through with politics." Nevertheless, the pesticides program's brief tenure in Atlanta had wide-ranging effects on

CDC's other activities. When Simmons was transferred from the Technology Branch to the pesticides program, many of the programs he once directed were grouped in the ecological investigations program, headed by Dr. Tom D. Y. Chin of the Kansas City Station. This put Chin, in Sencer's phrase, "on the same level of assault with Alex [Langmuir]." The Technology Branch was reduced to little more than the Technical Development Laboratory in Savannah. About a third of the lab's budget came from the *Aedes aegypti* eradication program, and when this was ended, for both budgetary and scientific reasons, the laboratory suffered a severe blow. In the summer of 1974, the Savannah field station was declared surplus to CDC's needs and was turned over to Chatham County and the Savannah Board of Education. Simmons, in retirement, could not understand it. He had a sentimental attachment to the laboratory he had built, but it was more than that. He did not see how CDC could ever get another hundred acres so isolated that could be used for so many purposes.[12]

Putting all the field stations into the ecological investigations program was Sencer's way of giving them a unity they had not had before. The work done at Kansas City, Phoenix, Fort Collins (the laboratory in Greeley moved there), San Francisco, Hawaii, and Puerto Rico all had one central theme: man's relationship to his environment. When Sencer dedicated the new building at Fort Collins in September 1967, he underscored the importance of this new approach. "We are emerging from an era during which faith in 'magic drugs' and 'magic insecticides' blunted the critical senses of both scientists and laymen," he said. In the new era, emphasis would shift away from the single-cause theory of disease to the complexities of the environment. Certainly, encephalitis, the principal disease investigated at Fort Collins, illustrated Sencer's point. Mosquitoes carried the virus, which had a variety of wild vertebrate reservoirs in addition to man. Sencer thought the environment might be involved in the transmission of diseases like streptococcal infections as well. That histoplasmosis, Rocky Mountain spotted fever, plague, and schistosomiasis, all of which were under investigation at the field stations, were related to the environment was obvious.[13]

When the Foreign Quarantine Service, one of the oldest and most prestigious units of the Public Health Service, was transferred to CDC in 1967, few people realized the enormous implications the move would have on the Atlanta institution's future. It had a huge staff—some 660 people—located at every port and international airport in the nation, at 414 points along the borders of the United States, and in 36 locations abroad. Quarantine officers gave vaccinations, diligently supervised medical and psychological examinations for persons applying for entry into the United States, and compiled epidemiological data from around the world. At the time Foreign Quarantine was transferred to CDC, the staff had taken on the additional responsibility of keeping plague-carrying rats from coming in from Vietnam. Quarantine officers took much pride in their service, which had been under the control of the surgeon general since 1878 and could actually trace its roots to colonial times. The style of its uniforms changed frequently—one man in Washington did nothing but design them—and its officers wore them proudly. Like the venereal disease and tuberculosis programs, the Foreign Quarantine Service did not want to move to Atlanta. Its officers came protesting, bringing with them some of their old uniforms.

It made sense to transfer the Quarantine Service to CDC because quarantine was a means of controlling communicable disease. What did not make sense to Sencer was the way the Quarantine Service was run. It looked as if nothing had changed since 1900. Out of a very large budget, 92 percent went for salaries and personnel expenses, excluding such basics as travel. The medical officer in charge of the Mexican border, stretching from Brownsville to San Diego, had an annual travel budget of only $75. Men in the service spent their time boarding ships and checking chest X-rays and vaccination certificates. They greeted international arrivals at the airport and went down the aisles looking in the eyes for jaundice. They gave 186,000 smallpox vaccinations every year to people crossing the border from Mexico.

Shortly before the Foreign Quarantine Service was transferred, two independent studies came to quite different conclusions about its needs and policies. The Bureau of the Budget did a time and motion study that showed that the service was understaffed and needed 144 more officers. But the advisory committee on foreign quarantine activities—the Weir committee headed by Dr. John Weir of the Rockefeller Foundation—made such sweeping recommendations to reduce the scope of activities that Dr. Alan W. Donaldson, formerly of CDC, but then with the PHS's Bureau of State Services, wanted distribution of the report carefully controlled. The Weir committee recommended that the Mexican border be as open as the Canadian one. Vaccinating people for smallpox at the port of entry was too late to be effective and was, therefore, useless. "There is no way, and never has been, of building a wall around a country which is impenetrable to communicable disease, and yet which permits international traffic to continue," the report concluded. "Quarantine is essentially still using the concept of the 'thin red line.' It is bound to break down because it disregards the basic ecological facts about communicable disease in the 'jet age.'"[14]

A crisis developed soon after the Quarantine Service was moved to CDC. Congress had enacted a pay raise for the PHS, but Jim Kelly, HEW comptroller, would not release any new money to raise the pay of the Quarantine Service. Sencer, knowing that something had to be done in a hurry, settled on a commonsense time and motion study of his own.

Jess Norman and Joe Giardano were dispatched to John F. Kennedy Airport in New York to see the Quarantine Service in action. Within twenty-four hours, Sencer got a call. "Doc, you're overstaffed," Norman reported. There were three shifts a day, with sixteen people on each shift, but from midnight to 8 A.M. there was only one plane to check. This incident prompted a management study of every quarantine station. The most egregious offender was the one in Miami. Former assistant surgeons general were retired there; one doctor rode the Electra out to Cuba and back once a day, psychiatrists looked at X-rays, and radiologists looked at vaccination scars. Sencer determined on a reduction in force. At JFK airport, without reducing the program, he cut the staff by 35 percent, and in Miami by half. For the PHS, this was something quite new.

Sencer and Watson homed in on some of the problems within the Foreign Quarantine Service on a visit to the New Orleans station. The officer in charge, given a few hours' notice of their visit, told them on arrival, "We have the boats ready for you. You can go down and see the ships." The inspectors began to bite their lips when informed that the visitors only wanted to see the station. It seemed that nobody from higher up ever came for anything but to take a ride on the river. When Sencer and Watson checked out the front office, they found that one high-ranking officer spent most of his time going through invoices of small bills. He pointed out with some pride that he had disapproved a $13 tab for gasoline for the lawnmower, inappropriately assigned to transportation rather than maintenance. At the same time, he bought smallpox vaccine in small lots at a cost of $1 a dose. When Sencer returned to Atlanta, he asked John Barron, the procurement officer, if he could get a better price. "Will two cents do?" Barron responded. For Sencer, "It was fun; it was hilarious."

Better management made the first cuts possible, but better procedure was responsible for those made later. How should quarantine be done at the end of the twentieth century? The answer was epidemiology and surveillance. Better epidemiology provided an early warning system on the occurrence of communicable diseases anywhere in the world. Better surveillance within the states picked up any threats to health that slipped by.[15]

When President Johnson asked for a reduction in overseas personnel in order to balance payments, CDC closed the quarantine offices in Montreal and Paris. Then, deaf to the cries of Quarantine that the health of the nation was being undermined, Sencer applied the staff formula worked out at JFK to all airports. Everywhere procedures were changed. "We stopped vaccinating people at the U.S.–Mexican border," Sencer said. "We stopped boarding ships. We began backing out of all those things that were absolutely ridiculous, and with the savings we were able to staff the family-planning program, the smallpox program, and all these other activities. We cannibalized."

The Foreign Quarantine Service shrank steadily. Within a few years, it had only sixty inspectors, fewer than the tiny nation of Kuwait had. Eliminating six hundred quarantine positions without endangering the nation's health required a fine balance of disease-surveillance technology with the number of people meeting airplanes and ships, and it could not have been done without good relationships with state and local health departments. Smuggling those positions into other programs more important to the nation's health required the acumen of good bureaucrats. Sencer and Watson passed the test.[16]

Family planning was one of the programs that profited from the shrinking of Quarantine, and in Langmuir's opinion, it was none too soon. He thought that, if necessary, half of the country's health effort should go to solving the problem of the population explosion. "We in public health assume responsibility for the problems we create," he said. "And by preventing babies from dying, we have created the population explosion." He believed that advances in contraceptive techniques made it possible to establish effective population-control programs anywhere in the world. He had one officer assigned to family planning in 1964, ten in 1967, and he hoped to train twenty or thirty each year. To support these, he secured funding from the National Institutes of Health, the Food and Drug Administration, and the Bureau of Health Services. When an HEW committee checked on the family-planning program in the summer of 1967, it found more work under way at CDC than at any other agency of PHS, even those with clinical programs. "It was a feather in Langmuir's cap to have been that far-sighted," Carl Tyler remembered. Tyler, the second EIS officer in family planning, took over the center's family-planning program in 1968 and directed it during a period when legal abortion and the association of contraceptives and cancer became issues of national concern.[17]

The family-planning program was but one of the new interests that exploded at CDC in the late 1960s. A large-scale study of birth defects began with surveillance of the five-county metropolitan Atlanta area. Clark Heath, the EIS officer whose interest in birth defects grew out of their possible connection to leukemia clusters, called Atlanta his laboratory. He worked with Arthur Falek, a geneticist at Georgia Mental Health Institute on a project that in time furnished hard statistical data in an area where such information was scarce. Atlanta had a population of a million and a half, large enough to rule out the statistical flukes inevitable in repeated samples of a hundred births, the only measure of birth defects until the Atlanta study. Two pediatricians, Allan Ebbin and Godfrey Oakley, shortly reinforced Heath and propelled the study forward. The March of Dimes provided financial support in the wake of the widespread interest in birth defects caused by the drug thalidomide. Although thalidomide babies were born mostly in Europe and Japan, they pointed to the need for surveillance of birth defects in the United States.[18]

Sencer encouraged expansion into new areas while stepping up the attack on tuberculosis and venereal disease. Tuberculosis had steadily declined, and more and more people were treated as outpatients. With enough treatment, tuberculosis patients got well, and hopes were high that tuberculosis could be eradicated within fifteen years. The government provided funds for tuberculin tests for those in the most critical groups—first graders, school personnel, and potential dropouts in junior high school and the twelfth grade. One major obstacle to the success of the program was the waning interest of physicians. The TB program chief, Alfonso Holguin, found it ironic that the dramatic success in controlling the disease made many physicians lose interest in it.[19]

There was less optimism about venereal disease. The syphilis-eradication program, under way since 1963, had stalled, and there was no hope of achieving success by the 1972 deadline. Meanwhile, new and serious problems emerged in other areas. In the full-scale attack on syphilis, attention to gonorrhea and other venereal diseases lagged. In the 1950s, many believed that gonorrhea was all but gone, but in the late 1960s, there was a veritable epidemic. It was more prevalent than measles. The lack of suitable animal models made gonorrhea research difficult, and drugs that had once effected immediate cures had to be given in larger and larger doses. The problem was compounded by an authentic import, oriental gonorrhea, which one in every four servicemen brought back from Vietnam. It was resistant to penicillin and exaggerated an already growing trend towards drug resistance of routine gonorrhea cultures.[20]

Most of the budget for venereal disease went to epidemiology, but the difficulty of control shifted attention to the part that research could play. The venereal disease research laboratory at CDC was one of three in the country working on a syphilis vaccine. By 1969 that work had hit a snag. More promising was the development of a better test for detecting gonorrhea, making early treatment possible.[21] The hope of bringing venereal disease under control, however, was dimmed by the very success of work done at CDC. A new sexually transmitted disease, herpes Type 2, was discovered, which has since been associated with cervical cancer.

Until 1967 all herpes viruses were thought to be the same, no matter where they occurred on the body. Virologist Walter Dowdle began to doubt this universal truth. As he worked on growth patterns of the virus, it became obvious to him that there was more than one type of herpes. With the assistance of Frank Pauls, a doctoral student from North Carolina studying with him, he confirmed his suspicions by devising a test differentiating between the two types. "We did not have a clue what it meant," Dowdle said, but he and Pauls determined to find out. They collected herpes strains from all parts of the body and from as many sources as possible, including Atlanta's Grady Hospital, where Dr. André Nahmias, former EIS officer and professor of pediatrics at Emory, practiced. Dowdle and Nahmias did a blind test. When this was done, Nahmias broke the code. One group had all been transmitted by genital contact; the other group was the simplex type associated with the mouth. At first, nobody believed it, but then there was an explosion of interest, first among scientists, and later with the public.[22]

The battle against any disease for which there is no vaccine is complicated, and this is especially true of diseases that are sexually transmitted. Social changes in the 1960s compounded the problem and tempered the earlier, perhaps naive, expectation that syphilis might be eradicated and other sexually transmitted diseases controlled. Although initial progress was made, a combination of factors made eradication almost impossible. The sexual revolution, the women's liberation movement, and the emergence of gay rights changed the social climate. The crowded living conditions associated with urbanization and the ease of national and international travel increased sexual interactions. In the late 1960s, the slope of the curve for sexually transmitted diseases turned sharply upward.

Eradication of syphilis in the United States, of *Aedes aegypti* mosquitoes in the Western Hemisphere, and of smallpox in the world might have qualified as ambitious enough goals for a single institution in any decade, but President Johnson wanted even more programs to fulfill his vision of the Great Society. When the president signed into law the Community Health Service Act in August 1965, he called on his advisors to develop "very ambitious, but obtainable and realistic, goals and objectives for this Nation in terms of improving the life and health of our people." A few days later there was a hurry-up call to Atlanta to send along ideas from CDC. In two days, a six-point program, "Dramatic Goals for the Next Ten Years," was sent to Washington. Besides the work on syphilis, smallpox, and mosquito control, the staff cited three other programs: virtual elimination of measles and rubella, isolation and identification of the virus of infectious hepatitis, and a sharp reduction in the incidence of tuberculosis.[23]

Success was not going to be achieved in all these areas, but CDC nevertheless played a role in the Great Society idea. The riots that swept many American cities in the summer of 1965 indicated that something was wrong, and the search for reasons turned up, among other things, rats. The first time a rat control bill came up in Congress, the House of Representatives refused even to consider it. Amid much jocularity, congressmen compared the dangers of two- and four-legged rats, discussed discrimination against country rats in favor of city rats, and recommended cats as a proper solution. One congressman said the "rat smart thing" to do was to vote down the bill "rat now." To approve it, they agreed, would be money down a "rat hole."[24]

Two months later, in answer to the outcry that followed the less than serious way in which the bill was treated, Congress approved a Rat Control Act. This bill differed from the earlier one in that the program would be part of an ongoing one administered by the Public Health Service rather than a new one in the Department of Housing and Urban Development. Rat control was assigned to CDC, where it was tacked on to the *Aedes aegypti* eradication program. "It was all political," Sencer said.

The program began with courses on rat control for hundreds of students. CDC asked for seventy new positions to support its small expert rat-control staff. The cost of the program for two years was put at $40 million. To succeed, the project had to include better housing and improved sanitation as well as extermination efforts, so in making grants to local communities, emphasis was on "people management." Many unskilled people got entry-level jobs looking for rat holes. In 1970 the program was moved to the National Center for Urban and Industrial Health, but it came back to Atlanta a couple of years later when it was put in the State and Community Services Division. Dr. Donald Millar, director of that division, had trouble every year justifying it. Except for affecting the stress level, it had nothing to do with health. Yet the rat-control program was an issue of esthetics and community pride, and CDC was glad enough to be involved.[25]

The programs of the Great Society proved insufficient to quiet the massive unrest of 1968 that followed the assassination of Martin Luther King, Jr. In May, thousands of America's poor staged the "Poor People's March" on Washington and camped in "Resurrection City" awaiting the outcome of their demands. As many as one hundred thousand were expected to stay for the summer. It was a situation ready-made for disaster, and health officials kept a vigilant watch. The District of Columbia Health Department was in charge, but it had an instant line of communication, day or night, to CDC in Atlanta.

On May 21, a health official, probably the public health advisor on the scene, reported that skin tests were under way and blood tests were being done as needed amidst a scene of *"utter confusion."*

> Now more than 2000 people in tent city; 5000 by week-end. May set up second city.
>
> Measles and DTP or TB beginning Wednesday. Polio?
>
> 1/4 to 1/3 under age 16; many young adults; few older.
>
> The representative from the Human Rights Medical Services seems to have disappeared. The DC Health Department has set up a round the clock medical center (8 A.M. to midnight) in Municipal building. No need for CDC yet.[26]

Just in case, the EIS was on instant call, and both jet injectors and vaccines were available.

The Poor People's March threatened the health of thousands, but the return of influenza that same year threatened millions. On July 29, a batch of influenza specimens arrived at the CDC laboratories from Dr. W. K. Chang in Hong Kong. A careful check showed that the flu virus was related to the A2 strain, but it had rearranged the proteins on its coat, altering its molecular personality. It showed little affinity for antibodies to any of the thousand strains of the flu virus in CDC's deep freezers. This was the first major change in the flu virus since the shift that had caused the influenza pandemic of 1957–58. Influenza immediately went to the top of CDC's agenda.

A radically different virus did not necessarily mean that there would be an epidemic, but it certainly called for precautions. At the time it was believed that flu went in cycles, and 1968 was supposed to be a "hot year." "Does the *virus* know that?" someone quipped, but precaution was the better part of wisdom. CDC sent virus cultures to the Division of Biologics Standards at NIH, which grew the virus and shared it with vaccine manufacturers.

There was speculation on when the first case would appear in the United States, but CDC did not have to wait long or look very far. By Labor Day, the virus was in Atlanta. One of the neighbors of Dr. Walter Dowdle, director of the WHO International Influenza Center for the Americas, came down with flu-like symptoms on a flight from the Far East. Dowdle went to see him and arranged for throat and nasal washings. Soon the man's wife was ill, too. In both patients, Hong Kong flu, as it was popularly dubbed, was isolated.[27]

The advisory committee on immunization practices met in Atlanta on September 4. Besides the regular members of the committee, the meeting was attended by Surgeon General Stewart and Dr. H. G. Pereira, director of the WHO Influenza Center in London. At the end of the meeting, the surgeon general announced that an epidemic could be expected. A new strain of Asian flu had hit six hundred thousand people in Hong Kong in July, and the virus would spread through air travel. Fortunately, the disease was more unpleasant than serious. A monovalent vaccine tailored specifically to the new virus would not be available for some time, and the current vaccines were virtually useless.

The first American town struck by the epidemic was Needles, California, where nearly five hundred people were ill by late October. In November, influenza had spread to seven states, and in January 1969, all but eleven states were affected. Flu-related deaths rose above the epidemic threshold in January, but a month later, the epidemic curve turned downward and CDC declared the epidemic over.

Epidemic control had gone well. Everything learned since 1957 was applied to good effect. The lead time was short, but good surveillance provided several large study populations to test the vaccine, and the communications network functioned well. The epidemic revealed several truths: the technology to produce mass quantities of virus did not exist; there was no way to ensure that those most in need of vaccine got it; and influenza control defied simple solutions. An influenza epidemic could not be stopped in its tracks. A world conference on Hong Kong flu held at CDC in November 1969 found no good answer to the most puzzling aspect of the epidemic. Why was it so much worse in the United States than elsewhere? It struck more than 53 million Americans, and there were 19,500 excess deaths, a mortality rate much higher than that of other countries. Langmuir wanted more statistics. "As an epidemiologist, I am still hungry," he said, citing the lack of quantitative measures of incidence, age- and sex-specific attack rates, and the character and severity of complications.[28]

Influenza, even if imperfectly understood, was a familiar adversary. In July 1968 a puzzling call came from Pontiac, Michigan. Nearly the entire staff of the Oakland County Health Department was ill. The janitor got sick on Monday, July 1. By Friday, sixty other staff members were ill. The Michigan Department of Public Health called for help, and three people left for Pontiac, two from epidemiology, one from the laboratory. They worked through the weekend in the County Health Department building with the air-conditioning turned off. On Monday, when it was turned on again, all of them got sick, and the investigation was turned over to new recruits from Atlanta. There were sanitary engineers, zoologists, veterinarians, industrial toxicologists, bacteriologists, and a mycologist. They learned the disease was highly infectious, but it did not spread. Members of the victim's family did not get sick.

Dr. Michael Gregg was among those who went to investigate what everyone called Pontiac fever. He suspected sabotage (did anyone have a grudge against the Health Department?), but he also kept thinking about the air-conditioner. He and Tom Layfield, an engineer, made an inch-by-inch examination of the attic, a space four feet high that served as a warm-air return for the air-conditioning system. For two days they crawled along the attic floor with flashlights. They found bird skeletons and rat excretions, and, certain this must be the cause, sent to Atlanta for an ornithologist and a mammalogist. But the ornithologist said the birds had been dead for years, and the only animal they caught in the traps was one stray house cat.

Deciding the disease had to be airborne, they kept returning to the air-conditioning. They inspected the ducts and found nothing, but when they cut a window in one of the ducts near the cooling tower, they found a pool of dirty water over which all the air circulated. They tested it with smoke candles, and almost immediately, acrid smoke appeared in every room. Mechanical defects in the system had allowed the pool of water to develop.

Clearly, this was the source of Pontiac fever, but the exact cause remained a mystery. Guinea pigs placed in the Health Department building were apparently healthy two weeks later, but tests showed that nearly all of them had lumps on their lungs. A culture of the lumps showed something—a virus, bacteria, rickettsia?—but nobody knew just what. Was it a new disease? "It appears to be a common organism that's gone astray because of its route through the air-conditioning system," Gregg said, "but there's still the medical excitement of thinking we may find a new disease." The cultures went into the deep freeze. They stayed there more than seven years before the answer came (see chapter 18).[29]

Sencer believed that good epidemiology and disease investigation were the best guardians of public health. He had little faith in legalism and regulation, although it was he who encouraged congressional approval of a measure that gave the CDC the only licensing power it ever had. At stake was the quality of the work done in the nation's medical laboratories. The uncertain quality of laboratory tests, brought to light some years earlier, surfaced again within a year after Sencer became director of CDC. Congressman Fogarty asked for an investigation.

Secretary Gardner appointed a committee with Sencer and Dr. Alan W. Donaldson as co-chairmen. The committee found that laboratory personnel were years behind the knowledge attained by research, that physicians were poorly equipped to evaluate laboratory results critically, and that there was a lack of standardized procedures and reagents. The efforts CDC made to improve laboratory performance through its national laboratory improvement program were salutary but not enough. As Dr. Marion Brooke, who headed the program, diplomatically observed, "Our function is not to control or regulate the state public health laboratories but to help those that want help in any way we can." The proposal presented to Congress in 1967 was for a grant-in-aid program to the states to demonstrate what could be done.[30]

Sencer's testimony before the Senate Judiciary Committee was sensational. He said that about a fourth of all laboratory tests used for diagnosis were faulty and, since this figure was derived from performance evaluation programs, "it may represent the *best* which laboratories can do." One irate Atlanta physician asked if Sencer were the "Lord High Sheriff of Medical Science," but the bill caught the public's attention, especially after one Straybourne Betz got a license as a medical technologist. Betz was a ten-year-old mongrel dog. The Clinical Laboratory Improvement Act of 1967 required all laboratories and laboratory personnel involved in interstate commerce be licensed. The act made CDC a regulatory agency. Except for quarantine, this was its first and only venture in federal control.[31]

Sencer was a persuasive advocate for his institution on Capitol Hill. Well informed and articulate, he prided himself on being ready for anything. "Lyle," he said to the epidemiologist Conrad in a telephone call from the Senate cloakroom, "I need the name of the EIS officer in Oklahoma, and tell me in twelve minutes the essence of that hepatitis epidemic he investigated ten days ago." Thus armed, Sencer was ready if the senator asked what the Communicable Disease Center had done for his state lately. The details of CDC's budget, which more than doubled during Sencer's years as director, posed no problem for him. He passed out copies at the hearings, but always answered questions about it from memory, giving, if necessary the page on which the item appeared.

He saw no limit to what the scientists, the engineers, and public health advisors of the CDC could do. His "we can do it" attitude was contagious, and the staff tackled project after project with serene confidence. His commitment to public health and to the institution he headed was total. He thought of himself as the first director to feel loyalty to CDC, although Larry Smith might have argued with him about this. Disarmingly bright, Sencer was seen by many on his staff as the "wisest man in public health with the best reflexes and judgment." He ran CDC as a family, as a benign autocrat. If his staff had a certain fear of him, they also had enormous respect.

In the early years of CDC's history, the ideas that came to fruition were often those of Joseph Mountin. Beginning in 1966, they were those of David Sencer. The institution became his lengthened shadow.

Immunization:
The Second Crusade

Measles, the most common and most infectious of childhood diseases, was the target of the second immunization crusade. The vaccine was licensed in March 1963, and the techniques of control honed in the campaign against polio could be adapted. It might be possible even to eradicate this disease, which was far more widespread than polio and, if complications developed, as deadly. James Goddard, never timid, announced eradication of measles as an attainable goal at the immunization conference in New Orleans in the spring of 1965. The barriers to widespread immunization against measles could be surmounted: the relatively high cost of the vaccine, the misconceptions concerning the seriousness of the disease, and public indifference. "Within three years," he predicted, "measles will be as rare as smallpox."[1] He did not take into account changed political priorities, which could alter the best-laid plans.

Before the vaccine was licensed, nearly half a million cases of measles were reported each year in the United States, and that was probably only a tenth of the true number. "Having measles" was just part of growing up. Although most cases were mild, some had serious complications. Encephalitis occurred in one case per thousand, leaving one-third of these victims mentally retarded. One measles patient in every two or three thousand died, one in two hundred had pneumonia, and one in twenty got middle ear infections.[2] These personal losses were compounded by the high cost of hospital and medical care and time lost from school.

Renewal of the Vaccination Assistance Act in 1965 added funds for measles vaccine to those for diphtheria, whooping cough, tetanus, and polio. Thus, a disease previously given little thought worked its way to the top of the health agenda. It was unconscionable that as many as a thousand children had died needlessly from measles since the licensing of the vaccine two years before. With more epidemiologists, a lot of energy, and a detailed plan, measles could be stopped.

CDC's subsequent measles chase did sharply reduce the number of cases, and it radically altered the course of the Epidemic Intelligence Service. Langmuir saw the fight against measles as an opportunity to do well by the EIS and at the same time do good for public health. The amount of money involved in the measles immunization program was quite large for the time, and it was natural for everyone to try to get some of it. D. A. Henderson, Langmuir's chief assistant, saw the possibility for EIS and called it to Langmuir's attention. Henderson talked often with Bob Freckleton of the immunization program, and he knew that a cadre of public health advisors was being trained for service in that and other units. If enough epidemiologists could be secured, they could join forces with the PHAs, and together they might make dramatic progress in the campaign against measles. Langmuir was receptive to the idea, and both Goddard and Sencer encouraged him. They were anxious to see the EIS program prosper; the need for trained epidemiologists was great.

Indeed, the need was so great there were never enough epidemiologists to go around. In the early years of the EIS program, many officers were assigned to state health departments because it was such good training. Langmuir quoted Mountin as saying, "Every commissioned officer in the PHS should be required to serve as a local health officer long enough to see at least one budget through the board of supervisors." But over the years the EIS had gradually gotten away from the practice of assigning officers to the states. Instead, they went for extra study in the valuable, but expensive, Career Development Plan, and when they got back, they were more interested in polio surveillance, influenza, the staphylococcal crisis, or in the rise of hepatitis as a disease of national importance than they were in assignments to the states. Langmuir acceded to their views and let the importance of state assignments dwindle.

When the possibility of eliminating measles surfaced, Langmuir saw that the creation of a field service division in the Epidemiology Program could serve both epidemiology and immunization. Dr. John Witte was just back from study at Harvard and was interested in measles control. Dr. Lyle Conrad, a former Peace Corps volunteer who had been fighting measles in Africa, wanted to establish a national epidemiology network with state epidemiologists as preceptors. Conrad knew that measles could not be controlled by people working in Atlanta; more people had to be in the field. Using measles as a mode, he vowed that he would make the new EIS officers the "best damned epidemiologists possible. We will chase measles up and down the country for the next couple of years and get rid of [it]."

Witte, Conrad, and all the epidemiologists in the newly created field service division got joint appointments in Epidemiology and Immunization, their salaries coming from two different budgets. They spent half their time fighting measles, the other half on general surveillance. Conrad and Witte thus joined Henderson, Bob Kaiser, and Clark Heath in the "EIS Diaspora."[3]

There had to be many more epidemiologists if the fight against measles was to succeed. Goddard approved an EIS class of seventy-five for 1966, more than double the size of that the year before. In 1967, there were sixty-nine. Bob Freckleton had the money, and Langmuir had the positions, and it worked out well. It did not bother Langmuir that a pyramidal chart could not show exactly where these EIS officers belonged, but it troubled the personnel officer, who wanted a more orderly procedure. All queries were waved away. "This is the way Dave Sencer wants it. It's working. Leave it alone." For Langmuir, the system was an administrative triumph. He had many more EIS officers but almost no additional duties. "I controlled the recruiting. [I] got my licks in during the EIS course and could draw on the state assignees when needed."[4]

Success of the immunization campaign rested on the measles vaccines, the first of which was developed by Professor John F. Enders of Harvard. In 1954 he obtained throat washings from a prep school student named David Edmonston on the first day of his measles eruption, and he successfully inoculated the virus into human kidney culture. Transferred serially to other tissue cultures and finally for fourteen passages in chick cells, the virus became the Edmonston B vaccine virus strain. The first field trials showed that about half the children receiving it developed fevers as high as 103° F. Many got a rash, and the trials showed that almost all of them developed measles antibodies. Reaction to the vaccine was substantially reduced by the administration of gamma globulin. A further attenuated vaccine, which did not require the use of gamma globulin, was developed later, as well as an inactivated vaccine. The latter, however, gave immunity of shorter duration and lesser magnitude.

Sencer ordered the Edmonston B strain and the gamma globulin to go with it for initial use in the immunization campaign. This brought searching letters from scientists, including Enders, who asked why he had made that choice when the Schwarz strain, a further attenuated vaccine requiring but a single inoculation, was available. Part of the reason was cost, Sencer explained, and part just good public health practice. The difference in price between the two vaccines was enough to make the vaccine available to almost three million additional children. "Many people have looked upon our action only as a way of saving money," Sencer wrote Enders, "but I prefer to look at it as more children being vaccinated at the same cost." High reaction rates to a vaccine dampened public acceptance of it and increased the work load for medical personnel, who had to make follow-up visits. Inoculation of five thousand children in Catawba County, North Carolina, in the spring of 1966 determined the standard dose of gamma globulin needed with the vaccine. A few days later, a measles epidemic in the Imperial Valley, California, was stopped by inoculating eight thousand children.[5]

The EIS had its first measles-fighting teams in the field by August 1966. They planned, promoted, and conducted immunization programs, investigated epidemics, and, as always, did surveillance. A few weeks later, CDC announced its national measles-eradication campaign. Bruce Dull read the position paper at the meeting of the American Public Health Association in November 1966. He confidently stated not once but twice that "eradication can be achieved in this country in 1967."[6] Langmuir thought it could be done, perhaps in as little as six months. They based the prediction on the soundest principles of epidemiology. The infection spread quickly by direct contact from person to person or was airborne among susceptibles in closed spaces. Its epidemiologic pattern could be explained fully by the balance of immunes and susceptibles in the population. With a high attack rate, the supply of susceptibles became exhausted in only a few generations of cases, so that even if a new case were introduced, another outbreak would not occur until another group of susceptibles was garnered, usually two or more years. That was the theory. If the susceptibles could be reduced to a low rate through immunization, measles would be conquered.

Measles is an epidemiologist's dream. It is highly infectious, has a predictable incubation period, and results in lifelong immunity. It is possible to construct a model of what will happen. Dull, Langmuir, and Sencer (who also signed the paper) cited the famous data on measles gathered by A. W. Hedrick in Baltimore over a thirty-year period from 1897 to 1927. Hedrick's study showed the importance of herd immunity: if the level of immunity was more than 55 percent, epidemics did not develop.[7]

In a country where smallpox, diphtheria, and poliomyelitis had been brought under effective control by immunizing a fairly high proportion of susceptibles, but by no means all of them, "so also can measles be controlled with the attainment of immunity levels that are reasonable and wholly practical to achieve." They believed this to be between 60 and 80 percent. When that was done, measles should totally disappear.

The plan for measles eradication had four essential components: routine immunization of year-old infants, immunization of other children upon entry to school, surveillance, and epidemic control. A single case of measles in a previously uninfected area constituted an epidemic. Control required that the diagnosis be verified, the source of infection traced, unreported cases detected, and susceptible contacts identified. A crash program of immunization based on this information should contain the epidemic. Older children and those in the lower socioeconomic groups were the most vulnerable. Five to ten million additional doses of vaccine were needed in those groups to bring their immunity levels up to those of suburban children.[8]

Surgeon General Stewart challenged health professionals to make eradication a reality. The American Public Health Association gave the campaign a ringing endorsement, and other health agencies followed suit—the American Academy of Pediatrics, the American Medical Association, and the American Association for Health, Physical Education and Recreation. The AMA was especially active in the area of publicity. What had been a campaign of public health professionals became a public crusade with President Johnson's announcement in March 1967 that measles would be eliminated that year. Sencer pledged that CDC would not let the president down. The press gave the campaign a good send-off with headlines like "Good-by to Measles," but it would take more than the endorsement of the president, the enthusiasm of public health professionals, and a good press to ensure success. The people had to be convinced that measles was a *serious* illness as well as a preventable one. That would not be not easy. The campaign against polio and diphtheria was just barely holding its own.[9]

Charles Schultz, creator of the popular comic strip *Peanuts*, used the first seven strips of 1967 to get measles shots for Charlie Brown and his friends and to spread the word: "Happiness is no more measles." A cartoon and a coloring book featured Measles, the bad guy, out to catch Billy. In the classic struggle of good versus evil, Dr. Immunity eventually mastered and tamed the villain. Kimela Fisher, the poster child from the National Association of Retarded Children, who had had measles encephalitis at age two, came to Atlanta to make television spots promoting the immunization campaign. New York City launched its effort with a circus in Madison Square Garden.[10]

Because immunization was aimed especially at the millions of children in lower socioeconomic groups, assistance from the Office of Economic Opportunity was especially welcome. OEO director Sargent Shriver offered the services of Volunteers in Service to America (VISTA) and Job Corps trainees. Children in the Head Start program could be immunized while at school. The federal government supplied $3 million for purchase of measles vaccine for state and local health agencies. Another $4 million was distributed to states and communities in supplies, educational materials, or personnel—EIS officers and the popular PHAs. Grants were made to forty states and fifty-four cities and counties for immunization of year-old children, and to twenty-nine state and city-county programs for immunization of children in kindergarten and the first and second grades. Grants went only to programs with a potential for success. Freckleton was upset when Michigan, in an end run around CDC, got $100,000 from the Children's Bureau for the purchase of vaccine, when it had been unwilling to organize a full four- or five-disease program or commit itself to an adequate maintenance program.[11]

The remarkably successful campaign made measles more prominent than any disease since polio. More than seven million previously unprotected children were immunized, and the incidence of measles dropped 70 percent in one year. A measles epidemic was halted in Mason County, Kentucky, with the vaccination of children in just the first and second grades, proving for the first time that the epidemic spread of measles could be stopped by vaccinating only a limited group. Epidemics might be stopped, but measles could be permanently controlled only by an intensive program of surveillance. This depended on the cooperation of physicians, many of whom were not anxious to add a reporting chore to their other duties. EIS officers in the field were instructed to counter this reluctance by demonstrating that surveillance works, that "ring" vaccination could stop an epidemic. "Demonstrate epidemic control! Nothing can encourage and improve reporting like *action* on your part."[12]

This action campaign received marvelous results. In 1965 there were 261,904 cases of measles in the United States. In 1968, there were only 22,000, an all-time low. In the three-year period, the massive vaccination program prevented an estimated 8.5 million cases of measles, 850 deaths from such complications as encephalitis, 2,800 cases of mental retardation, 500,000 days of hospitalization, and 17 million days of absence from school. By then 90 percent of the American people were covered. There were problems, of course. It was difficult to reach all those who most needed to be reached. In Atlanta an estimated 40 percent of the children in low-income areas were still susceptible to measles in 1968, so volunteers went door to door encouraging parents to have their children immunized. Epidemics sometimes broke out in areas where no organized health department existed, making control more difficult.[13] The most serious difficulty, however, arose with what should have been good news. A vaccine against rubella (German measles), on which so many birth defects were blamed, was licensed, distracting attention from the measles campaign just when there seemed to be the best chance of success.

The rubella vaccine, developed at the National Institutes of Health, became available in 1969, just before rubella was expected to make its cyclical return. Understandably, there was much interest in getting widespread use of the vaccine as soon as possible. The last epidemic of rubella had occurred in 1964–65, and the disease was known to run in cycles of six to nine years. After the epidemic of 1964, twenty thousand children were born with severe birth defects—about three-quarters of them were deaf—and there were thousands of wasted pregnancies. That epidemic was still a vivid memory five years later. Children born in 1964–65 to mothers who had had rubella in early pregnancy were ready to go to school. Public education programs for children with impaired hearing were swamped. Small wonder that there was so much interest in rubella that other programs fell by the wayside.

The scenario that led to such an intense interest in rubella at the expense of all other immunization programs began in Washington where, under the new Republican administration, HEW initially decided to let the Vaccination Assistance Act expire without any request for renewal. The Vietnam War drained the nation's resources, and many programs to improve life at home were shelved. When national voluntary health organizations pressured the HEW to set up a separate program for rubella immunization, Senator Kennedy introduced legislation reviving the Vaccination Assistance Act. He was intensely interested in rubella and almost singlehandedly turned the fight against measles into a campaign to conquer rubella. The authorizing legislation specified that funds should be used for rubella and for no other disease, and for a year and a half the immunization program was, in effect, the rubella program. With little money to fight measles, but with $25.6 million to fight rubella, the CDC field force that had worked so effectively to bring down the incidence of "red" measles turned its attention to German measles instead.[14]

The campaign began in June 1969, the same month the vaccine was licensed. CDC quickly made grants to forty-eight states and twenty-four localities to get rubella-control programs under way. The largest, for more than $1 million, went to California; the smallest, for $12,850, to the Saginaw, Michigan, City Health Department. Under the government's "Partnership for Health" plan, states were expected to supply 70 percent of the funding. Certainly the federal grants were not sufficient to the need, and states scrambled for additional funds. Where they were successful, as in the District of Columbia, which bought more than four times as much vaccine as the federal government furnished, the campaign worked well. In states like Alabama and New Mexico, which depended entirely on federal funds, the programs had difficulty getting off the ground. Harold Mauldin, deputy chief of the immunization program, said it was "unrealistic that the federal effort is so small." In Washington, Assistant Secretary for Health James H. Cavenaugh disagreed. "[F]rom the readings taken to date," he said in October 1969, five months after the campaign began, "I think the program is moving ahead well both in terms of resources and children."

At CDC the main concern was that the campaign be both "intensive and orderly," with full attention given to surveillance. Fifty million children, primarily in nursery school, kindergarten, and the early grades, were targeted. A formula was established to allocate the vaccine, at first in short supply. It allowed one and a half doses for each birth, not enough for some states, too much for others. A major problem was how to handle the young women who insisted on having the vaccine. While most were already immune, all would have to be tested.

The test was not foolproof and too complicated for all laboratories to do. CDC conducted seminars in Atlanta and around the country to train laboratory workers who, in turn, would teach others.[15]

A year after the campaign against rubella began, thirteen million children had been inoculated, mostly in public health clinics. Where vaccination rates were high, rubella declined by 37 percent; where they were low, the disease increased by 54 percent. "With continuous, judicious use of the vaccine and good surveillance of rubella," John Witte said, "we may never have another national catastrophe [such] as occurred six years ago."[16]

Gratification over the success of the rubella campaign was tempered by the upsurge in measles. Lyle Conrad was furious that the war on measles was being abandoned just when victory seemed assured. As funds for the measles program dried up, the incidence of the disease rose. In 1970, a year after funding for measles immunization virtually ended, there were forty thousand cases (almost a 100 percent increase over 1968), and in 1971, seventy-five thousand. An immunization survey showed that only 57.2 percent of the nation's children were immunized against measles, and in areas of urban poverty, the number of children protected was only 41.1 percent. Armed with these alarming figures, Sencer interceded with officials in Washington to get the rubella mandate broadened to once again include measles and to add mumps, for which a vaccine had been licensed. Again the measles curve turned down, and it stayed down until the swine flu episode of 1976 funneled the attention of all epidemiologists into a single channel. When everybody in the field was turned into a "swine flu-ologist," the measles curve turned up once more.[17]

Almost two decades after the intensive campaign against measles began, Langmuir looked back to see why his confident prediction that measles would be eradicated in six months had not been realized. The problem had seemed so simple. Just encourage widespread immunization to the point of elevating immunity well above the epidemic threshold and the virus could not survive. "Where did we get derailed?" he asked. He concluded that he had grossly overinterpreted the doctrine of herd immunity, that measles was an exception to the epidemic theory that disease spreads at a certain rate by close personal contact. He thought measles must be airborne in character and that a single dangerous spreader could contaminate the air of enclosed spaces in an hour or perhaps minutes, a "far cry from progressive person-to-person spread."

In retrospect, he decided epidemiologists had "sinned grievously in ignoring a continued scrutiny of field epidemiology." William Firth Wells, who argued in the 1930s that measles was airborne, should have been given more attention and respect. More shoe-leather epidemiology and more humility were called for. At the entrance of the "Territory of Epidemiology," Langmuir warned, there should be a sign: "Caveat praedictor."[18]

CHAPTER 13

Over Oceans and into Space

Several forces converged in the 1960s to turn CDC's attention to international health. The boom in jet travel increased the possibility of introducing exotic diseases from abroad. Veterans of the Vietnam War brought home both "oriental" venereal disease and a strain of malaria resistant to known forms of treatment. Even germs from outer space were a frightening prospect in that decade when man first went to the moon, a possibility, however remote, given vivid expression in Michael Crichton's novel *The Andromeda Strain*.[1] Of equal importance was the moral necessity to keep earth germs at home.

Any international traveler could be at risk. The German physician who developed smallpox shortly after he returned home from India had exposed everyone aboard the plane (which had continued on to America), all of whom had to be tracked down. Soldiers in Vietnam picked up diseases all but unknown in the United States.[2] Americans traveling abroad were warned against cholera, which had spread from India and Pakistan as far west as Iran. To keep these diseases out, CDC increasingly fought disease at the source. It extended its mandate overseas.

Rescue missions, mounted occasionally in the 1950s, became commonplace. CDC responded as readily to an overseas distress call as to one from the states. The number of calls in 1963 was unprecedented: poliomyelitis in the Marshall Islands, British Guiana, Barbados, and the Dominican Republic; hepatitis in England; cholera in the Philippines; diphtheria in Jamaica; malaria in Indonesia; rabies in Mexico and Canada. Smallpox-vaccination assistance was needed in the South Pacific,

Canada, and Sweden. Most requests were straightforward enough, but one from Bolivia in 1967 had political overtones. Bolivian troops hunting the Cuban revolutionary Che Guevara in the low-lying Riberalta region became ill with what appeared to be hemorrhagic smallpox. When the virologist John Noble responded, he found yet another disease, hemorrhagic exanthem of Bolivia. It was caused by a virus carried by black flies common to the Riberalta, to which soldiers from the Altiplano region had no immunity.[3]

Occasionally CDC provided aid for a single overseas victim. None was more grateful than Atlanta's Mayor Ivan Allen, who developed sleeping sickness while on a hunting trip in Africa. CDC supplied the proper drug from its rare-disease stockpile. The mayor recovered and returned home full of praise for the hometown institution. CDC, in turn, presented the mayor with a tsetse fly neatly embedded in paperweight. The specific culprit, David Sencer remarked wryly, had been found only with difficulty.[4]

The Vietnam War stimulated renewed interest in malaria research, which had virtually ceased at the end of the Korean War. Only at CDC and NIH was any work at all being done. The Army renewed its interest in the disease when troops were sent to Vietnam, an interest that grew in intensity every year. Returning soldiers brought back *Plasmodium falciparum,* the most deadly form of malaria, one resistant to both chloroquin and primaquin. At the same time, Peace Corps volunteers serving in West Africa introduced *Plasmodium ovale* to the United States. The search for new treatments began.

With the escalation of the Vietnam War in 1965, the number of cases of malaria rose steadily. Anti-malarial drugs offered some protection, and troops were issued head nets and insect repellent, but these were not used consistently. Head nets cut down visibility; insect repellent alerted the enemy. By 1967 malaria took more men out of action than wounds. This meant more malaria at home, too. Whereas there were only 59 cases of malaria in the United States in 1959, there were nearly 700 in 1966, and in both 1967 and 1968, more than 2,000 cases were imported. The need for surveillance had never been greater. In 1966, CDC appointed Dr. Hans Lobel as its first full-time officer for malaria surveillance. Although Lobel doubted that malaria would spread through the population, he thought caution advisable. Cases of malaria in four teenagers who had attended a drive-in movie near Opelika, Alabama, was proof enough that the danger existed. The drive-in was surrounded by ponds where anopheline mosquitoes bred, and the area was home to a number of foreign students at nearby universities and to thousands of Vietnam veterans.[5]

The rise in malaria once more stirred interest in the possibility of malaria eradication, first broached at the meeting of the Pan American Sanitary Conference in 1954. The decision then had been that eradication should be achieved before anopheles mosquitoes became completely resistant to insecticides. The conference urged governments to switch from control of malaria to its eradication, and the changeover began in 1955. The campaigns presupposed, unrealistically, that the means for wiping out the disease existed, that financial and human resources were sufficient to the task, and that wherever eradication was achieved, those areas would be protected against reinfection. The work of MCWA provided one of the best examples of a successful eradication program. Similarly successful programs had been carried out in Canada, Italy, and Greece. President Johnson was committed to malaria eradication, and Congress provided funds for grants and loans. These went directly to countries through the Agency for International Development (AID), and indirectly through the World Health Organization (WHO) and the Pan American Health Organization (PAHO). The need was urgent: malaria was the leading cause of mortality in economically underdeveloped countries. Success of the eradication program in India lent hope that it would work elsewhere. In 1965, after eight years work, great progress had been made. Much of the population was protected against malaria at a cost of only nine cents a person a year.[6]

Not everyone believed malaria could be eradicated. Dr. Justin Andrews, CDC's former chief and one of the world's experts on malaria, had doubts. He knew it was technically feasible to eliminate malaria in spite of insecticide-resistant mosquitoes and drug-resistant strains. What concerned him were "resistances" from administrative, educational, and financial sources. He thought that WHO and AID should seek advice from the most knowledgeable authorities in the social sciences as to how these "resistances" might be overcome.[7] Andrews proved to be a prophet.

CDC inherited the malaria-eradication program in March 1966, the same month that Sencer became CDC director. The Agency for International Development turned over the program to the Public Health Service, which in turn designated CDC to handle it. Eradication was to be accomplished in four phases: preparatory (geographic reconnaissance and surveys); attack (insecticidal spraying and increased medicinal treatment to stop transmission); consolidation (withdrawal of spraying operations when there was less than one case per thousand); and maintenance (no indigenous malaria for three years).

Even before the transfer was made to the PHS, Surgeon General Stewart spotted potential problems. Malaria eradication would not succeed without the assignment of more professionals from the United States, and this would be objectionable to countries that operated their programs on loans. In Ecuador, the integrity of the program had been maintained solely through the autonomy of the U.S. malaria advisor. If his salary came from loan funds, he would lose his authority, and the program would falter.

Donald Martin, head of CDC's Training Branch, was convinced that success depended on training. He blamed the failure to eradicate malaria on deemphasizing the training of malariologists, parasitologists, epidemiologists, and entomologists. Residual spraying, no matter how extensive, and reliance on suppressive drugs were not enough. Although malaria had virtually disappeared from the United States, the Training Branch had kept abreast of developments, and officers charged with malaria control in Vietnam came to CDC to study. The Training Branch provided the military with a complete entomological key to the 169 species of mosquitoes found in Vietnam. Martin wanted his branch given total responsibility for overseas training in malaria eradication.[8]

When CDC took over the malaria-eradication program, Donald J. Schliessmann, a sanitary engineer with a quarter century of experience at MCWA and CDC, was put in charge. When he retired a year later, Dr. Robert Kaiser was spun off from Epidemiology to take his place. Nobody believed that success would come soon, for eradication demanded perfection in everything from the top administrator to the spray men on the route. This was too much to expect. With its sections for operations, evaluation, training, and research, the organization looked right. The plan of action—reconnaissance and attack—was well established. But there were so many places for things to go wrong.

Success depended at least in part on the effectiveness of insecticides. CDC's Oatland Island laboratory was the principal U.S. agency working on insecticides to control disease vectors. By 1967 it knew that twelve anopheline species were resistant to DDT and that another thirty-four were resistant to dieldrin. The staff looked for other more effective products, greatly improved the quality of hand sprayers, and searched diligently for inherent biological weaknesses in mosquitoes that might be exploited.[9]

About six months after CDC assumed responsibility for malaria eradication, Sencer went to Asia to inspect programs under way there. It was a quick trip—"I was a malariologist in four countries in five days,"—but a revealing one. He found the program in Pakistan in danger of being phased out when only half complete because it absorbed too much of the national health budget. If Pakistan pulled out, worldwide eradication of malaria would be undermined, but AID/ Washington planned no action.[10]

Loss of interest was the major stumbling block in malaria eradication, but other things were involved as well. Many countries had poorly developed health structures; inflation steadily escalated costs; and some countries achieved eradication only to be reinfested from neighboring nations. As Martin had predicted, there was a desperate need for more training. Personnel from CDC's Training Branch were dispatched to the Eradication Training Center in Manila, where malariologists from around the world came to study. Much more research was needed, too. Six months after CDC took over the program, it proposed an increase in the research staff from 40 to 117. All the problems fell into two categories: administrative and technical. Whenever programs were prolonged because of administrative and logistical difficulties, technical problems were sure to follow. Most of these stemmed from vector resistance to insecticides, so time was of the essence.[11]

The leadership at CDC—Sencer, Langmuir, Schliessmann and Kaiser—wanted to give the malaria-eradication program an epidemiological cast. Langmuir put a pool of EIS officers on temporary assignment to find where malaria transmission was taking place and to narrow the focus of the program. The concept of substituting epidemiology for broad application of insecticide was hard to sell, and WHO did not make it official policy for several years. Funds for the program came to CDC from the Agency for International Development through a Participating Agency Service Agreement. The two agencies saw things quite differently. When CDC wanted to assign eight people to the eradication program in Central America, AID insisted on only four. AID thought the programs should be carried out by the countries themselves, with U.S. personnel acting only as monitors. CDC wanted active involvement and day-to-day evaluation. Complicating this basic disagreement was the fact that AID budgets in the countries were not for specific programs like malaria but rather for generalized items like technical assistance or capital assistance. Kaiser wanted much more specific control over the budget. Sencer complained that AID had no uniform policy on priority and support for malaria eradication, and that it had not accepted the terms of the agreement with PHS "either philosophically or operationally." He did not think that malaria eradication could be achieved unless the PHS had control of the program and resources.[12]

The administrative changes Sencer wanted were not made. Thousands of people were hired in the eighteen countries where CDC was involved in malaria eradication, but it had little control over them. Quite early, CDC had the largest payroll in Haiti, where hundreds of people were hired to spray mosquitoes. CDC furnished tons of DDT and whenever possible, some guidance, but the U.S. Embassy in Haiti was essentially in charge. People who came to work drunk or did not come at all were not fired. This was the responsibility of the host country, which usually was loath to exercise authority. Among the more constructive aspects of the malaria-eradication program was the development of the Central American Malaria Research Station in El Salvador. The first long-range comprehensive research on malaria ever done in that region was done at this CDC station.[13]

The malaria-eradication program was analogous to work with the states. The center's deputy director, John R. Bagby, explained to an officer in the State Department that CDC assisted states—"often surprisingly similar to imperial nations"—with communicable-disease problems, but the states made CDC an active partner in the process. CDC assumed that countries would welcome its participation in malaria-eradication projects and would work in partnership on the technical portions of those programs. CDC saw itself "as responsible for producing salutary changes in these programs—improvements which are significant and measurable."[14]

Sencer thought that malaria eradication was too caught up in the bureaucracy of AID to work properly. "It was not the CDC program that failed, but the whole malaria-control program that failed," he said. "Bob Kaiser and his staff were never able to influence sufficiently the larger program." Billy Griggs, director of CDC's Office of International Health, never believed that malaria eradication was "doable" with the resources and will put into it. "Perhaps with unlimited resources it could have been done," he said. In Africa, CDC worked only in Ethiopia. The countries of West Central Africa, where malaria is highly endemic, recognized that malaria would never be eradicated with the resources people were willing to commit to it.[15]

Progress in international health depended on trained workers, whether it was in malaria eradication or in fighting other ills of mankind. Peace Corps volunteers, much in demand for work in disease control, often trained at CDC before leaving for their assignments, and Peace Corps physicians were oriented to their new jobs in an intensive training program in Atlanta. It was foreign visitors, however, who composed the largest part of those training at CDC in international health. In 1968, 625 health workers from ninety-four countries enrolled for courses.

For years all those training at CDC found whatever housing they could in Atlanta, seldom easy in a city where the vestiges of segregation lingered, and especially difficult for visitors from Africa. For them, housing was often available only within the inner city, and sometimes this was substandard. Transportation to the Clifton Road headquarters was complicated, and life away from the center lonely. The loneliness and alienation proved too much for one foreign trainee in the mid 1960s, who took her life. Churches—primarily Presbyterian—not the government, provided a solution to the housing problem.

The sequence of events that led to building Villa International Atlanta (VIA), a center where foreign visitors might find housing and friendship within walking distance of CDC headquarters, began shortly after the woman's death, when a representative of the State Department contacted the Board of World Missions of the Presbyterian Church U.S., outlined the critical need for CDC's visitors, and asked for help. The Board of Missions in turn contacted the church's Board of Women's Work in Atlanta, which explored possibilities and began to make plans. In cooperation with the Protestant Radio and Television Center, the decision was made to build a center that would provide housing for foreign visitors to CDC, the TV center, and neighboring universities. In 1970 the Presbyterian Women of the Church donated their birthday offering of $287,339.63 to Villa International Atlanta. This covered the cost of the building, which opened in 1972, but funds for furnishings, landscaping, and equipment came from local foundations and companies. "Friends of the Villa," which included groups and churches other than the Presbyterians, was organized in 1971 to provide continuing support. From the day it opened, VIA nearly always was filled to capacity, and 70 percent of its guests studied at CDC.[16]

An institution steadily expanding the scope of its activities, as CDC was in the 1960s, was almost certain to get involved in the most exciting, glamorous, and technically difficult challenge of the decade, the exploration of space. In 1964 the National Aeronautics and Space Administration (NASA) approached CDC for help in working out methods that would ensure that germs from earth did not get transported into space. Dr. Goddard, then director of CDC, was immediately interested. So was Dr. Simmons of the Technology Branch. "Dr. Simmons could smell money anywhere and got some for the Phoenix Lab to do that," David Sencer recalled.[17] But it was more than just getting more money for research. Simmons and his staff were already working on ways to keep hospitals as free as possible of staphylococcus, and the attempt to protect the planets from contamination was an extension of that effort. Like many aspects of the space program, these efforts had tangible benefits for daily life.

At first, CDC's space efforts centered on making certain that interplanetary craft like the Mars-bound Voyager did not carry earth bacteria with them. The scientific community strongly recommended that an effort be made to determine what, if any, organisms lived on Mars, and this could be done successfully only if the spacecraft itself was sterile. Otherwise, not only would earth's microorganisms be carried into space, undesirable in itself, but the craft would test its own bacteria, making it impossible to know the truth about Mars. Because NASA had no laboratory for microbiology assay, it contracted with CDC to do the work. NASA's charge to CDC was to reduce the chance of releasing living organisms on Mars to less than one in ten thousand. Technology Branch laboratories at both Oatland Island and Phoenix were involved, as well as a laboratory at Cape Kennedy.[18]

The first task was to develop a means of detecting the microscopic life that workers building the spacecraft, being human, shed in the ordinary course of their existence. The second was to figure out how best to kill these microorganisms. This work was done primarily at Oatland Island, where volunteers spent a lot of time in a specially built stainless steel tank, seven feet high and three feet wide, so that the number and kinds of bacteria they shed could be ascertained.[19] Viruses posed no danger, because they reproduce only in specific cells, and fungi are readily killed by moderate heat, but bacteria are another matter. They are numerous and heat high enough to kill them would wreck the delicate components of the spacecraft. Research at Oatland Island proved that specially designed clothes reduced the number of bacteria shed, and that a combination of dry heat and ethylene oxide gas killed those that remained.

In Phoenix, a team headed by Dr. Martin Favero was to determine if all the components of the spacecraft itself were bacteria-free. The team built special labs with special equipment to monitor the presence of bacteria in all phases of assembly, making certain that bacteria did not become embedded in metal or plastic from which they might subsequently escape. These painstaking microbiologic assays were forerunners of the critical sterility tests that became standard procedure for hospitals.[20]

It was Jim Goddard who decided that the earth must be protected from contamination from the moon, and, at his insistence, a committee was formed in 1965 to work out the protective measures. Goddard was committee chairman, but when he moved on to the Food and Drug Administration, David Sencer inherited the job. The Interagency Committee on Back Contamination (ICBC) also had representatives from the Departments of Agriculture and Interior and the National Academy of Sciences. The committee determined that contamination might come either from the astronauts themselves or from the moon rocks they brought back, and it ordered protective measures.[21]

The elaborate procedure to keep the astronauts from bringing back moon germs was followed to the letter. They left their boots and gloves on the moon, vacuumed the lunar module before reentering the command ship, vacuumed and dust-sealed that vehicle, and breathed air filtered through lithium hydroxide canisters on the trip back to earth. When they landed in the Pacific, they donned decontamination suits, were sprayed with an iodine solution, and climbed immediately into the Mobile Quarantine Facility—an Airstream trailer minus wheels—for the three-day trip by ship, plane, and tractor trailer to the Lunar Receiving Laboratory in Houston. In this $11 million facility, they lived with doctors, technicians, and a cook behind biological barriers until the twenty-one-day quarantine was over. During that time, they provided specimens for culture on a variety of plants and animals, including germ-free pine trees, Japanese quail, and oysters from the Southern Hemisphere.[22]

Quarantine of the astronauts sparked a spirited debate in the scientific community. Some argued that the procedure was not rigid enough, others that it was unnecessary and ridiculous. Among CDC's staff there was a good bit of levity about the presumed dangers, but the position of the ICBC was that while the chance of contamination was slim, it was not zero, and they could not afford to take chances.

The ICBC met in Atlanta on Sunday morning, August 11, 1969, reviewed all the test results, and announced an end to the quarantine a few hours short of the allotted three weeks. At that moment, the isolation of quarantine gave way to rigid surveillance. For months the astronauts and all those in contact with them were watched closely for the slightest sign of health problems. Meanwhile, the moon rocks continued under investigation. Dr. Walter Dowdle was among those assigned to protect the earth from the dangers of moon dust. "I never felt so silly in my life," he said as he recalled all the talk about alien creatures that might escape. "Maybe they were right, but the moon environment was so alien to every creature we had on earth that it was amazing to me that anything would grow better here than there or even grow at all. I'll never forget [that] when they started inoculating some of the ground up moon dust into conventional tissue culture, everything died. Of course everything died. When you put dirt in tissue culture, it dies. That was a wild time."[23]

Although the astronauts posed no danger to earthlings nor moon rocks to the environment, the possibility of a previously unknown threat to health became a reality when two strange and terrible African fevers burst on the scene (see chapter 15). Both Marburg and Lassa fevers were vivid reminders of the constant challenges, both new and old, to public health. Ironically, the Airstream trailer in which astronauts and moon rocks moved in isolation from the landing in the Pacific to the security of the Lunar Receiving Laboratory found far longer service as a standby isolation unit for victims of these strange, terrible, and earthly fevers.

CHAPTER 14

The Crusade against Smallpox

The significance of international health to the United States found its best expression in the global campaign to eradicate smallpox. When the effort began, malaria eradication was entering its second decade, with no end in sight, and there were nay sayers who thought the attack on smallpox would fare no better. But, in little more than a decade, small-pox, a disease that had terrorized mankind for 10,000 years, was gone. The campaign succeeded where others failed because it was based on the scientific principle of surveillance. CDC played a starring role in the fight; elimination of smallpox became one of its proudest achievements.

Formal commitment by CDC to eradication of smallpox began in 1966, but work that led to that commitment was five years or more in the making. In 1961 Alexander Langmuir told Dr. J. Donald Millar, his newest aide-de-camp, "to keep an eye on smallpox around the world. See if you can make any sense of what's happening." Millar was a brand-new EIS officer, excited about being picked as Langmuir's "per-sonal valet." That order from his boss led to the most exciting work of his life.

Millar had never seen a case of smallpox, the last outbreak of the disease in the United States having occurred in the Rio Grande Valley in 1949. In his search of the medical literature, he charted five outbreaks in the British Midlands and Wales, all traced to importations from Pakistan. Most of the victims were unvaccinated hospital personnel. When he learned that many workers at Atlanta's Grady Hospital had not been vaccinated in thirty years, he knew American health-care workers were at risk. He and D. A. Henderson, chief of the surveillance section, investigated suspected cases of smallpox in the United States. All proved to be false alarms, but there was a genuine scare in the summer of 1962 when a Canadian boy developed smallpox after returning home from Brazil by way of New York's Idlewild Airport and Grand Central Station. Hundreds of New Yorkers who might have had contact with the youth were vaccinated and put under surveillance.

It was that incident that led to the establishment of the smallpox surveillance unit with Millar in charge. Four physicians were recruited to work with him—Drs. Ronald R. Roberto, John M. Neff, Thomas M. Mack, and J. Michael Lane. "We were all young, naive, and very enthusiastic," Lane recalled. "We got increasingly entranced about doing something about smallpox." They began with a study of smallpox vaccinations, the best way to do these, and the danger they imposed. They learned that vaccinations caused seven to ten deaths a year in the United States and set off a debate on the wisdom of vaccination that was not settled for almost a decade. They studied particularly how smallpox was introduced into the developed countries from the Third World. Langmuir often called their attention to the faith William Farr had in the logic of epidemiology. The famed nineteenth-century medical statistician believed that "natural laws govern the occurrence of a disease, that these laws can be discovered by epidemiologic inquiry and that, when discovered, the causes of epidemics admit to a great extent of remedy."[1]

While the smallpox unit increased its store of knowledge, developments in medical technology made it feasible to think about eradication. The Army developed a jet injector for subcutaneous shots just after World War II, and in 1962, Aaron Ismach, a civilian employee of the Defense Department, fitted this injector with an intradermal nozzle, making it suitable for smallpox vaccinations. CDC tested it for the next two years both in the United States and abroad. The first injectors were powered by electricity, difficult to maintain, and unsuitable for use in the underdeveloped countries where smallpox was most likely to flourish. At CDC's suggestion, Ismach developed the "ped-o-jet," operated mechanically by a foot pedal. It weighed less than twelve pounds, could be operated anywhere, and could give a thousand injections an hour. Equally important, the jet injector did not waste vaccine, which had been greatly improved. In the 1950s the Lister Institute in England had developed a freeze-dried product that could be stored for up to two years at body temperature. The combination of a stable vaccine and a rapid method of delivery made the eradication of smallpox technically feasible.[2]

In the summer of 1963, CDC tested the jet gun and vaccine in the Pacific island nation of Tonga. Some 65,000 people lived there, none of whom had ever been vaccinated. Isolation from the rest of the world had protected them against smallpox, but as new Asian markets opened up for its copra and bananas, smallpox, endemic in much of Asia, might be imported. Prince Tungi, Tonga's 350-pound leader, came to CDC to ask for help. The cameras rolled when this commanding figure was vaccinated with the new jet gun. Later the film was shown over and over again in Tonga to bolster the courage of the Tongalese people. For ten weeks in the spring of 1964, a four-man team from CDC—William Higgins and Drs. William Foege, Ronald Roberto, and Pierce Gardner—went from island to island and from village to village vaccinating the people. For comparative studies, they divided the population into four groups, three of which were immunized with the ped-o-jet. It worked well and the optimal vaccine dilution was determined. The "take" rate among the 45,000 people vaccinated was 98.4 percent. For the Tongalese people, the campaign meant protection against smallpox; for CDC the *Miracle in Tonga*, as the movie of the campaign was called, was a prelude to far larger projects.[3]

A few months later, Millar and Neff were invited by the Pan American Health Organization to work in an area of endemic smallpox in Brazil where conditions were very difficult. The disease was proceeding uncontrolled across the Brazilian jungles and had already crossed the border into Peru. The ped-o-jet worked well, and Millar and Neff made progress, but they were convinced that smallpox had to be eradicated in Brazil if other South American nations were to be protected.[4]

The smallpox unit attracted little attention until May 1965, when a woman from Ghana, who had been in the United States only two weeks, was hospitalized in Washington, D.C., with what appeared to be smallpox. Millar, Neff, and Lane were called in to examine the patient. They had serious doubts that she had smallpox, but the CDC laboratory, using the immunofluorescence (IF) technique, confirmed the diagnosis. Alexander Langmuir described what happened next: "We closed down Washington, D.C." More than a thousand persons who had had some contact with the patient, directly or indirectly, were vaccinated and placed under surveillance. All over the city, work schedules were disrupted; the whole thing was very public. When the patient recovered and no other cases appeared, the CDC laboratory announced results of a longer, more complex test. The woman had chicken pox. This embarrassing experience prompted an investigation of all smallpox tests. They were all flawed. In the best tradition of profiting from the Mountin dictum "Ignorance must be exploited," CDC began immediately to develop a pox-virus laboratory, which, under the direction of Dr. James H. Nakano, in time became the most prestigious in the world.

Although the Washington incident attracted much attention, it was only a blip in the record of the smallpox unit. It had steadily acquired the knowledge and skill to eradicate smallpox, but could do nothing until the social and political climate was right. The unit was, in Millar's words, "all dressed up with nowhere to go!" until D. A. Henderson tied smallpox eradication to the measles immunization program already under way in Africa. That gave CDC the chance it wanted. Millar called Henderson's idea a stroke of genius.[5]

In Africa, measles posed a greater threat to health than smallpox. The disease ravaged much of the continent, striking nearly all children and killing at least 10 percent before their fifth birthdays. The newly independent African nations, anxious to improve the quality of life, were keenly interested in the measles vaccine being developed in the United States. On a visit to America in 1960, ministers of health of four of the new nations talked with Dr. Harry Meyer, who was working on the attenuated Edmonston B strain of vaccine at the Division of Biologics Standards, then part of NIH. The health minister from Upper Volta immediately saw the potential value of the vaccine in his country, where one child in four died from measles. At his request, a field trial was conducted in Upper Volta. It was so successful the Agency for International Development provided enough measles vaccine for seven hundred thousand young children. From November 1962 to March 1963, Upper Volta mothers brought their children to the vaccination centers. A year later, Upper Volta had no deaths from measles, and the number of cases was sharply reduced.

Six more former French colonies—Dahomey, Guinea, the Ivory Coast, Mali, Mauritania, and Niger—asked for and received AID funds for demonstration projects in 1964. NIH was so taxed by these projects, it asked CDC to help. In December 1964, Dr. Lawrence K. Altman left for what he thought would be a six-week observation trip. His assignment stretched to six months, and he sent back vivid accounts of the problems the immunization campaigns faced. In countries where the roads were poor, the vehicles ill designed for the task, and electricity nonexistent outside the largest cities, the job of mass immunization was incredibly complex. Problems with equipment, administration, and communications added to the difficulties.

AID was nonetheless enthusiastic about the programs, and when four more countries were added to the original six—Cameroon, the Central Africa Republic, Chad, and Togo—Dr. A. C. Curtis of AID asked CDC to send in some teams. Nine medical officers were assigned for six months. What they learned proved useful in the smallpox-eradication campaign.[6]

The experience of the team in Togo was typical. In the village of Tchamba, four CDC epidemiologists, assisted by Peace Corps personnel, did simultaneous vaccinations for measles and smallpox. The government supplied a place for them to work and mechanics for their rented vehicles; the village chief persuaded mothers to bring their children for vaccinations and to return daily for two weeks to be checked. The CDC team did the rest. When the work in Tchamba was done, the team moved on to the village of Scoboboua and repeated the process.

In the district of Atakpame, they conducted a mass measles demonstration project. They divided the district into eighty-three vaccination areas, and each day teams consisting of one American, two Togolese, and a chauffeur set out to give measles vaccine to as many children as they could.

A typical day began at 6:45 A.M., when teams departed for the assigned villages. Each team usually worked four centers a day, often far apart. No Togolese doctor worked with them, and publicity was a problem. The difficulties that Altman had pinpointed earlier proved only too real, but AID continued to be enthusiastic about measles control and asked CDC for more and more teams.[7]

These calls presented both a problem and an opportunity for CDC. Henderson wanted to provide international experience for as many EIS officers as possible, but the design of the African measles campaign was flawed. Despite its obvious success, it reached only about a quarter of all the African children and promised to extend into the indefinite future. If, however, the measles campaign could be combined with one to vaccinate the entire populace against smallpox, then the project would be of inestimable value. For only a tiny additional cost, smallpox could be eradicated from all of West and Central Africa while measles was curbed. Smallpox vaccine cost but one thousandth as much as measles vaccine, and only one extra jet injector would be required for each team. Henderson proposed a joint smallpox-measles program in Africa, an idea that as much as anything else launched the global smallpox-eradication program.[8]

Eradication of smallpox was not a new idea. Fred L. Soper, who had directed Brazil's successful assault against yellow fever in the 1930s, persuaded the Pan American Sanitary Bureau to approve a smallpox-eradication campaign for the Americas in 1949, and within ten years it achieved notable success. In 1958 the World Health Organization adopted a resolution of the Soviet Union that a global eradication effort be made, but no deadline was set and there was no specific support. By 1965, advanced technology, an improved vaccine, and the success of CDC's smallpox unit in Brazil greatly enhanced the possibility of global eradication, even though many politicians and scientists remained skeptical. Why should the effort to eradicate smallpox succeed when that against malaria had failed? When the Agency for International Development kept asking CDC for more and more help in the African measles campaign, however, Henderson decided that the time had come to broaden the base.

First, Henderson had to persuade the PHS, and ultimately the president of the United States, that this was a good idea. His patient backstage persuasion worked. In May 1965, President Lyndon Johnson told the 18th Assembly of the World Health Organization: "This Government is ready to work with other interested countries to see to it that smallpox is a thing of the past by 1975." By August, CDC had a draft of a five-year program for measles and smallpox vaccination in West Africa that would, in time, be fully integrated into WHO's global smallpox-eradication plan. Its cost was an estimated $35 million. Compared with that of malaria eradication, the amount was modest indeed.

CDC was to begin work in 1966 in Cameroon, Chad, Dahomey, Guinea, the Ivory Coast, Mauritania, Mali, Niger, and Togo. At the same time, plans were made to extend the program to the Central African Republic, Gabon, Gambia, Liberia, Senegal, Sierra Leone, and Upper Volta. Henderson was convinced that only a regional endeavor would succeed, so two more countries, Nigeria and Ghana, would be added in a year or so. A regional office would be established somewhere in West Africa, with overall direction coming from the smallpox unit in Atlanta. The object was to give measles vaccine to all children from six months to six years of age and to vaccinate all individuals against smallpox. Henderson called the combination of the smallpox and measles campaigns "politically desirable, humanely urgent, and economically feasible."[9]

The United States was already spending $20 million a year to guard against the introduction of smallpox, so the African campaign was justified on the grounds that it protected American health. The White

House announced the program in November 1965. It would protect 105 million people from smallpox and measles in eighteen African countries. The Agency for International Development would contribute technical assistance, vaccines, jet injectors, field supplies, freezers and other refrigeration equipment; participating countries would pick up the local costs and operational personnel. From the old smallpox unit, CDC created the Smallpox-Eradication Program (SEP) in January 1966, with Henderson as its chief.

The commitment of the United States and CDC to the eradication of smallpox in West and Central Africa encouraged the World Health Organization to increase its support for the global program. In 1965, when WHO budgeted $63 million for malaria eradication, it allocated only $233,000 for smallpox eradication, a 300-fold difference. In 1966 both the United States and the Soviet Union proposed that WHO allocate more money for smallpox. By the narrowest of margins, a $2.4 million budget was approved—about $50,000 for each of the fifty countries where the work would be done. The greatest spur to the campaign's eventual success was the effort in West and Central Africa and the contribution by the Soviet Union of millions of doses of vaccine. The other members of the United Nations gave only modest support to the international effort, in all less than $1 million during the next seven years. Their singular lack of enthusiasm may have stemmed from the failure to eradicate diseases in the past. Beginning with the campaign against hookworm in the American South in 1906, which eventually extended to six continents, and including the global efforts against yellow fever and malaria, the concept of eradication had everywhere failed. Small wonder that there was little enthusiasm for the campaign against smallpox for which Henderson had such high hopes.[10]

It was one thing to decide on a program, another to get it going. For months Henderson operated without the able assistance of Don Millar, who had headed the smallpox unit from its inception. Millar was studying at the London School of Hygiene and Tropical Medicine as part of CDC's Career Development Program, and when he got back to Atlanta, the Smallpox-Eradication Program was well under way. Early on, Henderson secured the help of people who would play a vital part in the program's success. Bill Watson, CDC's executive officer, recommended that Billy Griggs, who had major responsibilities for operations in the Venereal Disease Program, take over administration of SEP. Griggs then sold Henderson on the idea that he should send public health advisors, the "685 Series type," to Africa along with the epidemiologists. This would ensure managerial and logistical expertise in each country. These "operations officers" proved crucial to the success of the program.

Besides recruiting and training the teams that went to Africa, Henderson negotiated agreements with each country involved. Even as President Johnson was announcing the program, Henderson and three staff members from CDC and AID were on the way to West Africa to work out details.[11] At the first stop in Upper Volta, they met with health ministers from former French colonies in West Africa, who pledged their support. Next, the Americans attended a meeting of a parallel group in Central Africa and again got approval for the program. They also visited and worked out suitable arrangements with Nigeria and Sierra Leone, former British colonies, and with Liberia, independent since 1847. Fourteen of the countries involved in the Smallpox-Eradication Program were former French colonies (Cameroon, the Central African Republic, Chad, the People's Republic of the Congo, Dahomey, Gabon, Guinea, the Ivory Coast, Mali, Mauritania, Niger, Senegal, Togo, and Upper Volta). Four former British colonies (the Gambia, Ghana, Nigeria, and Sierra Leone) plus Liberia brought the number of countries in the program to nineteen. The structure of the eradication program in each country was influenced by its British or French background. In the former British colonies, tribal chiefs had important authority and the health structure was decentralized. In the former French colonies, the traditional highly centralized French superstructure prevailed. The eradication program was tailor-made for each country to work within these very different frameworks.

Success of the campaign was threatened by the attitude of U.S. officials in the African nations, many of whom viewed foreign aid in terms of economic growth: better health depended on increased gross national product and per capita income; special projects were unnecessary. This philosophical problem was compounded by an economic one. Some countries where smallpox was endemic were so poor it was hard to fund local campaigns. The World Health Organization finally picked up some of the cost of gasoline, the most expensive item not covered by AID.[12]

Within a week after the Smallpox-Eradication Program was created at CDC, Henderson was in Geneva to consult with WHO officials. Dr. Marcolino Candau, director general of WHO, wanted him to direct the worldwide effort, and Henderson agreed that the post should go to someone at CDC, even though the program was barely off the ground in Atlanta. Don Millar might fit the bill for the post in Geneva if he were five or ten years older, but Henderson knew that "the prestige of age" played a dominant role in WHO. Millar would almost certainly not be acceptable.

WHO's overall approach to smallpox eradication was dominated by the malaria dogma of "around the block, house by house" and gave only lip service to the concept of surveillance. This disturbed Henderson, who knew that it would take time for "education and demonstration [to] persuade." On his trip to West Africa, he learned that advice from WHO, whether good or bad, carried much weight. He wrote CDC's chief:

> The preposterous statement by the Expert Committee on Smallpox that 100 percent of the population should be the target in vaccination if eradication is to be achieved was alluded to on repeated occasions [as] evidence that eradication in Africa would be difficult to impossible. Clearly then, we must have a WHO attitude at least sympathetic if not parallel or identical to our own in the evolution of the overall program.[13]

Henderson was convinced that surveillance was the key to success in eradicating smallpox. When the eradication effort began, he had worked for a dozen years with Langmuir, to whom surveillance was the sacred writ of public health. "One does not spend 12 months, let alone 12 years, with Langmuir without obtaining a point of view," he said. "What was applicable to infectious diseases in the United States seemed logical to try to apply on an international scale in smallpox."[14]

The master plan for eradication of smallpox in Africa, worked out by the team in Atlanta, had to be approved by all the participating agencies before the program could begin. A special program was also developed for each country, known in CDC jargon as E-1, and these served as the basis for program agreements with each country. In the early months of 1966, Henry Gelfand, Ralph Henderson, and George Lythcott, a black American pediatrician recruited to direct the regional office in Nigeria, traveled from country to country developing these plans. They were to be signed by October 1, 1966, but none was. Nigeria, the largest country involved and key to the success of the program, was especially recalcitrant, despite the enthusiastic support of its principal medical officer, Dr. Adeniji Ademola. Two coups in seven months had left the government in turmoil, and eradication of smallpox was not high on the list of priorities. Lythcott spent six weeks in Nigeria and could not even get an appointment with the chief of state to discuss the agreement. Only when he found a "friend of a friend" was he able to negotiate a meeting and get assurance that the project agreement would be signed. Senegal was the last; it did not sign its agreement until March 1967, five months after the deadline.

Meanwhile, in Atlanta, a smallpox-eradication staff was recruited. The administrative officers came mostly from the ranks of public health advisors; the epidemiologists were recruited from outside. Dr. Donald Hopkins, who joined the program in its second year, had never heard of EIS, but he was attracted to the smallpox program, where the impact of one's work could be easily seen. Typical of the recruits, Hopkins was young and enthusiastic.[15]

When Millar returned to CDC from London in the summer of 1966, training of the teams headed for Africa was well under way. The medical officers took the EIS course; the operations officers learned how to repair and maintain the Dodge trucks. Later they changed places, the medical officers taking a brief course in mechanics, the operations officers one in epidemiology. Everybody studied elementary statistics and learned something about management and laboratory operation, as well as how to repair and maintain jet guns. They also studied African history and customs, and the tribal tongues of the regions for which they were headed. Team members and their wives going to former French colonies also took a crash course in French.

They were ready to go before the countries in Africa were ready to receive them. Week after week passed before the necessary basic agreements were signed. It was left to Millar to explain to eager team members who had closed their homes, stored their furniture, and were living in crowded conditions in a run-down Atlanta motel that they must be patient and wait. When the first groups were supposed to leave for Africa in October, not one of the agreements had been signed, but as these trickled in, the teams left one by one. There was an operations officer for each country, plus one for each of the four regions into which Nigeria was divided. A medical officer was sent to each of the larger countries, but in the case of smaller countries, one medical officer served two or three. Some teams were still in Atlanta in January 1967 when the program in Africa officially got under way. Their goal was to reach "zero pox" in five years.[16]

In mid October 1966, as the anxious teams waited for the "go" signal, there was a changing of the guard in Atlanta. D. A. Henderson went to Geneva to become chief of the WHO smallpox-eradication program, and Millar took his place. "Welcome to the NFL," Billy Griggs said to him with admirable directness as soon as the appointment was announced, and for Millar it was "a chaotic time." The staff included people from his old smallpox unit plus those Henderson had brought into the program: Dr. Leo Morris, a veteran of smallpox activities in Brazil, and Drs. Henry Gelfand, Ralph Henderson, and Bernard Challenor. The Atlanta staff had to coordinate the multinational African campaign, digest the collective experience, and make certain that no important opportunities were missed. That meant frequent trips to Africa.[17]

The CDC teams left for Africa with the din of "naysayers" in their ears. The textbook writers, the international experts, the ex-colonialists said it could not be done. They even had a slogan to express the futility, "W.A.W.A., West Africa Wins Again!" But even when they discovered the smallpox problem to be much worse than they had expected, the eager teams from CDC were not disheartened. Only a tiny fraction of smallpox cases had been reported in northern Nigeria, and Sierra Leone had the highest incidence of smallpox in the world, nine times greater than India. Worldwide, WHO reported 131,418 cases of smallpox in 1967, but the real figure was 10 to 15 million. CDC hoped that vaccinating 80 percent of the people of West Africa would reduce the number of cases to fewer than 5 per 100,000 of population, and improved surveillance would do the rest.[18]

The incidence of smallpox was highest in the youngest of the newly independent African states. They had the least sophisticated health services and the worst communications. Roads, if they existed at all, were terrible. Some religious groups ritually infected people with the smallpox virus. Among the Yorubas in Nigeria and some of their neighbors in Dahomey and Togo, Shapona, the god of smallpox, was still a powerful force. Many people resisted vaccination lest they anger the Overlord of the Earth. In Western Nigeria one vaccination team was met with drawn knives when publicity posters circulated prior to their arrival asked the population to make war on smallpox. In the local language, the word for smallpox was the same as the name of the local earth god, and the people were incensed that they were being asked to make war on the deity.[19]

Everywhere the physical difficulties were enormous, the living conditions often miserable. The Dodge trucks could provide only part of the transportation. Motorcycles, bicycles, horses, donkeys, and camels were pressed into service, and in the more rugged areas, teams traveled on foot. Local workers operated the ped-o-jets; native leaders got people to the vaccination sites, which might be anywhere. At a trade fair, many thousands might be vaccinated in a single day. In remote regions, the teams reached a few people at a time.

In spite of the commitment to surveillance and the best principles of epidemiology, the initial approach was to vaccinate as many people as possible in the least amount of time. Henderson himself was the chief advocate of this course in order to take advantage of a rare coalescence of political, economic, and cultural forces. WHO was committed to the project; the United States and the Soviet Union supported it financially; manpower and technology were available to get the job done. Strict attention to the principles of epidemiology and surveillance came in a mid-course correction.

The mass vaccinations proceeded rapidly. The twenty-five-millionth vaccination was given to a young schoolgirl in Accra, Ghana, only a year after the first teams arrived. Music and dancing amid clouds of dust marked the occasion. Among the guests were Sencer and Millar from Atlanta, George Lythcott from the regional office, Surgeon General Stewart, and numerous African dignitaries. Just eight months later, without fanfare, the fifty-millionth vaccination was given, probably to a child in northern Nigeria, where one and a half million people were being vaccinated every month. Everyone believed there would be a dramatic decline in smallpox the next year.[20]

Coordination and direction of the African program came from Lythcott's regional office in Lagos, Nigeria, and from Atlanta, where Millar and a staff of about twenty-five oversaw everything. They made certain that the jet guns, vaccines, and trucks got to Africa, dealt with AID in Washington and WHO in Geneva, recruited and trained reinforcements, and analyzed streams of data coming in from the field. Three members of the staff—Drs. Michael Lane, Henry Gelfand, and William Foege—carved up Africa and took pieces of it as their personal responsibility. All of them made numerous trips to Africa to observe the work firsthand. Lane, who spoke French, took responsibility for the francophone countries, and added Guinea, Liberia, and Sierra Leone when those countries started their programs a year later. He remembers the "daily sense of excitement—the constant joy of coming in early and staying late and working on nights and weekends just because it was fun." The daily cable, nearly always announcing progress, made the work enormously satisfying.[21]

There would have been no victory reports without a potent vaccine, and supplying that was a real problem, especially in the early months of the campaign. Little satisfactory freeze-dried vaccine was being pro-

duced anywhere. Some vaccines were not potent when they were re-
constituted, and others lost their potency quickly under field conditions.
Almost none of the vaccine produced in the endemic countries met the
basic standards set by WHO. The campaign was already under way
before two widely separated laboratories—one in the Netherlands and
the other in Canada—agreed to serve as international vaccine reference
centers. Because the amount of vaccine needed would have cost more
than was budgeted for the entire program, WHO decided not to buy
any vaccine at all but to ask for donations. The most populous countries
were asked to produce their own vaccine. In Nigeria, CDC and WHO
provided support for the government vaccine-production laboratory at
Yaba, near Lagos, with the expectation that it might manufacture
enough high-quality freeze-dried vaccine to meet the needs of Nigeria
and perhaps other countries in West Africa. The task was plagued with
difficulties, and the vaccine produced there did not reach international
standards until 1974. The Soviet Union donated 140 million doses of
vaccine a year, the United States another 40 million. Eventually, more
than twenty countries donated some vaccine to the program.[22]

The ped-o-jet worked well for vaccinating large numbers of people at
a single location, but it was not suited for use house-to-house. The
campaign was barely under way in Africa when the simplest of instruments, the bifurcated needle, was added to the arsenal of weapons. It
was as effective as David's slingshot. The needle held exactly the right
amount of vaccine, suspended by capillary action, between its two
prongs. The needle was touched to the skin and the vaccination performed by 15 strokes of the needle through the droplet. It was cheap,
easy to use, and effective. The reuseable needles cost only $5 a thou-
sand, almost anyone could be taught the technique in a few minutes,
and the "take rate" was 98 to 100 percent. The bifurcated needle, used
experimentally in 1967, and introduced officially the next year, became
a mainstay of the eradication program.[23]

Nigeria was the hub of the African campaign. When the CDC team
arrived, they were welcomed by Dr. William Foege, a one-time EIS
officer and a medical missionary with the Lutheran Church. They had
been there only a brief time when there was an outbreak of smallpox in
the area where Foege worked, so he quickly became an active partici-
pant in the campaign. One day in the spring of 1967, just before the
people of eastern Nigeria—mostly members of the Ibo tribe—seceded
to form the independent country of Biafra, Foege and his fellow vaccinators had an experience they would never forget. As they approached
a roadblock guarded by nervous young soldiers with machine guns, the

brakes on their big green AID vehicle failed and there was a moment of panic. Foege recounted what happened next.

> Because [the driver] was not going to go into the roadblock, he turned off the road, [and] we went across a ditch, flying up the other side. We hit a tree and knocked it down, and the vehicle came to a rest against a house [without damaging it]. . . . A crowd began to gather around the vehicle. People called for a chief and an interpreter. The chief explained to me what damage I had wrought. He said that the tree was a juju god—a tree that they worshiped. He did this in a long oration with every few sentences being interpreted. At the end of this talk, he said that the village would now have to have a sacrifice [a chicken] to the juju god . . . which would cost ten shillings and we would have to pay for it.
>
> I had listened throughout this and at the end breathed a sigh of relief because I had expected something much more damaging than giving out ten shillings for a chicken. But, then I thought I would part with a little message of my own, still expecting to pay the ten shillings, and I tried to make a long oration. . . . I said that I understood that they had different customs from ours and I wanted to honor their customs. I'm sure they would feel the same way about the country I came from. We had our own juju gods. One of them, in fact, was this vehicle which had now been very offended to find a tree in its way. I would have to sacrifice to the juju god also, and would sacrifice a goat which would cost twenty shillings. . . . There was absolute silence for a short period of time—enough time for me to think I had made a real mistake. Someone started snickering. Then . . . everyone was laughing. No money changed hands, and pretty soon, I was on my way.[24]

The Nigerian-Biafran war began in late May 1967, and the CDC team had to leave the war zone. The church evacuated Foege's family, but he stayed behind as an advisor to the Biafran government. Later, when Biafra would not admit him on his return from a conference, he joined the Smallpox-Eradication Program and was shortly transferred to Atlanta.

Despite the war, the smallpox-measles campaign continued on both sides of the line with marked effectiveness, but the famine that followed in the wake of war brought a new dimension to CDC's activities. The Red Cross moved in to help refugees, and in the fall of 1968, Foege returned to Nigeria as an advisor. An intended stay of six weeks stretched to six months as he implemented a unique system for determining the prevalence of malnutrition and directed resources to the areas of greatest need. The principles of epidemiology, long used to determine the prevalence of infectious disease, were for the first time used to measure the prevalence of malnutrition. CDC devoted a great deal of effort to famine relief in Nigeria. About two dozen people were sent in to work on the problem, and the nutrition-surveillance information they garnered from the war zone became a classic in the annals of nutrition. Their work began CDC's interest in worldwide malnutrition, an interest that ultimately resulted in a new method of doing nutritional surveys. It applied the principles of science to famine relief (see chapter 16).

When Foege told Secretary of State Henry Kissinger about the number of people starving in the region and described the edema rates, the secretary commented, "For me, those are numbers; for you, they must be faces."[25] Indeed, they were. For all those who worked in Africa, seeing the faces of victims of disease and starvation made the experience an intensely personal one. The personal cost to CDC was high, too. When a plane carrying Dr. Paul Schnitker, a new EIS officer assigned to Nigeria for famine relief, attempted to land at Lagos, it exploded and burned. Schnitker was CDC's first fatality in the field.

The smallpox-eradication campaign achieved success earlier than anticipated because of a mid-course correction in the method of operation. The correction grew out of an experience in the Ogoja district of Nigeria, where there was a smallpox outbreak in December 1966. The mass supplies for the eradication effort had not yet arrived, so Foege, David Thompson, and Paul Lichfield, who rode to the area on motorbikes, took the practical course of stretching their supplies as far as possible. They used the techniques of surveillance and containment, getting the vaccine into as many contacts of victims as they could. By the time large quantities of supplies arrived a few months later, the outbreak was contained. Although less than half the population had been vaccinated, smallpox was gone.

It took a while to learn from the Ogoja outbreak, but the technique that had worked there eventually was applied wherever outbreaks of smallpox occurred. Foege was still turning the matter over in his mind when he returned to Atlanta. The concept was incorporated into the training course for the campaign's new recruits in the summer of 1967, and the following October, Foege spelled it out in a memo to Don Millar. By then he was calling the idea "eradication escalation," quickly dubbed "E-squared" or "E^2" by Mike Lane. Foege knew that by the summer of 1968, almost half the population of Africa would have been vaccinated. Surveillance data could be used to determine which half of the remaining population needed to be included. He divided the countries into three groups: those that required no special attention; those that required consultation to improve surveillance but not an all-out drive; and those like Togo and northern Nigeria that required supplements of equipment and personnel.[26]

The idea was presented at one of the daily staff meetings early in 1968. The program's attack phase was barely a year old and was working well. Millar was not enthusiastic about change, but he was willing to give it a try. A seasonal slump in smallpox cases occurred every October, and Foege wanted to take advantage of it. He believed that if all cases of smallpox were diligently sought out and their contacts vaccinated, the back of the disease would be broken. According to Millar, smallpox workers in Africa viewed the idea as a "typical cracked brain head-quarters scheme, completely out of touch with reality," and they gave it a cool, if not hostile, reception. There was one major exception, Dr. Donald Hopkins, who was then working in Sierra Leone. He and Jim Thornton, his operations officer, put the search-and-destroy plan into effect in August 1968. Within nine months, when less than 70 percent of the population of Sierra Leone had been vaccinated, smallpox was gone. Their success encouraged seven countries where smallpox out-breaks still occurred to try it.[27]

Project E^2 brought an early end to smallpox in West Africa and became the method of choice in WHO's campaigns elsewhere, steadily pushed in that direction by D. A. Henderson. WHO refused to use the term *eradication escalation,* however, probably because it was too sug-gestive of terminology used by the U.S. military in Vietnam. Instead, it evolved a new name: first, *selective epidemiologic control,* and finally, *surveillance/containment.* Don Millar admitted this was "probably more descriptive, but certainly less graphic."[28]

Implementation of Project E^2 required a small amount of extra money at a time when there was growing public resentment of foreign aid. The countries involved had to be convinced that the "search-and-destroy" plan would work, and there was the problem of finding all the smallpox cases. Newspapers, radio, letters, mission stations, and health and volunteer agencies were all used to track down outbreaks. The original case had to be found and lab specimens collected to verify the diagnosis. Then all those in areas contiguous to the patient, both geo-graphical and sociological, were vaccinated.

The concept of eradication escalation was superimposed on the over-all plan of mass vaccination, which continued unabated. The number of smallpox cases dropped steadily. July 1969 was the first month in which no case was reported. By October, every country had reached "zero pox" except Nigeria. Two months later, the importance of the role played by the African people in the campaign was symbolized in a ceremony in the little village of Boubon, Niger, when M. Issa Ibrahim, Niger's minister of health, gave the hundred millionth vaccination to a small boy carried on his mother's back. In May 1970, when the last smoldering outbreak of smallpox was extinguished in Nigeria, the whole region of West and Central Africa was declared smallpox free. The campaign had achieved success a year and a half ahead of schedule, but the event went largely unnoticed. Although there were no bands and flags to mark the event, achieving zero pox in West Africa set the stage for global eradication.[29]

The end of the African campaign meant the end of outside funding for CDC's Smallpox-Eradication Program. Millar moved out of the unit to take charge of CDC's Division of State and Community Services, but Sencer was unwilling to let the SEP die. He put William Foege in charge and committed domestic funds to keeping the truncated program alive. The health infrastructure of African nations, to which SEP had made important contributions, needed nurturing. These could be the nucleus of comprehensive childhood immunization programs, improved disease surveillance systems, and epidemic control. An abrupt halt to the program could endanger the smallpox-free status of West Africa and negate the progress made towards measles control.

The measles campaign also had a mid-course correction, not unlike that of E^2 for smallpox. The initial plan to vaccinate children for measles over a three-year period was changed to a cycle of six months to a year. It worked so well that Gambia interrupted measles transmission and kept itself free of indigenous measles for four years, something no other country in the world has ever done.

There was other work to do, too. The SEP unit became the center for malnutrition studies, an extension of famine relief in Biafra. It also waved the flag for smallpox eradication around the world, and acted as a kind of fire brigade against the disease. When a smallpox epidemic broke out in Yugoslavia after a Muslim pilgrim returned from Mecca with the disease, CDC answered the call for help.[30]

In the midst of the West African campaign, the Smallpox-Eradication Program made the controversial recommendation that vaccination for smallpox be abandoned in the United States. Lane and Neff studied the side effects of smallpox vaccination and concluded that universal vaccination was more dangerous than the modest benefits it brought the country. They were not the first to have thought of this. Dr. C. Henry Kempe, professor of pediatrics at the University of Colorado Medical School, insisted earlier that smallpox vaccination was dangerous and even caused some deaths, but he had not quantified the data and put them into rates. When Lane and his colleagues did this, they decided

Kempe was right, that the time had come to stop vaccinations. It was very controversial, and from 1968 to 1971 there were many debates about it. "We were in some places pilloried for our thoughts," Lane said. With some embarrassment, Sencer asked Lane to put a statement on the paper he and Millar wrote for the *New England Journal of Medicine* that this was not the policy of CDC. Even the Advisory Council on Immunization Practices recommended that vaccinations be continued. Asked to explain the division of opinion in his own agency, Sencer said: "In medicine there are no absolutes. Knowledge is often expanded through discussion of differing viewpoints. An organization which does not allow for open discussion of differing viewpoints will deservedly lose its most capable people."

When the brouhaha broke, Lane was in a thatched hut in the Southern Celebes of Indonesia working on smallpox outbreaks, so he knew nothing about the outburst for several weeks. For him, the recommendation that vaccinations be stopped was no trial balloon. The data were compelling, and he was surprised that three years passed before anything was done. Not until 1971 was the ACIP ready to recommend that routine immunization of children be discontinued. Sencer wanted a consensus in the medical community before the public announcement was made, and no one wanted to jeopardize the global eradication program by inadvertently encouraging some countries to stop vaccination prematurely. The arguments to discontinue vaccinations in the United States were convincing. The reservoir of smallpox was steadily dwindling, so the risk of importation was small. If a case were imported, rigid surveillance would prevent its spread. The surgeon general, following the recommendation of ACIP, issued a statement in September 1971 that routine smallpox vaccination was no longer necessary in the United States.[31]

In 1967, when WHO began its intensive smallpox-eradication program, a world map showed five major areas where smallpox was endemic, embracing thirty-one countries: South America, where the disease was still a problem in Brazil; West and Central Africa; eastern and southern Africa; southern Asia from Afghanistan to Burma; and Indonesia. While CDC was most heavily involved in West and Central Africa, it answered calls for help elsewhere, especially in Brazil and Southeast Asia. Its success in West Africa bolstered the hope that the program would succeed. The SEP staff—particularly Millar, Foege, and Lane— acted as "evangelists" to preach the gospel of surveillance and spread the good news. They made the circuit of WHO regional meetings to tell the Africa story. As chief of CDC's smallpox program, Foege attended the meeting of the Asian nations in 1973 and encouraged them to redouble their efforts. He was horrified when a representative of the Indian government suggested postponing the date of smallpox eradication for an additional five years. Foege jumped up and gave an impromptu speech, the essence of which was "it can be done" if they would but try harder. Physically impressive (he stands 6 feet, 7 inches) and passionately committed to the cause, Foege persuaded them that they could indeed eradicate smallpox within the time originally allotted—if only *he* would come and help.

There was nothing to do but accept the invitation and the challenge. Foege and his family left for India to direct one of the last and most important phases of WHO's global eradication effort. D. A. Henderson in Geneva was decidedly relieved. The year before, with WHO's program foundering in India and Bangladesh, he asked Foege, "Is there not *one* single person who could be seconded from CDC?" Lane took over direction of the Atlanta headquarters, and recruited and trained people for short-term assignments so that Foege would have enough "bodies" to do the job. Bill Watson was the first to go, and he was followed by other managerial types, mostly public health advisors, and, in turn, by most of CDC's epidemiologists. Sencer found the money and the positions in the Quarantine Service. By July 1974, twenty representatives from CDC were in India, where 130,000 cases of smallpox were reported. Lane knew that he would have to put more people in India later that year, and still more in 1975, because, as he put it, "While things are getting better, they aren't getting better fast enough." Economic chaos, famine, and political instability in India made the work difficult. The target for global eradication was 1976, and time was running out.[32]

E^2 was used with good effect in India. Foege knew that in surveillance there was need for redundancy: it was many times harder to find *every* outbreak than to find *most* outbreaks. Beginning in October 1973, every village and every house in it were visited once a month. In the village marketplaces, team members handed out smallpox cards showing the picture of a smallpox victim and offering a $12.50 reward to anyone who reported a new case. Towards the end of the campaign, this tactic proved to be the most effective one in Foege's arsenal.

Whenever a case was found, a containment team went to the village, confirmed the diagnosis, listed all the residents, vaccinated them, and traced the source of infection. Guards were placed at every house where there was a case, and some team members remained behind to vaccinate newcomers. Next came a search of all the people who lived within a radius of ten to twelve miles around the village. Two weeks later the search was repeated.

Foege played many roles in India, one of which was the "man with the money bags." He hand-carried cash to consulting epidemiologists so they could buy whatever they needed on the spot. He stuffed thousands of dollars into a money belt or briefcase and made his way from team to team. When he read about people who had been killed as they left the bank with much smaller amounts, he felt vulnerable. It was his secretary who persuaded him to stop. He knew that whenever Foege was on a train, at least six people in the regional office knew not only which train he was on but which compartment he was in. He feared that the temptation might be too great for someone, so a more orthodox system for delivering the money was worked out.

Foege was never aware of any danger while carrying large sums of money, but twice on a single day as he was traveling with his seven-year-old son, there were genuine threats to his life. For his son's sake, he conquered his fear and remained calm. In the morning as they were crossing the Ganges on a small ferry with a jeep, five horses, some bags of grain, and about twenty people, the ferry sprang a leak and everyone began bailing. Later that same day, jeering students, demonstrating against political corruption, stopped their jeep, rocked it back and forth, and demanded money. Foege passed out smallpox recognition cards and offered money to any of them who brought him a case. "They . . . became so confused by the fact that they could not talk to me without getting a smallpox recognition card that they finally dispersed and let us go."[33]

The all-out war against smallpox in India was so intense that Foege feared he was losing perspective. "The non smallpox world is ceasing to exist," he wrote Sencer at Christmas time 1974. There were forty outbreaks a week in India, fewer than in the past, but frustrating because some of them were blamed on the bad work of a half dozen epidemiologists. Many had occurred in a district where in order to improve his record on paper, the epidemiologist closed outbreaks without checking them. The transmission rate was high, and Foege lamented that they were paying for every recent mistake. "We have tightened up containment and will finish up despite the transmission potential but the last 6 weeks have been like a slow motion nightmare as we have not been able to move fast enough to keep up with the problems." Nevertheless, he thought the job would be done by February 1975 "unless our problems become of Bangladeshian size."[34]

By February, the goal was not yet accomplished, but it was in sight. Foege took advantage of a visit to India by Dave Sencer to stage a ceremony announcing the impending victory and to get a public commitment to the concept of surveillance from any doubters among Indian health officials. Sencer talked of a "masterful organization" of "surveillance and containment," which had brought the disease to its lowest level ever. The fact that these concepts were poorly understood was reflected in a report published by the *Times of India*. The editor urged caution in accepting such an optimistic report: "First of all, can it be confidently claimed that the 590 million people in this land have all been immunized or that they will regularly get revaccinated? Are the social and religious taboos related to vaccination removable overnight? Finally, is officialdom organized and efficient enough to ensure national protection?" Despite such skepticism, the goal was reached in May 1975. Orthodox Hindus gave thanks to Shitala Mata, their goddess of smallpox. Others acknowledged the hard work of the World Health Organization and of the Indian government, which spent $18 million on the campaign. A few may also have thanked CDC.[35]

The greatest threat to the success of the Indian campaign came from neighboring Bangladesh, where the most devastating kind of smallpox, *Variola major*, still existed in 1975. CDC's Dr. Stanley Foster directed the work there under conditions made more difficult by war and monsoon floods. Some twenty thousand Bengali and international health troops, armed with two-pronged vaccination needles, searched for cases from the rice paddies and tea plantations in the north to the resettlement camps outside Dacca in the south. They rode on tops of trains to vaccinate hordes of beggars; they even checked cemeteries for undetected smallpox. To anyone reporting a new case of smallpox, they paid $20, about a month's pay. In September 1976, there were only sixteen reported cases and the epidemiologists established a pool betting when zero pox would be reached. Many bet on the middle of October. It was a good choice. Bangladesh became smallpox-free that month. The last victim was three-year-old Rahima Banu. She survived what proved to be the world's last case of the severe form of smallpox.[36]

Thanks in large part to systems of surveillance, the world was gradually becoming smallpox-free. The CDC's Dr. Leo Morris introduced surveillance to Brazil in 1967, and four years later smallpox was gone from that huge nation. Mike Lane taught the Indonesians how to do surveillance, thus providing the key to success there. Nepal was smallpox-free until cases were imported from India, so India's victory was also Nepal's. In Sudan, smallpox was conquered by 1973, leaving Ethiopia and Somalia as the last countries in the Africa where smallpox still existed. With victory in India and Bangladesh, these countries on the Horn of Africa were the only ones in the world where smallpox was found. CDC's role in this area was relatively small, but when there were widespread outbreaks of smallpox in the region in southern Somalia in the spring of 1977, WHO worked out arrangements for a team of epidemiologists from the United States to work there. Among them were Dr. Stan Foster, who had spent four years battling smallpox in Nigeria and another four in Bangladesh, and Dr. Jason S. Weisfeld, who had worked in both India and Bangladesh. Dr. Weisfeld investigated the last case of smallpox to occur in the world. A twenty-three-year-old Somali cook named Ali Maow Maalin became ill on October 26, 1977, with *Variola minor,* the milder form of smallpox prevailing in the region. Like the little girl in Bangladesh, he recovered. Although his was the last case of naturally occurring smallpox in the world, two women in England died from smallpox ten months later when the virus escaped in a laboratory. Don Hopkins has called this accident the virus's "defiance," and the subsequent death by suicide of the laboratory director, one of the world's foremost authorities on smallpox, its "ultimate salute."[37]

While surveillance was the key to victory over smallpox, success could not have been achieved without the work of the laboratory that had to diagnose and confirm smallpox cases. No nation could be declared smallpox-free until the laboratory confirmed it. Before 1974, about 300 specimens a year were sent to the laboratory to be checked, but as smallpox became rarer, the work of the lab steadily increased. Nearly every case required laboratory diagnosis, and specimens came in by the thousands. In 1978, when WHO certified one country after another smallpox-free, the CDC smallpox laboratory processed more than four thousand specimens, all of them negative. It was the definitive sign that smallpox had been conquered.

The work of the laboratory was complicated by the possibility that an animal reservoir for smallpox existed. In India, one and perhaps two performing Macaque monkeys (*Macaca mulatta*) picked up smallpox from the households in which they lived. In Atlanta, the virologist John Noble showed that the virus could indeed be transmitted from one monkey to another. The disease never went beyond the sixth generation, however, and the transmission never went from monkeys to humans. Not once in the entire global smallpox-eradication campaign was smallpox traced to an animal source. Two diseases that looked like smallpox, but were not, also complicated the task of ascertaining if the world was smallpox-free. Monkeypox, clinically indistinguishable from smallpox, was first found in Africa in 1970, and, until it was diagnosed as something other than smallpox, posed a threat to the credibility of the eradication campaign. The whitepox virus also produced a disease in African green monkeys similar to smallpox and monkeypox. The position of these variants of the monkeypox virus had to be clarified. Studies of the genetic structure of these viruses ultimately showed they posed only a minimal threat to man. The final debate over smallpox was whether or not to keep some of the virus for research. The decision was yes, if for no other reason than to distinguish diseases in the future that might look like smallpox from that ancient foe. CDC is one of the two repositories for the virus, the other being the Research Institute for Viral Preparations in Moscow.[38]

Two years from the day the last case of smallpox appeared in Somalia, the Global Commission for the Certification of Smallpox Eradication declared Somalia and the world smallpox-free. Don Millar, a member of that international team, was there for the final exciting scene; the impossible had been done. The cost to the United States of the ten-year campaign was only $32 million. It would cost that much every two and a half months just to keep smallpox at bay.

David Sencer saw another dimension to the victory over smallpox. He remembered the dozens of eager young public health advisors and epidemiologists who went to India on three-month assignments. "It had a marvelous effect on them because it changed their lives," he said. "They saw what public health could do and they became believers."[39]

Euphoria, loosed by victory over smallpox, permeated CDC, bolstering the hope that stubborn health problems at home could be overcome and new threats to health vanquished. This optimism was put to immediate test. The outcome shook CDC to its foundation (see chapter 18).

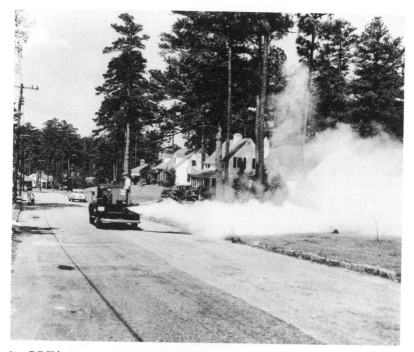

1.   DDT being sprayed from an MCWA truck during the 1940s in an effort to control malaria by eliminating the anopheline mosquito.

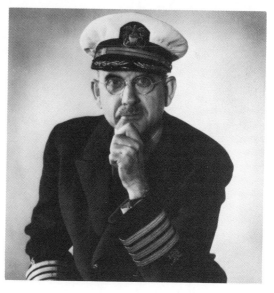

2.   Dr. Joseph Mountin, chief of the Public Health Service Bureau of State Services and founder of CDC.

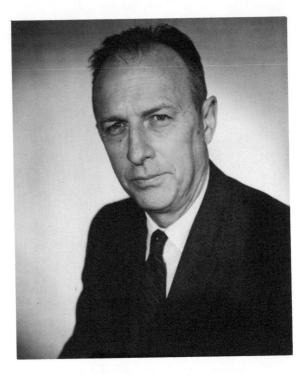

3. Mark Hollis,
CDC chief, 1946.

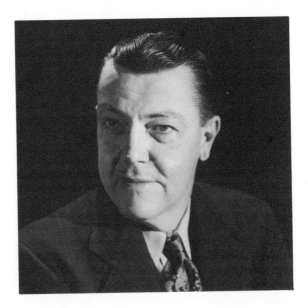

4. Dr. R. A.
Vonderlehr, CDC
chief, 1947–52.

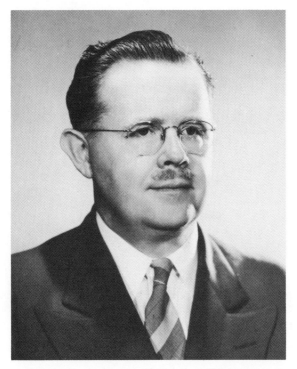

5. Dr. Justin Andrews, CDC deputy chief, 1946–52; chief, 1952–53.

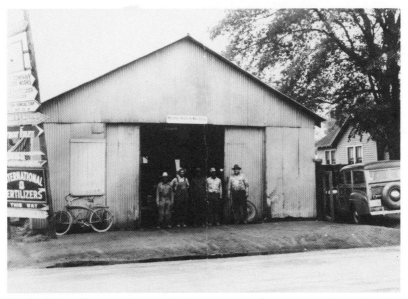

6. MCWA office in a Savannah, Georgia, warehouse, circa 1946. Bicycles were a main mode of transportation.

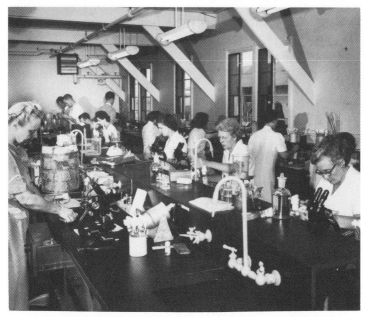

7. Early CDC laboratory, circa 1950, Chamblee facility.

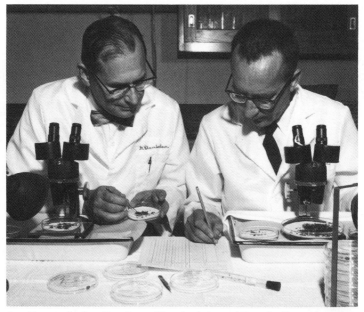

8. Entomologists Drs. Roy Chamberlain and Dan Sudia at the Montgomery Laboratory determined which birds acted as a reservoir for eastern equine encephalitis. They fabricated much of the equipment used in their research. Circa 1952.

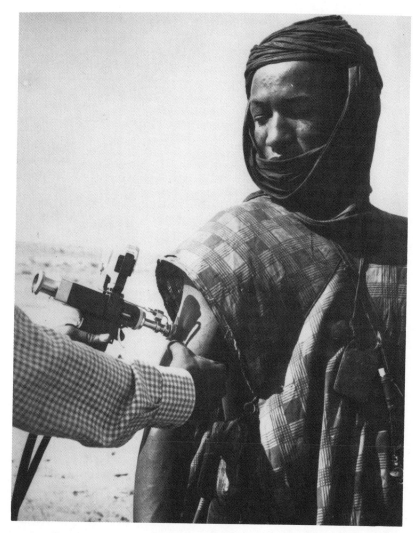

9. Smallpox eradication. A Tuareg nomad receiving smallpox vaccination, Mali, circa 1967.

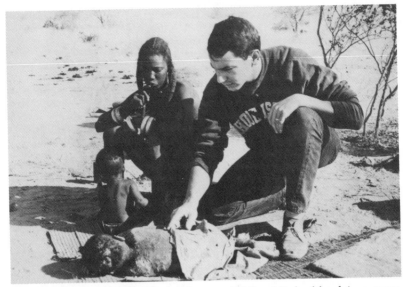

10. Smallpox eradication: Tony Masso, a CDC public health advisor, examines a child with smallpox, Niger, 1967.

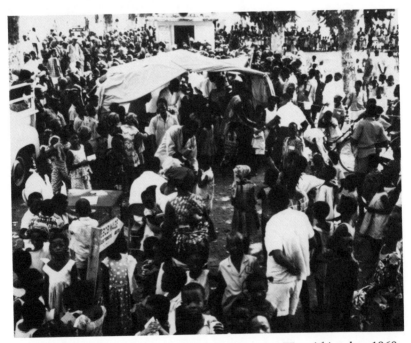

11. Smallpox-eradication program vaccination site, West Africa, late 1960s.

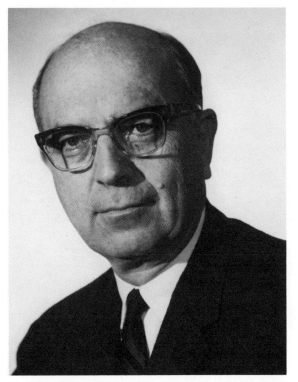

12.   Dr. Alexander D. Langmuir, founder of the Epidemic Intelligence Service.

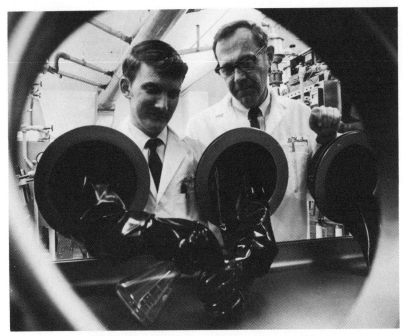

13.   Bill Gary, chief technologist, demonstrating the use of glove ports in Class III cabinets of the Maximum Security Laboratory. At right is Dr. Robert E. Kissling, chief of the virology section, who was in charge of the Maximum Security Laboratory, circa 1971.

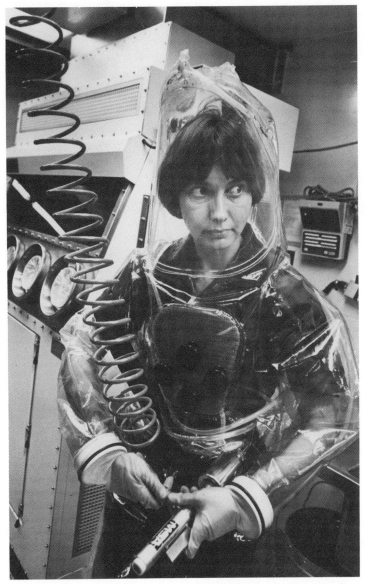

14. Senior laboratory technician Luanne Elliott adjusts positive pressure suit used as protection from contamination in the first "permanent" maximum containment laboratory, about 1977. This was the portable laboratory obtained from NIH, also called Building 9.

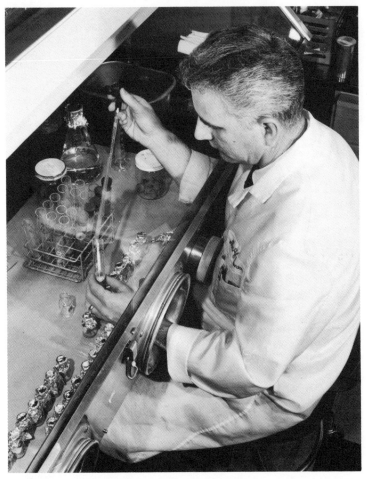

15. Laboratory technician working with nutrient medium in a Class I cabinet with glove ports in Building 9.

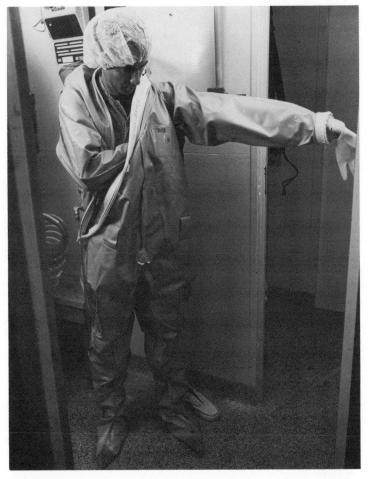

16. Donning positive pressure suit prior to entering Maximum Containment Laboratory, 1984.

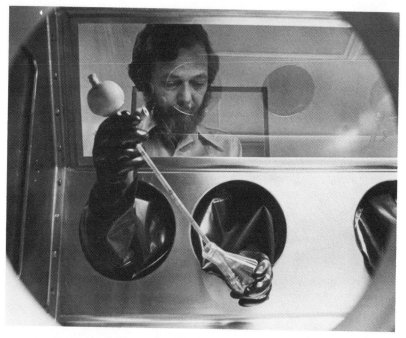

17. Dr. Karl Johnson in the Maximum Containment Laboratory working with highly dangerous Machupo virus, which causes Bolivian hemorrhagic fever. (While working in the field he contracted the disease himself.)

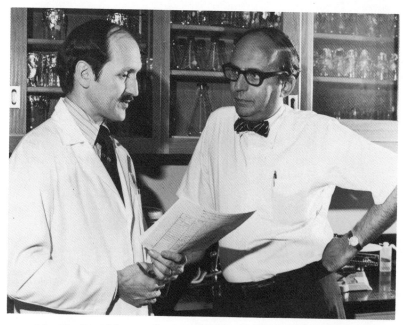

18. Dr. David Sencer, director of CDC, 1966–77, right, with Dr. Gary Noble in the late 1960s. Noble was then chief of the Respiratory Virology Branch, Bureau of Laboratories; in 1990 he is assistant director of CDC for HIV/AIDS.

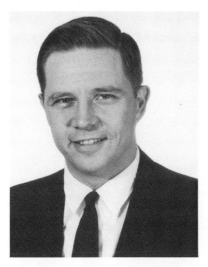

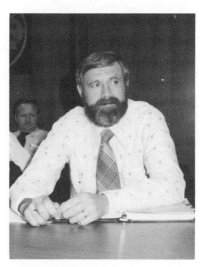

19. Dr. D. A. Henderson, first director of CDC'S Smallpox-Eradication Program; later director of the World Health Organization's global smallpox-eradication program.

20. Dr. William H. Foege, director of CDC, 1977–83.

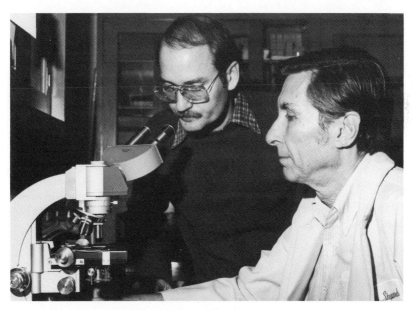

21. Dr. Charles C. Shepard (right) and Dr. Joseph E. McDade at microscope after isolation of the organism (now called *Legionella pneumophila*) that was apparently the cause of the Legionnaires' disease outbreak in 1976.

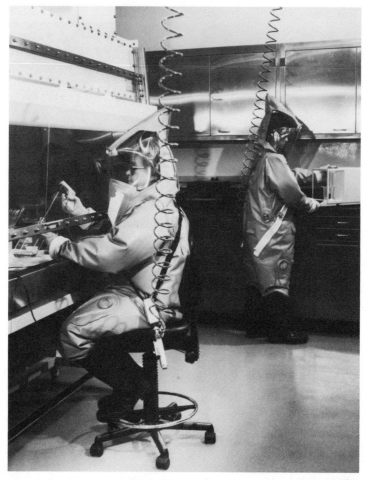

22. A worker uses living cells to culture a virus in a laminar-flow biosafety cabinet in the biosafety Lab IV facility of the Viral/Rickettsial Diseases Laboratory, 1988. This laboratory, opened in October 1988, is the only civilian biocontainment laboratory in the United States approved for both Class III and Class IV biosafety levels of research. (Class IV viruses—such as Lassa, Marburg, and Machupo viruses—are those for which there is no vaccine or specific cure.) At level IV, workers wear one-piece plastic suits for protection from potential contamination.

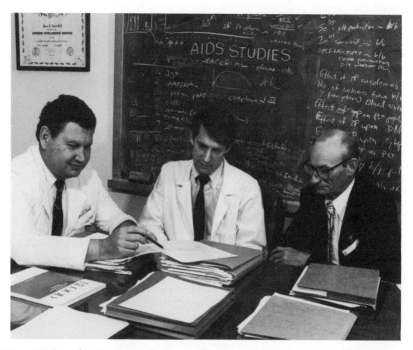

23. AIDS study. Dr. Bruce L. Evatt, director, Division of Host Factors; Dr. Steven J. McDougal, chief, Immunology Branch, and Dr. Onno van Assendelft, chief, Clinical Medical Branch (all in Center for Infectious Diseases) in conference on AIDS/HIV research.

CHAPTER 15

Africa's New Challenges

While the campaign to eradicate smallpox was under way, daunting new challenges came from Africa. During a ten-year period, three previously unknown fevers, always terrifying and often swiftly fatal, originated on that continent. CDC was called to help.

MMWR reported the first of these in early September 1967: a disease of unknown etiology had appeared in persons having contact with African green monkeys. Initial symptoms included severe prostration, nausea, vomiting, diarrhea, and muscle aches. Later the heart, liver, and brain became involved, and death usually occurred in seven to twelve days. An accompanying editorial note said that an international investigation was under way.[1]

The malady first appeared in mid August among laboratory workers in Marburg, West Germany, and a few days later at a laboratory in Frankfurt. In both institutions, African green monkeys were used in the production of Salk and Sabin polio vaccines. Within a month, twenty-eight people were stricken with "green monkey disease" and seven died. German health officials invited CDC to participate in the investigation on September 1, and three days later, two staff members from the Foreign Quarantine Service—epidemiologist Dr. James W. Mosley and veterinarian Dr. John H. Richardson—arrived in Frankfurt as members of an international team. Their report concluded that the disease originated in green monkeys shipped to Germany from Uganda, that laboratory personnel who worked with minced tissues were most susceptible, and that the infected monkeys probably showed no signs of illness to alert animal handlers to danger.

That was a cause of real concern. The monkeys were shipped to

Germany by way of London and spent some time at Heathrow Airport. Where had the monkeys acquired the infection? Had there been a cross infection with another species of primates at the airport? Had anyone there been exposed? Mosley and Richardson thought not, but they knew that in any laboratory where green monkeys were used, workers were at risk.[2]

CDC had no laboratory facilities secure enough to work on what was soon dubbed Marburg fever, and constructing a new building would take too long. As a stopgap measure, a specially built laboratory trailer secured from the National Cancer Institute was set up on the back lot. There Dr. Roslyn Robinson, then the director of the Laboratory Branch, and the virologist Dr. Robert Kissling cultured the organism in baby hamster cells and identified it as a very large virus with a bizarre cylindrical shape. It was ten times as big as any virus ever seen before. Its bullet shape seemed to put it in the class of the agent that causes rabies. German scientists quickly confirmed the work done in Atlanta.[3]

The need for a more secure laboratory was recognized even before the appearance of Marburg fever. On the roof of Building 5, Dr. Telford Work had a small facility called "The Penthouse." It provided a safer environment for his work on Venezuelan encephalitis, which is especially dangerous to research workers because it becomes an aerosol in the laboratory. Even though the Penthouse had special air controls, it was never entirely satisfactory and certainly it was totally inadequate for Marburg fever research. The smallpox laboratory, even if it had been available, was not sufficiently secure. In fact, there was not a maximum security laboratory in all of the Public Health Service where an unidentified highly infectious agent could be studied safely.[4] The need was so great that after the researchers had worked for a year in the National Cancer Institute's trailer, a small laboratory building 40 by 80 feet was constructed behind Building 5. When it opened in 1969, it contained two labs. One, directed by Dr. Kissling, provided space for biological containment of equipment needed for work with tissue cultures, eggs, or small animals. The other, headed by Dr. Charles B. Reimer, chief of the Biophysical Separations Unit, was unique. It provided the microbiological containment necessary for purifying, concentrating, or characterizing dangerous agents. Work was done in specially designed biological containment cabinets that had negative air pressure, and all air was filtered before being exhausted from the building.[5]

Building 5-A was not complete when still another frightening disease appeared in Africa. Early in 1969 at a mission station in Lassa, Nigeria, an American nurse died of a strange unidentified malady marked by high fever, pharyngeal ulcers, pneumonia, and gastrointestinal hemorrhage. The nurse who cared for her also became ill and died. Her nurse, Lilly Pinneo, was stricken in turn, but survived. She was evacuated to the United States, and her struggle to live initiated important new studies at CDC. The disease that almost took her life was the first mystery investigated in the new maximum security laboratory.

CDC's involvement in the case began in late February 1969, when Dr. Herman Gray, a medical missionary and EIS alumnus, brought his patient to Lagos from the Jos Plateau, to which she had been evacuated from her mission station. He wanted her admitted to the Lagos Teaching Hospital, but when that hospital refused to accept her, Gray contacted Dr. Stan Foster, director of the smallpox-eradication program in Nigeria. Foster put the desperately ill woman in the smallpox hospital, and he and Gray talked. Foster wanted Dr. Lyle Conrad, who was in Nigeria working on famine relief, to look at her. Conrad brought along Dr. Karl Western, who was there on a short-term assignment. The four EIS alumni who examined Pinneo that Saturday morning had more than twenty years' experience in West African tropical medicine. They all decided it was a new disease, probably caused by a virus. Western thought it should be called Lassa fever, since it was customary to name arboviruses after a nearby town or river. Gray spoke for the mission, which wanted Pinneo evacuated to the United States. Conrad agreed to go with her if she could be kept alive until Monday.

The mission bought three first-class tickets on a Boeing 707, and Conrad and a nurse turned the left-hand side of the first-class compartment into a hospital. Conrad carried along an "interesting bucket of specimens" in formaldehyde. They were from the first two victims of Lassa fever. Pinneo herself was a kind of living test tube taking back specimens for study. The red tape of quarantine was handled by a simple letter written on Foster's stationery and signed by both Foster and Conrad: the patient was in the third week of an illness with an infectious disease, but she was not contagious. Since she did not have a quarantinable disease like yellow fever or cholera, quarantine passed her through without difficulty. Earlier the mission had contacted Dr. John Frame at Columbia-Presbyterian Hospital in New York City, where Pinneo was admitted. Conrad's bucket of specimens went to Dr. Jordi Casals at Yale University, the nearest arbovirus laboratory.

When Conrad got back to his office in Atlanta, he confronted a furious David Sencer. "What do you mean bringing back missionaries from overseas with dangerous infectious diseases?" he demanded. Conrad assured him that it was done all the time, that this was a major health problem in Africa, and that CDC had to take a look at it. But Sencer would not be mollified. He pulled Conrad off the case and assigned Dr. Michael Gregg to follow it.[6]

Scientists at Yale University began to study the specimens from Lassa at once, and by August Dr. Casals and Dr. Sonja Buckley had news, which was first reported in *MMWR:*

> A virus has been isolated from sera of two nurses, who died, and from serum and pleural fluid of a third nurse, who recovered from a febrile illness. All three were American nurses who had been working for the Sudan Interior Mission in Nigeria. Their clinical disease included fever, pharyngeal ulcers, pneumonia, pleural effusion, rash with petechiae, albuminuria, leukopenia, azotemia, and in one instance, terminal gastrointestinal hemorrhage. A fourth case occurred in a laboratory investigator who was working with the virus.[7]

The fourth case was Casals himself. The virus escaped from his containment facility, and he became desperately ill and nearly died. A few months later a technician who worked on another floor was also infected, and he died. Yale closed down the laboratory, and the work came to CDC, where the new maximum containment laboratory was nearly complete. Work on Lassa fever got under way there in early 1970. The new laboratory, built for the study of Marburg fever, was already too small.

The picture of the causative agent of Lassa fever made in the Yale laboratories proved that the disease was indeed caused by a virus, but it was not insect-borne; it was something new. This was an *arena* virus carried by rodents. The first *arena* virus was discovered by Dr. Karl Johnson, a research virologist with the National Institutes of Health, who spent years at the Panama field laboratory of the Infectious Disease Institute. In his work on Bolivian hemorrhagic fever, Johnson discovered an entirely new kind of virus and, with the help of the CDC's Dr. Frederick Murphy—whom Johnson described as an "artist" with the electron microscope—pinpointed it accurately. To Johnson and Murphy, the virus of Bolivian hemorrhagic fever looked like the one found in house mice that causes lymphocytic coriomeningitis. That virus had been known for quite a long time but had never been classified. The virus particles look as if they have little grains of sand in them, so Johnson and Murphy named Johnson's discovery *arena,* from the Latin word *arenosus,* which means sandy. As soon as they saw the pictures of the Lassa fever virus, they knew immediately that it was an *arena* virus and, as such, had a rodent as its reservoir.

Conrad was delighted to learn the correctness of his early conjecture that a virus caused Lassa fever. He took even more satisfaction in the role that he and the other EIS alumni had played in what he called a "classic case" of the EIS pinpointing a new disease and getting out the warnings. "We take advantage of the accidents of nature."

After 1970 CDC was deeply involved in Lassa fever research, both in Atlanta and in Africa. There were outbreaks of the fever in Liberia, Guinea, Sierra Leone, and again in Nigeria. Each time, CDC sent people to investigate including Drs. David Fraser and C. C. (Kent) Campbell. Campbell was on his way home from Sierra Leone, where he had investigated an outbreak of Lassa fever in 1972, when he became seriously ill. He stopped in Ireland to interview nurses who had worked in the epidemic zone and while there developed such a high fever it was thought that he, too, was a victim of Lassa fever. No one would take the risk of moving him on a common carrier, so the Public Health Service borrowed from NASA a module once used to transfer astronauts to the quarantine station. The module was loaded on an Air Force C-141 and Campbell was flown in the module to Staten Island, where he was a patient in the PHS Hospital. Although he did not have Lassa fever, his case demonstrated the need for a germ-tight mobile quarantine facility. A few years later, CDC got one of the NASA modules for its very own.

The search for the carrier of Lassa fever began early. Armed with the knowledge that the virus was carried by a rodent, Tom Monath went to Africa, where he spent a couple of years catching all kinds of rats and studying them intensely. In 1972 he identified the carrier of Lassa fever as the rat *Mastomys natalensis.*[8]

In February 1975, an emergency call came to CDC from South Africa, where there was a suspected epidemic of Lassa fever. Three cases had been admitted to a hospital in Johannesburg, and before the hospital officials realized what the problem was, a nurse had been infected and numerous interns, residents, and staff had been exposed. The hospital had thirty-two people locked up. Sencer asked Lyle Conrad to go, but remembering the argument they had in 1969 when he escorted Lilly Pinneo home, added an admonition: "I don't want you to bring back Lassa fever." Within a few hours, Conrad was on his way, taking with him only a few essentials, including some Lassa fever serum made from the blood of recovered victims.

He arrived in Johannesburg at about five o'clock in the afternoon after a flight of eighteen to twenty hours. Dr. J. H. S. Gear, an expert on polio virus, as famous in South Africa as Sabin is in the United States, met him at the airport and invited him to go on rounds at the hospital in an hour. There was time only to stop at the hotel and put the serum in the freezer. The rounds extended into an hours-long discussion of the differential diagnosis of Lassa fever. Although dead on his feet, Conrad, remembering Lilly Pinneo, knew that the patients he saw that night did not have Lassa fever. He gathered specimens and sent them back to CDC for analysis.

Discussions about the epidemic went into the third day, and still the doctors could agree only on the basics. The first victim was an Australian hitchhiker, who had been traveling in Rhodesia with his girlfriend. He died, the young woman was quite ill, and she passed the disease to a nurse. To keep it from spreading further, the thirty-two doctors and nurses who had been exposed were still locked up. Conrad was convinced the patients did not have Lassa fever; Gear thought it was yellow fever, and if not that, then hemorrhagic hepatitis. When Conrad disagreed, Gear suggested that perhaps it was like the Marburg fever virus that had struck so many laboratory workers in Germany in 1969. They entered the differential diagnosis for Marburg fever. In Atlanta, workers in the "hot lab," as it had come to be called, confirmed Gear's hunch. Sencer and Murphy called Conrad in Johannesburg with the news. It was Marburg fever, the first time the disease had appeared naturally. The extraordinary size of the virus and its bizarre shape left no doubt.

Epidemiology of the three Marburg cases showed not a common source of infection but a person-to-person transmission at six-day intervals. Conrad got his worksheet and surmised that it was quite possible that the South Africans would want to go to Rhodesia to do some fieldwork. He asked Sencer's permission to go along. For a month, Conrad traveled with Margaret Isaacson of the South African Institute of Medical Research; Jimmy Johnston, a South African sanitarian; and Eric Burnett Smith, the Rhodesian minister of health. They traced every step of the hitchhikers. From the six-day incubation period, they knew that the young man who had died had picked up the virus somewhere along the road. He had been bitten by something that left a nasty lesion, but he could not identify what it was. Neither could Conrad and the South African team find any clues. They knew where the hitchhiker had been; they knew the source was there somewhere, but it melted away as suddenly as it appeared. Marburg fever subsequently struck twice in Kenya, but again left no clue as to the source. Of the three African hemorrhagic fevers, Marburg is the most elusive.

When Conrad got back to Atlanta, Sencer immediately quizzed him. "Did you bring back Lassa fever?" he asked. "You know very well I didn't," Conrad replied. He had brought back the Marburg virus instead. "But at least this time," Conrad said, "Dave was friendly."[9]

The mysterious appearance of Marburg fever in Africa underscored the already apparent need for a larger and even more secure laboratory for the study of "Class Four" viruses, those that cause diseases for which there is no vaccine or cure and that have a high fatality rate. Lassa fever was one of these, and increasingly it was recognized as a threat to international health. The disease showed up repeatedly in London among people coming in from West Africa and on several occasions spread to hospital personnel. It was terrorizing. Every time there was a scare, CDC got a call, and the staff did what they could to help. The great bottleneck was the inadequacy of laboratory facilities.

After the latest Marburg fever scare, CDC located a portable high security lab, designed and built by Robert J. Huebner of NIH, an expert on leukemia. He believed leukemia to be an infectious virus disease, and in case of an epidemic, he wanted a secure laboratory that could be taken down and moved anywhere. A model was built and set up in a building in Washington. Officials at CDC believed that with some modifications it could serve their needs and would increase the laboratory space available for work on the Class Four viruses by three or four times. The cost was not great, and it would save a trip to Congress to get money for a new building. The portable laboratory was moved to Atlanta.

At about the same time, a cutback in the budget of NIH had fortuitous results for CDC. After four years of threats to close Dr. Karl Johnson's laboratory in Panama, it was finally done in 1975. Johnson, who had discovered and named the *arena* viruses, came to CDC to direct the new "hot lab" being put together. The building was supposed to be complete by Christmas 1975, but in the summer of 1976, it was still not operable. The new lab was different from any other in the world. In half of it, workers wore space suits with air lines like umbilical cords tied to the ceiling. The system at once increased the security of laboratory workers and gave them more freedom. The Army had used space suits for laboratory staff working with animals, but never before had there been a complete laboratory built with space suits as an operating principle. There were skeptics, but Johnson believed in the concept. He thought it would make an incredible difference in both the nature and the quantity of work that could be done.[10]

As work on the new laboratory in Atlanta progressed, a field station for the study of Lassa fever was set up in Sierra Leone, and Dr. Joseph McCormick was sent out to run it. McCormick had already established a reputation as an expert epidemiologist. In the meningitis epidemic that swept Brazil in 1974–75, McCormick went to help. He learned Portuguese in a mere four weeks, took complete charge of managing the epidemic, and joined in the massive vaccination campaign mounted by the Brazilian government to guard against future outbreaks. He worked mostly in the Amazon forest, vaccinating people in isolated areas. He called it "a spectacular opportunity." When he returned to Atlanta, McCormick worked primarily on Lassa fever. For him the assignment to set up the field station in Sierra Leone meant a return to Africa. A decade earlier he had lived in Zaire for two years, teaching mathematics and science in a Methodist mission school. He taught his classes in French and became increasingly fluent, a skill that proved most useful in the emergency that developed almost as soon as he was settled in Sierra Leone.

In late August 1976, when many on the staff at CDC were totally immersed in the strange disease that had struck the American Legion convention in Philadelphia (see chapter 18), Johnson got a telephone call from the Tropical Institute in Germany with news of a strange epidemic that had swept across the southern part of Sudan. There was great panic among the people, and the caller wanted to know if CDC planned to do anything about it. Johnson replied that CDC could do nothing without an invitation, but he immediately informed Lyle Conrad that something was up. About a month passed before British scientists were allowed into the area, got some specimens, and passed some of them along to CDC. Within three days, Murphy had a picture of the virus and knew that it was not the elusive agent of Marburg fever, although it seemed to be closely related to it. Meanwhile, a similar epidemic broke out in Zaire and, at a single hospital, hundreds of people, including much of the staff, became acutely ill with a hemorrhagic fever and died. David Sencer was anxious for CDC to get involved, but when no formal invitation was received, he took matters into his own hands. He contacted the chief of the viral-disease section of the World Health Organization in Geneva, told him that he was sending his best people, and left it up to him to get them into Zaire. Johnson and Joel Bremen, an epidemiologist who had spent seven or eight years in Africa working on smallpox, left at once for Geneva, while Sencer, insisting "it was time to get going," pressured the U.S. Embassy in Kinshasa to use its influence. He was finally persuasive, and Johnson and Bremen boarded a plane for Kinshasa.

En route, Bremen told Johnson what they could expect in Zaire. The gentleman sitting next to them overheard the conversation, inquired if they were from CDC, and introduced himself. He was Dr. William Close, the personal physician to Zaire's president, General Mobutu Sese Seko. Sixteen years earlier, Close had gone to Zaire as a mission surgeon, and he had since become the closest thing that country had to a minister of health. He also ran Mama Yemo Hospital in Kinshasa, the largest one in Zaire. His friendship, good will, and savvy proved invaluable in the weeks to come. "Bill Close knew who was who, and what was what, and what was under this rock, and where you could get a barrel of oil and a whole lot of things," Johnson recalled. "If it had not been for that, I don't think that we could ever have done it."

What they did was analyze the third and most terrifying fever to strike Africa in a decade. Its victims ran high fevers, went into shock, and suffered massive external and internal hemorrhages. About 90 percent of them died. The epidemic was centered in the Catholic mission village of Yambuku in north-central Zaire, and before it subsided, almost as quickly as it had appeared, there were 318 cases with 280 deaths. The new malady was named Ebola fever after the nearby river. Johnson, Bremen, and others from CDC who went to investigate were part of an international team, which also included scientists from Belgium, France, South Africa, and Canada. Although they did not know it at the time, the epidemic was virtually over before their work began. It was centered in a hospital where, they subsequently learned, it was spread not only by person-to-person transmission but by dirty syringes and needles. These were used over and over again, not only on patients in the hospital, but on outpatients as well, particularly pregnant women who came to the clinic for vitamin B_{12} shots. When most of the staff were dead, the hospital had to be closed, and the epidemic subsided. There continued to be some person-to-person transmission in the villages, but not enough to sustain the epidemic.[11]

McCormick had barely settled into his Lassa fever work in Sierra Leone when he was called to Kinshasa and told to bring with him the field isolation unit, the only portable biosafety lab in the area. It took several days for him to get there, since travel between countries in Africa was difficult. On arrival, he learned that his assignment was to go overland eight hundred kilometers to Sudan to determine if there was any connection between the two epidemics. Having lived in Zaire earlier, McCormick knew the country well, and he did not believe that there could be any connection. The distance between the epidemic areas was great and embraced several tribal groups. The people did not speak each other's languages, there was no commercial travel, and no place to stay. Nobody believed him, so McCormick got a Land Rover, a driver, some diesel fuel, and K rations from the embassy dating from the 1940s and struck out into basically unknown territory. All along the route, he looked for evidence of transmission of Ebola fever and found none. When he reached the Sudan border, he talked his way across and reached a village where the disease was known to exist. He arrived there before anyone else. He made his investigation and left a note for his CDC colleague Don Francis, who was traveling with a team from the United Kingdom. He told Francis where the first case was, where the victim was buried, and where to find his wife and brother, who had survived the disease.

Investigation of Ebola fever involved a complicated transfer of staff, materials, and specimens between Atlanta and Africa. The New York Quarantine Station at John F. Kennedy Airport in New York was the transfer point, and the weather in the winter of 1976–77 was the worst in memory. Material arrived in New York daily from Atlanta, but flights to Africa went out only three times a week. On every flight from Khartoum and Kinshasa, there were specimens to be sent to CDC. To expedite delivery, every shipment from CDC to Africa and from Africa to Atlanta was "bird-dogged" except one. That was the only one that got delayed or lost.

When lab work on specimens from both epidemics was completed, McCormick's hunch that they were unrelated proved to be correct. The diseases are clinically the same, and the viruses that cause them look alike, but they are genetically and biochemically different. As Johnson explained, the minor, but important, "little footprints" they left were not the same.[12]

Investigation of Ebola fever was for Johnson and the members of the international scientific team a "galvanizing" experience. Many of them feared that this might indeed be the Andromeda strain. European airports nearly closed down to traffic from Central Africa, and in Africa itself there was near panic in those areas where the fever was present. When a Peace Corps volunteer whom Johnson had recruited to help with the laboratory work became seriously ill and had to be evacuated, the only country in the world that would take him was South Africa, which had already contended with Lassa and Marburg fever and was willing to accept the risk. After hours of negotiations by Lyle Conrad in Atlanta with officials at the Pentagon and the governments of Canada, Egypt, Great Britain, Germany, and South Africa, the arrangements were made. A U.S. Air Force C-141 flew from Madrid to Kinshasa, picked up the patient, Stan Foster, and Margaret Isaacson, who were caring for him, and flew to Pretoria. The plane was not permitted to fly over other countries, so it went out to sea and crossed back to South Africa. All the while, pots of boiling paraformaldehyde perked away in the plane to keep it sterile. Cost for the plane was $6,000 an hour. Weeks later, a bill for $170,000 arrived at CDC. "Now pay the bill," Bill Foege, by then CDC's deputy director, said as he dropped it on Conrad's desk. Conrad suggested sending it to the Peace Corps. The experience underscored the necessity of preparing for the worst. It was then that CDC secured the astronauts' mobile quarantine facility from NASA.[13]

Strangely, little attention was paid to Ebola fever in America. In 1976, Legionnaires' disease captured the attention of the public, and, by comparison, work done on an exotic disease in Africa seemed relatively unimportant. Yet the work done on Ebola fever was one of CDC's greatest success stories. It investigated every single case of the fever in Zaire and located the probable index case, a schoolteacher who had gone to the hospital. Epidemiologists quickly associated transmission of the disease with needles and brought a quick end to its spread; the laboratory staff isolated an entirely new virus and identified it as different from, but related to, the Marburg fever agent. They did much of the work in the first "hot lab," by then almost a decade old. (The "space suit" facility did not open until 1978.)

Ebola fever, like its cousin Marburg fever, subsided into the continent of Africa, making only sporadic appearances. Another epidemic in Sudan in 1979 gave McCormick, who went to investigate, one of the more dramatic experiences of his life. It was nearly dark when he arrived in the remote village and quite dark by the time he got to the airless huts where patients lay on mats. With only a few kerosene lanterns for illumination, McCormick took blood samples and separated these with a hand centrifuge. He wore a gown, mask, and gloves for protection, but when an old woman jumped as he was drawing a blood sample, McCormick stuck his finger. He knew that the death toll in Zaire from needle sticks was 100 percent, so McCormick had some tense moments and days. He gave himself some plasma, finished his work, packed the specimens, and gave them to the pilot who flew out at dawn for Khartoum. For days he watched the old woman intensely, but, it developed, she did not have Ebola fever after all. Whatever she had was not transmitted to McCormick.

If Marburg and Ebola fever were elusive, Lassa fever proved to be ever-present. The field laboratories in Sierra Leone (the main facility at Kenema and two small labs at mission hospitals twenty-five miles away) provided a wealth of material for study, although conditions in the laboratories were less than ideal. Only in Kenema was there a constant supply of electricity, and eventually, as the economy of Sierra Leone deteriorated, even that vanished. Failed radios made communication difficult, and laboratory equipment constantly broke down. McCormick, a "fix-it" person, did everything from rewiring centrifuges to repairing refrigerators, skills he did not learn at Duke University Medical School.

The work in Sierra Leone began with clinical and epidemiological studies, so McCormick, in addition to working in the lab, treated patients in the hospital and went to the villages. He also caught rats. In time, the combination of his work and the sophisticated virus and antibody studies done in the new "hot lab" in Atlanta yielded considerable knowledge about the disease. Lassa fever, so dramatic in its impact, is ever present in much of Africa and probably affects more than one hundred thousand persons a year. Many of the cases are as bad as those that struck down the missionaries, but others are much less severe. Even so, because so many are affected, Lassa fever causes several thousand deaths annually.

The disease yielded its mysteries gradually. The drug ribovarin reduces mortality, and control of the carrier, *Mastomys natalensis,* will prevent infection. Unfortunately, rat control in Africa is even more difficult than elsewhere. McCormick, the mammalogist who came to help him, and the Peace Corps volunteers who signed on learned that *M. natalensis* lives in houses, not in the bush or agricultural areas. The deadly Lassa virus is probably spread through urine, with any scratch or cut acting as a portal of admission. They learned there are no easy answers. Rat poisons are expensive, and in a protein-starved region, rats are part of the diet.[14] Not surprisingly, control of Lassa fever proved to be as much a social and economic problem as a medical one. And what had appeared to be a new disease turned out to be a very ancient one making a dramatic appearance on the world's stage.

CHAPTER 16

Acquisitions

CDC got a new name and its old initials back in 1970 when the National Communicable Disease Center became the Center for Disease Control. Its new name described its expanded mandate: a giant umbrella under which almost anything concerning the prevention of disease could be gathered. The old initials brought joy to old-timers. "It's CDC Again!" trumpeted the employee newspaper, *The Word*.[1]

By the time the long-rumored name change was announced, the Atlanta institution was already at work on nutrition. For some time, David Sencer had had his eye on PHS's nutrition program, and in the spring of 1969 there was widespread speculation in Washington that the Atlanta agency would take it over. In testimony before Senator George McGovern's Select Committee on Nutrition and Human Needs, Sencer said that the established procedures for gathering data, so essential to epidemic control, were applicable to a campaign against malnutrition. He proposed fifty community projects to seek out victims of malnutrition to demonstrate the effectiveness of the method. "We're not modest," he told a local newspaper. The administration bought the idea, and CDC moved quickly to work out details.

The idea, at least locally, fell on receptive ears. "[CDC,] that quiet miracle worker tucked in the suburban trees near Emory University . . . is about to be designated the agency to work on the hunger program," the *Atlanta Constitution*'s editor, Reg Murphy, wrote in a signed column a few weeks later. "If Congress will only act to designate it as the agency, the country may begin to alleviate malnutrition." The institution that had just wiped out smallpox in Africa "certainly has the staff knowhow to begin working on the program."[2]

Sencer seized the opportunity to move into the war on hunger when the Ten-State Nutrition Survey foundered. In 1967 Congress conducted hearings on the existence of hunger in the United States and authorized a comprehensive survey of malnutrition. The secretary of HEW was to report back in six months. He turned the job over to the reorganized nutrition program in the National Center for Chronic Disease Control. A random survey of every state in the union was impossibly large, so ten states, representing various geographic regions and cultures, were selected. Data collectors concentrated on urban ghettos, isolated rural communities, and areas with large numbers of migrant workers.

In January 1969, Dr. Arnold Schaefer, chief of the nutrition program, gave a preliminary report to Congress: nutrition could not be separated from health. Height and weight measurements, wrist X-rays, urine and blood samples all demonstrated a close connection. Malnutrition was evidenced in retarded growth, less efficient physiological performance, and lower serum and urinary excretion levels of certain nutrients. Only after prolonged deprivation did the classical deficiency diseases become evident. Schaefer emphasized that good nutrition depended on many factors—availability and price of food as well as personal preference. Even as he spoke, the detailed information on which he based his report was being put on computer punch cards. Those cards were the nutrition program's bottleneck and Sencer's opportunity. Schaefer's group had neither the facilities nor the expertise to analyze them. When they asked CDC for help, Sencer agreed, but only if the nutrition program were transferred to Atlanta.[3]

Dennis Tolsma never forgot the Washington meeting at which the transfer was announced. The young public health advisor was just beginning a new assignment in the center director's office when his new boss took him on a hurried-up trip to Washington. He met Joseph English, director of the Health Services and Mental Health Administration (HSMHA), a catchall agency that embraced roughly half the Public Health Service, including CDC, and English's deputy, Robert Van Hoek, who to Tolsma looked very official in his PHS uniform. Sencer mentioned that the Ten-State Survey was really in trouble and volunteered to fix it, and Tolsma assumed that was the reason they were there. The meeting was the next day.

We sat in this huge conference room at one end of the table. The meeting was to begin at 10:30. The door opened and in came Arnie [Schaefer] and his team, summoned for a meeting with the HSMHA director. I could tell by the looks on their faces that it dawned on them only at that instant what was going to happen to them. They saw Dave Sencer sitting there. It was extraordinary. The play of emotions on those faces was quite illuminating to a young public health advisor who had just moved to the Office of the Director and the first thing I am doing is raiding a program.[4]

Sencer had determined that CDC would have a different and broader mission, one that put activities dealing with primary prevention under one roof. "This was not the sort of plan . . . one puts in writing lest you be accused of empire building," he explained years later, "but . . . [with] a critical mass of epidemiology, laboratory and training capability, it made sense to bring the prevention agencies together." Takeover of the nutrition program was the first step.

For a few months, the headquarters for the nutrition study remained in Washington, even though the punch cards from the Ten-State Survey were moved to Atlanta immediately. It was not until January 1971 that the nutrition program was physically moved to CDC and workers had to decide between their jobs and a move few, if any, of them relished. Like their counterparts in the venereal disease and tuberculosis programs, many opted not to cast their lots with an agency they did not like, and they dropped out. As Sencer put it, "We lost the whole bunch."[5]

Results of the Ten-State Survey were published in a five-volume report, but the Senate Select Committee on Nutrition and Human Needs insisted on a preview. It was Senator McGovern's pet project, and Senator Ernest Hollings was also intensely interested. Senator Hollings, tipped off that the report would show that fifteen million Americans were hungry and malnourished, three hundred thousand of them in his own state, hinted at a cover-up by the Republican administration. The senator predicted it would take an act of Congress to get the cards out of CDC.

That was not necessary, but the analysis did require almost total dedication of CDC's then quite modest computer capabilities. The final report confirmed Hollings's worst suspicions about the state of nutrition in America: there were millions of poorly nourished people in the country, particularly preschool children and women aged eighteen to forty-four. Evidence of malnutrition was found most often among blacks, less often among Spanish Americans, and least often among whites. School lunch provided an important part of the nourishment of many children, especially if they were black; obesity was a significant public health concern; iron-deficiency anemia was widespread.[6]

At CDC nutrition was "housed" in the Smallpox-Eradication Program, whose staff had first applied epidemiologic principles to famine relief in Africa. For a year or so, it was hardly a program at all, its efforts being concentrated on getting out the Ten-State Survey, but in due time it emerged with an agenda; it would do surveillance of growth, obesity, and anemia. Dr. Milton Z. Nichaman was brought in from the Division of Chronic Disease in Washington to direct the work.

After nutrition surveillance defined the problem, remedial activity could begin. Since no single criterion characterized a person's total nutritional status, Nichaman suggested monitoring hemoglobin and hematocrit, height and weight. These measurements detected iron deficiency and nutritional problems reflected by growth, and were routinely performed procedures in many health-screening programs. Five states agreed to provide data; the nutrition program provided testing and measuring equipment, training, data analysis, and feedback.[7]

The "quick and dirty" ways of getting facts, first used in the Biafran famine, were adopted for nutrition surveillance. The level of malnutrition was determined by looking at several measurements—height for age, weight for height, and weight for age. Each person's place on the scale could be determined from the fifth percentile to the ninety-fifth. A simple computer system was developed so that individual states and other countries could handle their own data. This was CDC's classic pattern of service: simplify procedures and make them usable.

Findings of the survey, released in 1975, revealed much about the status of nutrition in the United States. The large number of obese children, as expressed in the weight-for-height measurements, indicated that the national problem of obesity had its roots in eating habits developed in childhood. In Louisiana nearly a third of the overweight children were less than 90 percent of the accepted height for their age. They got too many calories, but their diet was insufficient to make them grow.[8]

Both before and after its transfer to CDC, the nutrition program was active in the international field, especially on projects concerning vitamin A and iron malnutrition. These overseas studies produced information applicable to domestic situations and created a reservoir of goodwill for the United States. Wherever a famine existed, CDC was ready to send a team. William Foege, who pioneered the use of simple techniques to judge the degree of malnutrition, found in Biafra that famine afforded very valuable opportunities for study. In the usual situation, it is difficult to separate malnutrition from the things that cause it: lack of education, poverty, other forms of deprivation, or mental retardation. Famine deprives many groups of food, even those whose educational, social, and cultural backgrounds would not ordinarily lead to malnutrition, so much could be learned. In 1973 CDC began a regular response to the drought and famine crisis in sub-Saharan Africa. Its simple, inexpensive, and objective measures made the allocation of food more efficient.[9]

The nutrition program at CDC formally came to an end in 1973 with the reorganization of the Health Services and Mental Health Administration, one of the periodic restructurings of the PHS. Its admirers were distressed that this "open-eyed means of assessment" was no more. The PHS replaced it with a mammoth nutrition coordinating committee, which oversaw nutrition work in many different places. In spite of its loss of mandate, however, CDC continued its nutrition work much as before, although a slight effort was made to keep it from being so visible.[10]

In January 1972 the National Clearinghouse on Smoking and Health (NCSH) joined the CDC fold. Sencer welcomed the prevention agency, which had "brought about the conscious recognition that cigarette smoking *is* dangerous to health," and he asked his staff to demonstrate their commitment to the work of the Clearinghouse by banning smoking from classes, conference rooms, and elevators. "We at CDC believe in preventing disease. We have immunized our children, we have immunized our dogs and cats, and are screening for glaucoma. This demonstrates our commitment to preventing disease. Let us now demonstrate our belief that smoking is dangerous to health."[11]

Smoking was first recognized as a health hazard in the 1920s, when various researchers cited tobacco as a carcinogen, but no action was taken at that time. Interest first centered on cancer of the mouth and throat. Lung cancer, relatively rare in the 1920s, was encountered in the 1930s. In 1951 the American Cancer Society began a study of lung cancer and smoking, and its report was the biggest news at the meeting of the American Medical Association in 1954. Another decade passed before the surgeon general's advisory committee on smoking and health issued its famous report definitely establishing a link between cigarette smoking and excess morbidity and mortality.[12] The next year Congress appropriated $2 million to establish the Clearinghouse to collect and disseminate information on smoking and health, encourage educational activities on tobacco use, and conduct research on the behavioral nature of the smoking habit. Its director was Daniel Horn, a sociologist who was a member of the group that made the first report to the AMA.

Like other agencies transferred to CDC, the Clearinghouse on Smoking and Health lingered in Washington, its staff reluctant to move. Some thought the clearinghouse would lose its effectiveness away from the center of power, but Sencer was absolutely committed to spreading the word that smoking was dangerous to health. He was irate when three billboards advertising cigarettes appeared in Atlanta on which the surgeon general's warning about the hazards of smoking, required since 1970, was so small as to be unreadable. "[A]t best it can be called only tokenism," he complained to the Bureau of Consumer Protection. "Under no circumstances can the warning be read from the highway. Is this in compliance with the consent orders that the tobacco industry has signed?" He proposed that CDC staff, located in every state, act as watchdogs to see that billboards complied with the law.[13]

CDC's program of growth by acquisition leaped forward in 1973. At the beginning of President Nixon's second term, he asked for the resignation of the heads of all government agencies. Dr. Vernon E. Wilson, director of the Health Services and Mental Health Administration, duly turned in his resignation, and the president accepted it. Sencer was called to Washington to fill in temporarily. He presided over the disintegration of HSMHA, or "HSMA-ha-ha-ha," as it was irreverently called at 1600 Clifton Road, where many old-timers thought that it came close to putting the Public Health Service out of business.

Sencer's arrival in Washington coincided with one of the periodic reorganizations of the Public Health Service. The service had lost much of its authority to non-physicians in the Department of Health, Education and Welfare, and Dr. Charles Edwards, the assistant secretary for health, was determined to make some changes. As Sencer put it, he wanted to "fight off the department." The first step was to break up HSMHA. As a result, CDC moved up a notch in the department to become a full-fledged agency on a par with the National Institutes of Health and the Food and Drug Administration. The breakup of HSMHA sent the National Institute of Mental Health to NIH, and created two new agencies—the Health Services Administration and the Health Resources Administration—to pick up major portions of what was left. The reorganization coincided with sharp cuts in the budget, so Sencer's task as a temporary administrator was a thankless one. Rumors circulated that seven thousand people would lose their jobs; Sencer proposed closing the PHS hospitals, and he eliminated regional medical programs. Programs at CDC fell victim to the ax, too. Funds for the newly acquired smoking and health program vanished, the nutrition program disappeared, and as an economy measure, the highly successful Kansas City field station and the technical development laboratory at Savannah were closed. But even in adversity, Sencer saw an opportunity. The reorganization left three pieces of HSMHA homeless. Sencer scooped them up and brought them to Atlanta—the National Institute of Occupational Safety and Health (NIOSH) and, from the defunct Bureau of Community and Environmental Management, lead-based paint poisoning prevention and urban rat control.[14]

NIOSH had been in existence only two years when it was made part of CDC, but its roots were much deeper in the past. The government set up the Office of Industrial Hygiene and Sanitation in 1914, primarily to protect workers in such dusty trades as granite work. In 1937 the program became part of the Division of Industrial Hygiene at NIH, where it played an important role in protecting workers in war industries during World War II. In 1944, Industrial Hygiene was moved to the Bureau of State Services in the PHS. It had headquarters in Washington and field stations in Salt Lake City, Cincinnati, and later, Morgantown, West Virginia. In the PHS shakedown of 1968, Industrial Hygiene got a new name—the Bureau of Occupational Safety and Health (BOSH)—and new headquarters in Rockville, Maryland. When Congress passed the Occupational Safety and Health Act in 1970, BOSH, always an unfortunate acronym, gave way to NIOSH.

The evolution of NIOSH might have turned out differently. When asbestos was recognized as a health hazard, there was talk in Washington of creating an occupational health center in North Carolina's Research Triangle using CDC as a model. The politicians sought advice from industry on the proposal, and a representative from the DuPont Company went to Atlanta to look over CDC. Bill Watson met his private jet at the airport and spent the rest of the day showing him around. The DuPont executive was horrified that anything like CDC might be created for occupational health, and the idea of the North Carolina center soon fizzled.[15] Surely some industrialists were appalled when occupational health was moved to a center not "like CDC" but to CDC itself.

Even Sencer admitted that the transition was difficult. NIOSH had a legal mandate and a different constituency from CDC: NIOSH worked with labor, CDC with the state health departments. The basic principles of disease control were the same, but these different constituencies made for an uneasy union. Having just been elevated to the status of a national institute, NIOSH understandably wanted to keep its independence and visibility, and in the move to CDC, these might be lost. The physical move of NIOSH to Atlanta did not come right away (no move ever did). It took eight years, much persistence, and some political maneuvering to get that accomplished (see chapter 23).

Shortly after NIOSH became part of CDC, its director, Dr. Mark Key, resigned, and Dr. John F. Finklea took his place. With CDC's backing, Finklea pushed the staff hard and created a fair amount of resentment. But the work he began was important. Within months NIOSH was engaged in the first major federal effort to prevent occupational diseases and injuries. It focused on potentially dangerous toxic substances to which workers were exposed and, with the Occupational Safety and Health Administration (OSHA), developed standards designed to protect the worker. It tackled the most serious agents first—asbestos, benzene, beryllium, lead, mercury, silica, and noise—and responded to new threats like Kepone and vinyl chloride.[16]

The remnants of the Bureau of Community and Environmental Management—lead-based paint poisoning and rat control—wound up in Don Millar's care. He set up a special division on environmental health and put Dr. Vernon Houk in charge. Houk had been medical director of an expedition to the Antarctic; he was an authority on tuberculosis and a talented manager. It was the latter skill that got him the job of protecting the environment. He was, as Millar put it, "outrageously successful." When Houk took over lead-based paint poisoning prevention, it was a social and political issue rather than a health program. Created as part of the Great Society and aimed primarily at blacks, it had never worked. It made grants to major cities for blood tests on children to determine their exposure to lead. If the tests were positive, some effort was made to remove the lead from the premises. But it was never coordinated, and progress was measured by the inch. Houk tackled the problem as a health issue and organized a systematic program. Within months deaths from lead-based paint began to decline. For several years, there were none at all. Only when money for the program dried up and vigilance dropped did the problem surface once more.[17]

The lead-based paint project was never the congressional joke that the rat-control program was. Transfer of the latter to Atlanta in 1973 was a curtain call, since rat control had been part of CDC in the 1960s. While it was not the kind of program CDC would have started voluntarily, it had much public appeal and served a public relations function. If it did not get rid of rats, it gave poor neighborhoods a legitimate avenue of complaint and may have alleviated stress. Rat control, like the lead-based paint program, disappeared when Congress changed the funding scheme. Instead of allocating funds for specific programs, Congress folded many programs into "block grants" that gave communities a greater voice in how they spent the money. Many of them dropped rat control.

These two projects provided CDC with an opening to the field of environmental health, one it had ventured into before only to study leukemia clusters and birth defects. Water fluoridation was added to its responsibilities in 1975, when dental disease prevention was transferred to Atlanta. This was a modest start for a program that in a few years' time would report from Love Canal, Times Beach, and Mount Saint Helens, and, in the name of health, organize and win a campaign to remove lead from gasoline.

Getting people to take more responsibility for their own health was a public health trend of the 1970s. The National Clearinghouse on Smoking and Health had spread the word that smoking was linked to cancer, heart disease, and other ailments, but in its educational thrust it was virtually alone in government. President Nixon called attention to the need for a national program in health education in 1971 and appointed a committee to make a study. In September 1973, the committee recommended to the president that a National Center for Health Education be established in the private sector, and that within HEW there should be a focal point to make the government's involvement in health education more efficient.

Sencer was picking up pieces of HSMHA and moving them to Atlanta at the time, and he saw the opportunity the committee recommendation afforded: CDC would be the government's focal point in health education. He won the support of the assistant secretary for health, and, ignoring the protests of the National Clearinghouse on Smoking and Health, moved that program to Atlanta. He used its funds and positions to establish a Bureau of Health Education at CDC.

It was something new. In the past the PHS had put its health-education effort into categorical programs like rat control or prevention of lead-based paint poisoning, or had combined health education with offices of public information. The latter were poorly funded, short-lived, and mostly ineffective since they were based on the assumption that the simple transmission of information would cause behavior change. Sencer was not an enthusiast for these traditional forms of health education, but he did believe that individual, family, and community lifestyles were important determinants of public health. He also thought a Bureau of Health Education would strengthen CDC, and he recruited Horace G. Ogden as its director. Ogden represented both the old and new concepts in health education. He had spent much of his career in PHS public information offices, but he also had experience in adult education and community development.[18]

The apparent promise of health education was not immediately realized. The bureau remained quite small, tucked away in a little building that at one time had been a residence. Dennis Tolsma, who succeeded Ogden, called the location "institutional body language." Away from the center of action, the bureau was a stepchild. Even though the Clearinghouse on Smoking and Health was the nucleus of the organization, most of the staff did not move to Atlanta, so less attention was paid to the dangers of tobacco than to the general aspects of health education. It was not long before there were charges in high places that CDC had killed the Clearinghouse.

The change of administrations in 1977 brought a new secretary to HEW, who took immediate action to give the anti-tobacco movement more visibility. Joseph Califano, an ex-smoker with the zeal of a convert, moved the clearinghouse back to Washington to keep it under his own watchful eye. CDC's commitment to health education was secure enough by then, however, to survive what proved to be only a temporary loss.

The Bureau of Health Education launched a number of activities as diverse as the Berkeley Project to develop health curriculums for grade-school children and the kidney donor project. The first was very successful, the latter a failure. The oil embargo of the early 1970s put CDC into the business of matching kidney donors with those who needed transplants. As speed limits dropped to conserve gasoline, so did the number of highway fatalities and, consequently, the number of kidneys available for transplant. The shortage was severe in Virginia, which called CDC for help. Sencer saw this as a good education initiative. If the management techniques CDC had applied to so many other health problems could be used to match kidney donors to recipients, many patients would not have their lives disrupted by dialysis treatments, and the government, which was just beginning to pay for these, would be spared much expense. With considerable enthusiasm, CDC set up pilot projects in several cities to work out an orderly system. Sencer was certain CDC could make it work, but essential support from the medical community and the public was not forthcoming. Those involved with providing dialysis treatments, where big money was at stake, were not interested, and surgeons were reluctant to become part of such a disciplined system. "We could not get that off the ground," lamented Bill Watson. "We could not sell it as a policy. We finally just folded our tent and went away."[19]

In the game of musical chairs health agencies played in the mid 1970s, CDC inherited one of Joseph Mountin's pet projects and just as quickly got rid of it. In 1973, when huge cuts were made in the public health budget, the Arctic Health Center in Alaska was abolished and transferred to CDC in that order. Looking to the day when the inevitable population surge occurred, Mountin had envisioned a center that would concentrate on the health problems of the colder regions, but in spite of its talented staff, the Arctic Center was never a viable operation. Its chief claim to fame was the largest collection of black bear skulls in the world. When CDC acquired the budgetless center, there was nothing to do but close it down, and the job of breaking the news—"a very unhappy business"—fell to Bill Watson. The people were only slightly mollified when CDC set up a very small field station in Anchorage for epidemiologic and disease-surveillance work.

Telling the staff they were out of jobs proved to be easier than getting rid of the buildings. CDC tried to give them to the University of Alaska, which refused to accept them without money for heating and maintenance. The energetic Alaska congressional delegation managed to get $2 million tacked on to CDC's budget for that purpose. The money did not arrive until the first day of June, giving CDC just thirty days to get rid of it.

"We were wringing our hands," Watson recalled. "How do you do this?" When the grants and contracts people could offer no help, CDC's normally conservative general counsel suggested that Watson just give the University of Alaska the money. The suggestion did not follow any known government protocol, and Watson was hesitant, but the general counsel insisted that if Congress said the university could have the money, it would be quite all right to hand it over. And so it was done. The vice rector of the university came to Atlanta, and with a minimum of ceremony picked up the check.[20]

Acquisition of these diverse pieces of the PHS drew CDC into the vortex of many socially sensitive issues. Its relations with the public thus became both more complex and more important.

CHAPTER 17

In Pursuit of the Promised Land

As victory over smallpox in West Africa neared, David Sencer challenged Don Millar to take the lessons learned in Africa and apply them in America. Could he instill into CDC's domestic disease-control programs—tuberculosis, venereal disease, and immunization—the kind of magic that propelled smallpox eradication? Millar had nagging doubts. He knew this meant an aggressive approach to disease control unparalleled in the United States.[1]

Venereal disease was a particularly stubborn problem. The deadline set for the eradication of syphilis in the United States was approaching, and it was obvious that the goal would not be reached. In fact, except for a dip in the curve of incidence from 1965 to 1968, the number of cases of infectious syphilis had gone up instead of down, and in 1970 gonorrhea led the list of reportable diseases in the United States. Since 1957 its curve of incidence had moved steadily up, and by 1970 a true epidemic was sweeping the country. Yet control methods for both diseases were well known. If a nationally coordinated program of tracing contacts were implemented, if each index case were found, and if all the contacts were traced and treated in an ever-widening circle, it was theoretically possible to eradicate both diseases. The approach had clear parallels to E^2 and the eradication of smallpox.

The HEW secretary outlined the program to President Nixon. The federal government would provide leadership and coordination; state and local governments would pick up part of the cost. The proposal had implicit political advantages quite attractive to the Nixon administration. An initial investment of $16 million provided visible evidence of the administration's commitment to national social and health problems in the face of stringent economic restraints.[2]

Inspired by West African triumphs, Don Millar spurred on his troops with the fervor of a modern-day Moses leading the Israelites into the land of Canaan. We are looking into "a sort of promised land in venereal disease control," he told the Communicable Disease Control Conference in 1972. The financial resources as well as the public enthusiasm and support were all there. "I see my role here as that of a visionary, perhaps even a naive visionary. . . . We can no longer wail about the lack of funds, shortage of people, inadequate or unpopular therapy regimens, etc. etc.! Our time in the wilderness is finished. We are looking into the promised land," Millar said.[3]

The troops in Millar's army were primarily public health advisors who had succeeded in the fight against venereal disease whenever the financial support was there; it was a budget cut that sent the syphilis curve up in 1969. Millar thought the right approach would turn that curve downward once more. In two-thirds of the states, the rate of infection was so low that vigorous action should bring eradication. The long incubation time for syphilis made it possible to treat the disease before it spread, and the cure was known. Gonorrhea was more difficult; it raged uncontrolled. A short incubation period made pursuit of contacts difficult, and a changing organism complicated treatment. If a parallel were drawn between the smallpox-measles program in Africa and Millar's challenge for a renewed attack on venereal disease in America, syphilis was like smallpox, and gonorrhea was like measles. Although there was no vaccine for either, Millar viewed antibiotic therapy as the "vaccine" for venereal disease. Vigorous treatment of suspects and contacts was good preventive therapy.

In 1972 CDC launched a national effort against gonorrhea. For the public health advisors, it was the third major phase of their work in a quarter century. Organized to fight syphilis after World War II, they achieved such success by 1958 that the problem was assumed to be licked. Funding was cut, and many PHAs found other employment. The second phase was the syphilis-eradication campaign of the 1960s, which, with its first signs of success, also fell victim to budget cuts. Gonorrhea was the target for the 1970s. CDC made grants to the states for this all-out effort.

The work got under way against a backdrop of the sensational public disclosure of the Tuskegee experiment. In late July 1972, Jean Heller of

the Associated Press broke the story of the forty-year-old study of untreated syphilis in black males in Macon County, Alabama. The *New
York Times* ran it on the front page. The Tuskegee experiment quickly
became a cause célèbre; the press held it up as an example of the
potential for scientific abuse. The Public Health Service in general and
the CDC in particular were accused of being "un-American." Compar-
isons were made with Nazi Germany, and genocide was mentioned.

It was a former public health advisor who tipped off the press to the
Tuskegee experiment, which was virtually unknown outside medical
circles. Peter Buxton, hired as an interviewer in 1965 during the
syphilis-eradication campaign, overheard colleagues talking about it
and wrote to headquarters for reprints of the published articles. Disturbed about what seemed to be a lack of ethical concern, he pursued
the matter with Dr. William J. Brown, then head of CDC's Venereal
Disease Branch, who dispatched someone to San Francisco to talk to
him. Later Buxton was brought to Atlanta, where, he said, he was
harangued at a meeting of the top venereal disease–control staff. Buxton was not intimidated and pursued the issue even after he resigned as
a public health advisor. He was particularly concerned about the racial
implications of the experiment at a time when there was much racial
unrest in America and cities were erupting in race riots. All the participants in the study were black, and as Buxton wrote Brown, "Today it
would be morally unethical to begin such a study with such a group."
Brown showed the letter to Sencer, who called together a panel of
medical experts to review the study and make recommendations.

The panel met in Atlanta in early February 1969 and concluded that
the knowledge gained by the Tuskegee Study was great enough to war-
rant its continuation. Dr. Gene Stollerman, chairman of the Department
of Medicine at the University of Tennessee, was the lone dissenter. Like
Buxton, he raised the moral issues and urged that the men be treated.[4]

The panel was concerned with science, not civil rights, a stance
Sencer defended. Both the Alabama Health Department and the Macon
County Medical Society, by 1969 a mostly black group, agreed for a
variety of reasons to let the study alone. "There was some concern
about risks in treating [the men] and grave concern about creating
adverse publicity, not just for the PHS but for the people in Tuskegee,"
Sencer said. "Part of it was that they had all known about it, and they
had not done anything. Some of the guilt would come back on them."[5]

And so the study continued. The day after the story broke in the
press, CDC issued a background paper outlining the history of the

Tuskegee Study and reviewed the findings published in medical journals since 1936. In the early years of the study, the only treatments for syphilis were toxic substances like mercury and arsenic, which many physicians viewed as posing as great a risk as the disease. When penicillin became widely available in 1946–47, the decision was made not to recommend treatment for the men because there were no data that showed it to be effective in treating late syphilis, and the short- and long-term toxic effects of the drug had not been documented. Participants were treated for other medical problems as they arose, however, so that by 1972, seventy-five of the seventy-six syphilitic patients known to be living had received antibiotic therapy. In about 30 percent of these cases, the therapy was thought to be adequate for the cure of syphilis. The paper listed the groups that had supported the study over the years—the Milbank Memorial Fund, the Tuskegee Institute, and the Macon County Health Department. The paper concluded:

> Although this study has been widely publicized in professional circles since its inception, and although persons in the study group were informed they had syphilis, were informed that they could request and receive syphilis treatment at any time, and were treated appropriately for other medical conditions as they arose, it has been necessary throughout the course of the study to make judgments whether to recommend to all the syphilitic patients that they receive treatment. At no time in the course of the study has treatment been without risk, and the judgment has been consistently made that this risk has outweighed the benefits anticipated from treatment.[6]

The assistant secretary for health, Dr. Merlin K. Duval, called for an investigation and within a month convened a nine-member ad hoc panel to conduct a probe of the study. Five panel members were black. After months of meetings, the panel recommended that the study be discontinued and that the men participating in it be given appropriate medical care. It found that the study was "ethically unjustified in 1932," although it acknowledged that there may have been scientific justification at the time for a short-term study. In the panel's opinion, however, penicillin therapy should have begun by 1953.[7] Dr. Vernal Cave, director of the Bureau of Disease Control for the New York City Health Department, was a member of the secretary's task force and one of the most vocal critics of CDC and the Tuskegee Study. Sencer was particularly aggravated by Cave's criticism, because Cave had served as chairman of sessions at scientific meetings where papers on the Tuskegee Study were read and "he never said a word." After the task force issued its reports, Senator Edward Kennedy held public hearings before the Subcommittee on Health during which two of the Tuskegee Study survivors testified that the government should offer them compensation so that they could see doctors other than those provided by the Public Health Service.[8] The hearings dramatically underscored the need for federal guidelines on human experimentation.

It fell to CDC to track down survivors of the experiment and tell them that the government would pay their medical expenses for the rest of their lives. The government also picked up funeral expenses, previously paid by the Milbank Fund, but it did not offer a cash settlement, thus making a lawsuit inevitable. A year after the study became public information, a $1.8 billion class action civil suit was filed, but the case never came to trial. In December 1974, the government agreed to pay $10 million in an out-of-court settlement.[9]

The Tuskegee Study has been called unethical by numerous critics, but it also has its supporters. Among the critics is Allan M. Brandt. "The Tuskegee Study," he writes, "reveals the persistence of beliefs within the medical profession about the nature of blacks, sex, and disease. . . . There can be little doubt that the Tuskegee researchers regarded their subjects as less than human. As a result, the ethical canons of experimenting on human subjects were completely disregarded."[10] T. G. Benedek, on the other hand, has defended the study, although he found it methodologically flawed. It picked up the long-term Oslo study of untreated syphilis by Dr. Caesar Boeck from 1891 to 1910. Benedek observes that control groups are used in medical research to observe the natural history of disease, at least for short periods of time. He notes:

> The Tuskegee Study had been in progress for 12 years when the possibility of a dramatic improvement of treatment appeared, for 16 years when new insights into the ethical implications of research began to be advocated, and was 39 years old when it abruptly became the subject of severe criticism for ethical deficiencies. . . . The righteousness of the ethical critics fails to take into account that in the context of the 1930s thoughtful physicians could detect no ethical dilemma in an investigation such as [this] . . . and that very little would have been accomplished therapeutically by initiating penicillin treatment in the 1950s.[11]

Millar, like CDC, inherited the Tuskegee Study. It was totally unrelated to the national gonorrhea-control program that was the primary concern of the Venereal Disease Branch in the early 1970s, but the Tuskegee publicity cast a shadow on Millar's pursuit of the promised land. There would be others. Sencer decided to close the venereal disease research laboratory and spread its component parts elsewhere in CDC. The decision to close the most important venereal disease laboratory in the United States, if not in the world, was made primarily for economic reasons. Millar's division picked up the laboratory's outreach services; the rest went to bacteriology in the Laboratory Branch.

Dr. Albert Balows, director of the bacteriology laboratory, remembers the day in 1976 when two strains of penicillin-resistant gonococcus, an unheard-of phenomenon, arrived at CDC. The laboratory checked the strains again, and discovered that the original state reports were accurate. Both strains came from men recently stationed in the Philippines, where there was, as Balows put it, "a festering nest of resistant gonorrhea . . . growing on a daily basis among the prostitutes." In areas around military installations, as many as 35 percent of these women were infected, but this was not true elsewhere in the islands. The new strains of gonococcus were of great scientific and social significance. They provided the world's first evidence of penicillin-resistant gonorrhea, and made the job of controlling it much harder.[12]

The prospect of eradicating tuberculosis was brighter than that for venereal disease in the 1970s. For ten years, project grants to the states had financed outpatient treatment with new miracle drugs. Isoniazid was especially effective. It was cheap, had no serious side effects, and was taken orally, making it easy to administer. The incidence of tuberculosis steadily declined. Initially, there was hope only that TB could be cured, but this gave way to the even brighter prospect that the white plague could be eradicated. Among the believers in the dream was David Sencer. "When you have the disease way down as we do now," he said in 1969, "it is the time to accelerate the program and step on it and eradicate it."[13] His optimism was rooted in Africa.

A tuberculosis surveillance system was begun in 1968 to identify the estimated twenty million people in the United States infected with *Mycobacterium tuberculosis* and accordingly at high risk of developing TB. The next year, rates plunged by the greatest amount in a decade. As had often been the case in the past, success was accompanied by a decrease in direct federal funding. The Nixon administration was committed to the idea that the states should decide what their needs were. In return for the privilege of choosing how to spend the federal money allotted, the states picked up a larger portion of the tab. The success of outpatient treatment for tuberculosis had been demonstrated so effectively by the 1970s that many states used their federal funds to continue it. In due time, outpatient therapy spelled the end of expensive tuberculosis sanitariums, and the states closed them down. Surveillance demonstrated that mass chest X-rays and even skin-testing were inefficient means of finding tuberculosis patients, who most likely belonged in special population groups—older males in the cities, the poor, immigrants, blacks, Indians living on reservations, Eskimos. New cases nearly always appeared among those in close contact with an existing case. Seek out the existing cases, treat them actively, keep a close watch on their contacts, and theoretically, tuberculosis transmission could be stopped. With isoniazid used as a preventive, the prospects of eradicating tuberculosis seemed bright indeed.

Even so, it was dangerous to be complacent about tuberculosis, for it could strike anywhere. Its appearance on Capitol Hill in February 1970 made the point painfully obvious. In an eighteen-month span, tuberculosis occurred among seven employees on Capitol Hill. Three worked in the Senate restaurant; two died. Everybody on Capitol Hill had to be tested. It was the largest mass screening in years—13,586 people. Dr. Vernon Houk, then deputy director of CDC's Tuberculosis Branch, went to Washington to direct the work. Both skin tests and X-rays were used in the screening process. Those with X-ray abnormalities were referred to private physicians, and more than 2,300 others were started on isoniazid therapy. For the first time, a problem only hinted at in the past became obvious. In some people, isoniazid triggered hepatitis. Nineteen of the Capitol Hill group on isoniazid therapy developed hepatitis, two of whom died. "It dampened the enthusiasm for preventive treatment," observed the head of the Tuberculosis Branch, Dr. Phyllis Q. Edwards. "We can't just put [isoniziad] in the bread or the drinking water." The Capitol Hill episode was a learning experience. Through research, the high-risk groups for isoniazid therapy were identified.[14]

Of all the roads to the promised land, immunization seemed the most likely. Past experience proved that it worked, but after the initial success, interest lagged, and the incidence of disease shot up again. This was particularly true of measles, which requires a low number of susceptibles to fuel an epidemic. As funding for measles immunization dropped, the dream of eradicating measles faded.

By 1973 more than a third of the nation's preschool children were unprotected against preventable disease. Millar chafed at the roadblocks that kept the immunization program from being successful. It troubled him that Gambia achieved zero measles incidence in 1967 and kept it at zero for four years until AID support for its program stopped; it was the only country in the world ever to reach that goal. To boost interest in immunization in the United States, CDC declared October 1973 to be "Immunization Action Month," and a special effort was made to locate and immunize large pools of persons susceptible to a whole range of childhood diseases.[15]

Acquisition of environmental programs from HSMHA in 1973 gave Millar an additional assignment and another approach towards achieving the promise of public health. He moved Dr. Houk from tuberculosis control to the Environmental Services Division. Under Houk's leadership, the incidence of deaths from lead-based paint poisoning dropped to zero and the attack on another serious health menace, lead in gasoline, began. Studies Houk's unit did for the National Center for Health Statistics showed that the level of lead in the blood is closely related to exposure to lead in gasoline. People who live near highways absorb more lead than those living farther away. Those who live near lead smelters had very elevated blood-lead levels. Houk considered the threat to health so grave, he got out and vigorously marketed the information to policymakers and the public and made sure that they understood it. When they did understand it, he got action.[16]

"I am the person principally responsible for getting the lead out of gasoline in this country," he said. "I did not write the regulations—that was EPA—but we did the studies." The amount of lead in gasoline was reduced by half from 1976 to 1980. Blood-lead levels dropped by 37 percent. The statistical correlation was almost perfect—.95 out of 1— this could have happened by chance less than once in 10,000 times.[17]

About the time that CDC became an agency of the Public Health Service in 1973, Sencer appointed an in-house group to look at CDC and decide where it should go in the future. It was called the "Under 42 Committee." By definition its members were young. In theory, at least, they had fresh ideas and thought broadly. Don Millar was the chairman. The committee wrote a report suggesting among other things that CDC do more work on chronic diseases and that some reorganization was in order. To Sencer's dismay, Millar outlined the contents of the report to a good friend who was a reporter for an Atlanta newspaper. The reporter wrote an article that Sencer thought premature. Its release abridged the plans he had for the report, so he put it away, and it was forgotten in the rush of events that followed in the mid 1970s.

Sencer did not share the real purpose for the Under 42 Committee with Millar: his belief that in the future public health would apply the concept of prevention to environmental and lifestyle issues. He wanted CDC to move in that direction. The smoking and nutrition programs, recently annexed to CDC, were concerned primarily with this new concept of prevention. So were the programs that came to Atlanta with the breakup of HSMHA. Sencer was getting them under one roof.[18]

The expanded emphasis on prevention had to wait for a few years and a new director, but there was much solid accomplishment in the far-flung agency, both in the United States and abroad. As the epidemiologist Michael Gregg put it, "We took advantage of unique health problems, and we ran with the ball."

Hepatitis research was a case in point. When Gregg took over as director of Epidemiology's viral disease division in 1968, there were just two EIS officers working in the hepatitis section in Atlanta, and there was a small group, primarily laboratorians, working on hepatitis at the Phoenix lab, where, thanks to CDC's connection with NASA, chimpanzees were available for research. But that year CDC's work in hepatitis exploded. As several of those working on the problem put it, "We ran a hundred miles an hour."[19]

The impetus for this burst of activity was the detection of the Australian antigen of the hepatitis B virus by Dr. Baruch Blumberg in 1966[20] and the arrival in Phoenix in 1968 of Dr. James Maynard, who became director of the CDC laboratory there. A man of forceful personality, Maynard determined to push the Phoenix Laboratories to the forefront of hepatitis research, and within a few years, he succeeded. He knew what was going on not only in his own laboratory but in all the other hepatitis laboratories as well. The deputy director of the Phoenix Lab, Dr. Martin Favero, explains: "He made himself an expert on hepatitis and he kicked the door down at NIH. 'I represent CDC and we have our chimps. If you want to use our chimps, then we'll have a collaborative study.' He was the outsider and he forced his way in. . . . and would not go away. He forced them to do studies with us. He had some jewels, the animals." Maynard and Friedrich W. Deinhardt, a German researcher who was a consultant at NIH, were personal friends. Favero describes hepatitis research circles as having "a lot of good old boy stuff. We went in on [Deinhardt's] coattails."[21]

In 1971 the Phoenix labs discovered that hepatitis B was sexually transmitted. The initial announcement was made primarily on the basis of analysis of miscellaneous reports, but when serologic tests became available in the mid 1970s, it became clear that many hepatitis B cases are not transmitted by the standard blood routes. The findings were confirmed by the Phoenix lab's large study of homosexual men, which showed that they were uniformly at high risk. A later study of five widely isolated counties in the United States showed that hepatitis B is transmitted through heterosexual contact as well.

The serologic test for hepatitis B made possible the identification of infectious hepatitis—hepatitis A. When the cause of serum hepatitis was known, what was left over was hepatitis A. It was no accident that the Phoenix lab was the first to discover the hepatitis A virus from a naturally occurring epidemic. Favero explained, "CDC has its fingers on the pulse of outbreaks in this country, and the gold [for research] is the material of an outbreak."[22] Dr. Daniel W. Bradley, chief of the immunochemistry section of the Phoenix lab, spearheaded the research. Using fecal specimens obtained from a food-borne outbreak of hepatitis A in Phoenix, the lab got the first picture of the virus with electron microscopy. More accomplishments followed in quick succession. The lab developed diagnostic tests for hepatitis A, and did some renowned studies on transmission of non-A, non-B hepatitis, another manifestation of this complex disease.

The resounding success of the Phoenix lab made it possible for Maynard to argue that all hepatitis work should be transferred to Phoenix, and though the transfer brought no joy in Atlanta, this was done. It was a bit unusual for CDC to put all of its eggs in a basket two thousand miles away, but the decision not only fostered the work in hepatitis, but unwittingly provided a model for the reorganization of CDC. In Phoenix there was no formal division between the Laboratory Branch and the Epidemiology Branch, and harmony prevailed. Epidemiologists and laboratorians worked and ate together, and the friction that too often marked relations between their branches in Atlanta melted away under the blue skies of Phoenix.[23]

Living up to its new name, the Center for Disease *Control* expanded its work in disease prevention. It set up a program to find out specifically which practices used by hospitals to control infections worked and which did not. The Study on the Efficacy of Nosocomial Infection Control (SENIC) was the largest and most sophisticated medical survey CDC had ever undertaken. Sencer had great faith in it. He believed that hard scientific data would reduce the number of nosocomial infections, shorten the time spent in the hospital, and cut costs. The sensational disclosure in 1971 that some intravenous fluid from Abbott Laboratories, the nation's largest supplier, was contaminated, underscored the urgency of the problem. The results from SENIC sustained Sencer's belief. Effective controls cut the rate of hospital-acquired infections in half.[24]

Work of one of the newer additions to CDC, the National Institute of Occupational Safety and Health, established the danger to health of exposure to vinyl chloride. In 1974, the year after it became part of CDC, NIOSH investigated deaths from cancer of the liver of several workers at the B. F. Goodrich Co. in Louisville. Four workers died of this relatively rare disease in a five-year period. Evidence pointed to exposure to vinyl chloride as the cause, and NIOSH concluded that a new occupational cancer had been discovered.[25] Vinyl chloride was one of 350 toxic substances for which NIOSH and the Occupational Health and Safety Administration (OSHA) began to set standards. In 1975 a NIOSH report showed that nearly one-third of *all* diseases of factory and farm workers were work-related.

CDC applied the principles of disease control to natural disasters like floods and tornadoes. The same epidemiological principles applied. This was also true in handling famines. In the mid 1970s, CDC began its regular response to famine in the Sahel region of Africa, where drought, war, and political upheaval left the people desperate. It also answered special calls to Bangladesh and Nepal. Its "simplified field assessment of nutritional status" made the complicated job of making nutritional surveys easier.[26] CDC always looked for simpler approaches to a problem, sometimes with unexpectedly good results. Beginning in 1965, CDC staff were appointed to the Pakistan–SEATO Cholera Research Laboratory in Dacca, where they carried out the epidemiological aspects of cholera research. The Dacca laboratory used oral rehydration to save the lives of cholera victims in Bangladesh and India. The technique, developed by Commander Robert Allan Phillips of the U.S. Navy, used an "oral electrolyte cocktail" with a specific sodium-glucose ratio. Even desperately ill patients can absorb it and prevent death from dehydration. Like so many things learned abroad, oral rehydration had immediate benefits at home, where it has been used to treat diarrhea.[27]

The staff rallied quickly in the spring of 1975, when Saigon fell and thousands of Vietnamese refugees came to the United States. After a stopover in the Pacific, the refugees came to processing centers on the mainland. CDC was among the PHS units working on health aspects of the resettlement program, both to protect the refugees and to prevent the importation of disease. EIS officers and public health advisors checked medical records, looked for quarantinable diseases, and gave thousands of shots. They did the work competently, but also with kindness. One HEW regional director was astonished at the goodwill that prevailed among all the people—the Army personnel and the employees of various agencies of HEW. He had never seen anything like it. He described the scene at Fort Chaffee, Arkansas, where they worked twelve-hour shifts, seven days a week, and sometimes had to be forced to go back to their motels after fifteen or sixteen hours on the job. "The employees are caught up in the euphoria of helping others. Each employee has established a feeling of personal responsibility to these people—a feeling that is hard to describe and impossible to duplicate in their normal jobs back home." Some CDC staff got so involved they offered to sponsor Vietnamese families. Davie Newberry had committed himself when he belatedly asked how many people were in the family he invited. There were eleven. For a while, all of them crowded into the Newberrys' house, putting seventeen people under one roof.[28]

Like the new immigrants, CDC continued its own pursuit of the promised land throughout the 1970s. In both cases hope was often tempered by experience.

CHAPTER 18

1976

The year 1976 should have been one for celebration. As the United States observed its bicentennial, the Center for Disease Control marked its own special passages: it was thirty years old, its Epidemic Intelligence Service was twenty-five. Success bred confidence; the global eradication of smallpox was in sight, and measles, always a stubborn adversary, had reached its lowest incidence in history just two years before.[1] Celebration should have been in order for CDC's 4,104 employees, but it was not. Instead, the institution found itself at the center of a political storm.

In early February 1976, David Sencer was in Washington when he got a call from the home office. The laboratory reports from the influenza isolates sent from Fort Dix, New Jersey, had come back. Most were the familiar A/Victoria strain, but four were not. "Are you sitting down?" Walter Dowdle asked Sencer. "They are swine."[2]

The news was startling. The great influenza pandemic of 1918–19, in which 450,000 Americans died, was swine flu. Sometime before 1930, the virus found a reservoir in swine (hence the name) but except for an occasional case among persons who had contact with swine, there had been no human transmission of the deadly strain until the outbreak at Fort Dix. Although no one had ever seen the 1918 virus, survivors carried antibodies in their blood, so its structure was known. The virus at Fort Dix was antigenically related to it; all Americans under the age of fifty were susceptible. According to custom, the virus was named for the place and year it occurred, A/New Jersey/76 (Hsw1N1).

Sencer hurried back to Atlanta. In the laboratory, Dr. Dowdle, who headed the virology unit, repeated the tests in "clean rooms" and came up with the same results. Sencer scheduled a meeting for Saturday, Valentine's Day. In addition to CDC staff, there were Dr. John Seal, deputy director of NIH's National Institute for Allergy and Infectious Diseases (NIAID); Dr. Harry Meyer, Jr., of the Bureau of Biologics (BoB) in the Food and Drug Administration (FDA); Dr. Martin Goldfield of the New Jersey Department of Health, and Army influenza specialists.

Dowdle summarized: a large number of influenza cases occurred among recruits at Fort Dix, New Jersey; the State Health Department, unable to identify some of the specimens, forwarded nine of them to CDC, one of which came from a soldier who had collapsed and died after a forced five-mile night march. Four of the nine, including that from the dead soldier, were swine flu. When Dowdle reached the climax of his report, the chin of Dr. Philip Russell of the Walter Reed Army Institute of Research dropped, and others were as shocked as he. Sencer went around the room and asked for opinions. Michael Gregg remembers being very scared. For several years, he and other epidemiologists at CDC had played the "what if" game: What if a new strain of influenza came along and there was a pandemic? The symptoms of the New Jersey outbreak were classic. Like pandemics in the past, this one began in the military with person-to-person spread. Gregg thought his professor at Columbia University would have said, "The good Lord is telling you something."

Those at the Valentine Day's meeting agreed on surveillance at Fort Dix and a systematic search for other cases; the potential for a major epidemic was real. If there were any dissenters, they were circumspect. The next issue of the *Morbidity and Mortality Weekly Report* carried an announcement, one the editor, Michael Gregg, remembers as being quite hard to write. No one wanted to frighten the public, but the news was certain to leak out, and it was better to make an official announcement. Reporters were briefed on Thursday afternoon before the Friday publication date, the custom when there was news of great import. That same afternoon, a Baltimore paper informed CDC that it was running a story with the headline "Killer Flu Hits Military." *MMWR* beat the newspaper reports by a whisker.[3]

Sencer did not mention the pandemic of 1918–19 in the briefing, but it did come up in the question-and-answer session. The *MMWR* announcement was typically straightforward, although the accompanying editorial note hinted at an impending emergency.

To date, all other reported A isolates from the Continental United States have been A/Victoria–like. Because of the difficulty of characterizing the swine virus in the laboratory, some isolates may have been unrecognized as such. To determine if the A swine virus is causing other influenza in the U.S., CDC has sent all state health departments and WHO collaborating laboratories appropriate instructions and reagents for viral isolation and serologic testing.[4]

During the next week two meetings were held at the Bureau of Biologics in Bethesda to discuss what to do next. The first session was quite large and involved people from CDC, NIAID, and BoB, as well as the distinguished scientists Dr. Albert Sabin, of oral polio vaccine fame, and Dr. Edwin Kilbourne, of the Mt. Sinai School of Medicine, a leading expert on influenza. A few days later, at a smaller and informal session, Sencer and two of his staff, Dr. Michael Hattwick, of Epidemiology, and Dr. Dowdle of the laboratory compared notes with Meyer and Seal. Hattwick reported on the current status of influenza in the United States, and Dowdle said that all the isolates received so far at CDC were A/Victoria. NIAID knew about three patients who possibly had swine flu at the University of Virginia Hospital. (An EIS team left immediately for Charlottesville.) The BoB had already sent seed virus to the vaccine manufacturers, which had a six-week turnaround time. The next step was to advise members of the Advisory Committee on Immunization Practices.[5]

Planning for an influenza epidemic was based on both an understanding of the influenza virus and what was believed to be the rhythm of epidemics. Type A/influenza periodically sweeps over the world in pandemic form and may appear between times in epidemics large and small. Since 1890, pandemics had occurred at roughly ten- to twenty-year intervals, the two most recent being 1957 and 1968. The virus itself constantly changes. If the change is minor, as is the case most years, only the normal amount of influenza, resulting in about seventeen thousand deaths in the United States, might be expected; when a major shift occurs in either the hemagglutinin or neuraminidase antigens—proteins on the virus coat—an epidemic is possible because the immunity of the year before offers little protection. If both proteins change, immunity is virtually nil. The reversion to swine flu in 1976, like the appearance of Asian flu in 1957, represented a shift in both antigens.[6] What made the situation so unusual in 1976, however, was the appearance of the swine flu virus alongside the A/Victoria strain. The presence of two competing influenza strains made it extremely difficult to predict what would happen.

The Advisory Committee on Immunization Practices met at CDC March 10 in a session that lasted for seven hours. For the first time ever, a few members of the press were there including Harold Schmeck, medical reporter for the *New York Times.* Dr. Kilbourne also came and so did Dr. Martin Goldfield, epidemiologist for the state of New Jersey. The normal procedure for ACIP meetings was to present the surveillance findings and pass out a draft of CDC's recommended action. On that day, however, no draft was handed out, because, as Sencer recalled, "We literally did not know." The meeting ended with no recommendation, but there seemed to be a consensus, summed up by ACIP member Dr. Reuel A. Stallones, dean of the School of Public Health at the University of Texas: flu comes in pandemic cycles and it was time for a pandemic strain; isolates not seen for many years had the potential for a pandemic. More important, for the first time in history, there was time enough to develop a vaccine. The practice of good preventive medicine demanded action.

There were some dissenters. Dr. Russell Alexander, professor of public health at the University of Washington, an EIS alumnus and one-time CDC staffer, was reluctant to put *any* foreign material into millions of people, and suggested stockpiling the vaccine for use if needed. He expressed his reservations through questions. Goldfield, who later became the most outspoken critic of the mass immunization plan, spoke about the outbreak at Fort Dix from the vantage point of the home state, but if he had reservations, he did not express them. Sencer remembers that Goldfield said at that meeting, "Just give me the vaccine and in two weeks, I'll vaccinate the whole state of New Jersey. Let's go."

Sencer presided at the meeting but did not ask for a vote. Instead, he promised to call them the next day. As the session broke up, however, he signaled his own views in an unintentional pun. "It looks as if we are going to have to go whole hog." He then went directly to the office of Bill Watson, his deputy director, and told him, "There is a basic and risky decision to be made, and I am the one to make it."[7]

Minutes of the ACIP meeting reported a general consensus. Person-to-person transmission of swine flu at Fort Dix made an outbreak of swine flu likely the following winter. "It was, therefore, agreed that the development of vaccine must proceed. It was also concluded that if vaccine is produced a plan must be developed for its use. Stockpiling would not allow for a sufficiently rapid response after outbreaks begin and, in addition, public demand for the vaccine would undoubtedly be great."[8]

Force of personality doubtless played a role at the ACIP meeting, as in all the sessions that determined the subsequent course of action. Dr. Dowdle came out of these meetings shaking his head. "I could not believe the decisions that had been made. One or two people could sway the whole group. . . . It was a marvel to see how this happened." He saw swine flu as "more of a curiosity than a threat," but then it got outside the scientific realm and beyond CDC's control.

The day after the ACIP meeting, Jim Bloom and other members of CDC's management staff began to put together a document entitled "Action Memorandum" for Sencer. This paper subsequently was cited by critics of the swine flu–immunization campaign as the document that "put the gun to the head of the administration." It presented four options: (1) do nothing and let the marketplace prevail; (2) subsidize vaccine manufacturers but go no further; (3) launch an extensive immunization program with the government in complete control; or (4) make grants to the states to purchase vaccines and immunize the population at risk, using the resources of both the public and the private sector. Sencer favored the fourth option. The cost, at fifty cents a shot, plus expenses for administration, research, and surveillance, would be $134 million. The memorandum indicated there was a "*strong possibility* that this country will experience widespread A/swine influenza in 1976–77" (emphasis added). As he had promised, Sencer called the ACIP members and reached most of them, but not Alexander. All lent their support to option four.[9]

The memorandum went to assistant secretary for health, Dr. Theodore Cooper, who forwarded it to HEW Secretary David Mathews under his own signature. When HEW's top staff convened in Washington for their daily staff meeting on Monday, March 15, Dr. Cooper had left for a business trip to Egypt, so the assistant secretary, Dr. James Dickson, was in charge. It was Dickson who accompanied Sencer and the BoB's Meyer to a conference with Secretary Mathews later that morning. Sencer recalled what happened:

> We briefed the secretary who kept asking the probability. He wanted a number. We could not give him one. It was unknown. In terms of the smoking gun approach, I did say that many things force decisions but this is the first time that a rooster had forced your decision. Flu vaccine is made in fertile eggs, and without roosters you do not have fertile eggs. . . . If we were going to do it, we had to do it while the manufacturers were ready. If we waited six weeks or two months, we could not get it. He had to make a decision soon.[10]

Sencer was later accused of giving the secretary a hard sell, but he insisted that his was no "tear-jerk story with people dying in the streets." The campaign was good preventive medicine, and "if you believe in that you sell it."

Later that morning, the secretary sent a memo to James T. Lynn, director of the Office of Management and Budget. There were no qualifying phrases. It mentioned "a return of the 1918 flu virus. . . . when half a million people died." And it added "The projections are that this virus will kill one million Americans in 1976." From that point on, the decisions that guided the immunization program were more political than scientific, and it was an election year.[11]

President Gerald R. Ford, sold on the idea that something had to be done, wanted to consult the nation's health and political leaders before making an announcement. Sencer, Meyer, and Seal provided a list of about fifty medical specialists, manufacturers, mayors, and governors who were invited to a White House conference. Among them were Dr. Sabin, for whom the White House dispatched a plane, and Dr. Jonas Salk, Sabin's rival in the controversy over polio vaccine. The day before the meeting, Sabin wrote Sencer expressing his support for this "nonprecedented effort to get this vaccine into 'every man, woman and child' in the country." It would guard against a possible epidemic and afford an opportunity to learn more about acute respiratory disease.[12]

The cabinet room of the White House was a bit small for the session with the president. In fact, some of those most closely involved in the decision-making process were bumped so that their superiors could come. The president, flanked by Drs. Sabin and Salk, listened as Assistant Secretary for Health Cooper filled in the background. The president then asked for everyone's opinion in turn. Although both Drs. Sabin and Salk shook their heads when the other was speaking, at the end of the meeting there seemed to be agreement that a national immunization campaign must be launched. After everyone had a chance to speak, the president invited anyone who hesitated to express his doubts openly to speak to him privately. He retired to the Oval Office to wait. No one followed.

Bolstered by unanimity, the president made the public announcement in the press room a few minutes later. He asked Congress to appropriate $135 million to inoculate every man, woman, and child in the United States. The congressional hearings began the following week.[13]

That much was policy. The decision to immunize nearly everyone in the United States was made at the highest possible level. The logistics of how to do it fell to Don Millar, who thus once more got a special and

difficult assignment from his boss. As director of CDC's Bureau of State
Services, Millar had direct contact with state health departments, a
liaison vital to the success of the immunization program. Perhaps it was
symbolic that he got the assignment on the Ides of March, the same day
that Sencer first briefed Secretary Mathews. "It fell to my lot; maybe it
was karma—maybe I had to pay off some past sins or something," he
said. The first problem was an organizational one. Should a special
organization be set up within CDC to handle it? Millar thought not. He
wanted the job left within the Bureau of State Services, where he had an
army of a thousand people on whom he could call, but he did set up a
special task force to oversee the National Influenza Immunization Program (NIIP) just as there had been one for smallpox eradication. It
included representatives from all segments of CDC: epidemiology, laboratory, training, immunization, public relations, health education, and
Millar's right-hand man, Windell Bradford, a public health advisor and
one of CDC's most efficient managers. It took the task force only a few
days to identify the basic elements of the massive program—vaccine
manufacture and distribution, field trials, mobilization of health resources, encouragement of public acceptance, and surveillance of reaction to the vaccine. Immunization would begin in September, and everything would be done by the end of the year. Secretary Mathews was
kept apprised of plans.[14]

Millar put the existing public health systems on an emergency foot-
ing. As in any immunization effort, the states were in charge of local
details, while CDC supplied vaccine, jet injectors, and personnel. CDC
also provided informed-consent materials, which were used for the first
time. An emergency superstructure, which Millar likened to the Rocky
Mountain fur trade, was set up. He divided the country into six regions
and assigned a "brigadier" to each. These brigadiers rendezvoused with
health officials just as the nineteenth-century brigadiers had rendezvoused with Indians and mountain men to buy furs. The task force in
Atlanta met three times a week, sometimes joined by Bill Foege, who
had returned from India to become CDC's assistant director for operations. They identified potential problems with a PERT chart (Program
Evaluation Review Technique), a method originally designed for weapons systems. It enabled them to predict most, but not all, of the problems that surfaced in the campaign.

Planning for the NIIP was well under way by the time state health
officials, presidents of state medical associations, and other representa-

tives of private medicine gathered at CDC on April 2 to talk about the program and learn what their role would be. In the week after President Ford's announcement, rumbles of dissent appeared in the news, and journalists were ready for a bit of fireworks in Atlanta. They knew Dr. Martin Goldfield would have something critical to say, and as soon as he took his seat, the cameras moved in. What he said duly appeared on the evening news. "There are as many dangers to going ahead with immunizing the population as there are [in] withholding. We can soberly estimate that approximately fifteen percent of the entire population will suffer disability reaction."[15]

Sencer was surprised at Goldfield's defection, and others were annoyed at the stridency of his attack. A delegate from New Hampshire noted that perhaps "the New Jersey contingent . . . feel they own the virus and have a right to more public visibility." The Medical Society of Wisconsin, like Goldfield, had doubts about the program, but Sencer's commitment remained secure. He saw the swine flu program as serving a double purpose: to provide insurance against a possibly devastating epidemic and to boost state health departments. For too long these departments had been pressured to provide sickness care rather than to work for prevention, and the swine flu program could set them once more on the right track. In that sense, Russell Alexander agreed with him. He wrote Sencer that preventive medicine had much to gain from the swine flu program, although he was still hesitant to proceed. Without another swine flu outbreak, prudence dictated stockpiling vaccine instead. He sent "personal regards from your 'half-a-hog' colleague."[16]

Swine flu posed a threat not only to the United States but to the entire world, so the World Health Organization became involved. WHO informed ninety-five influenza centers of cases in the United States, but since swine flu did not appear elsewhere, no other nation made plans for massive inoculations. Increased surveillance would suffice. Millar, who attended the meeting of the WHO expert committee on influenza in Geneva, observed that no other country was in a position to carry out an immunization program, "but nobody was pounding the table that you should not do it if you had the vaccine."[17]

Congress quickly passed the $135 million appropriations bill, which President Ford signed into law on April 15. During the congressional hearings, there were hints that trouble lay ahead with the pharmaceutical manufacturers over the matter of liability, but no one paid much heed.

In Atlanta, the task force worked on the nuts and bolts of the operation. Vaccine production was the first problem. Four pharmaceutical companies were needed to produce the unprecedented amount of vaccine, a task complicated by the presence of competing strains of the flu virus in the population. Thousands of doses of A/Victoria vaccine had been produced before the swine virus emerged. These were made into a polyvalent vaccine for high-risk groups by adding the swine flu strain. Major emphasis was on the production of monovalent swine vaccine for everybody else. Not everything went smoothly. Millions of doses of vaccine were lost when the Parke-Davis Company used the wrong seed chain, and the field trials produced both good and bad news. The good news was that for adults over twenty-four years of age, it took only half as much vaccine as had been anticipated to get a good response (200 chick cell agglutination units), and there were few side effects. Young adults aged eighteen to twenty-four, however, got a poor response and children from three to ten did not respond at all, except to doses so high there were excessive side reactions, mostly fever and sore arms. A national immunization program could hardly succeed if children were left out. These problems provided the backdrop for Goldfield once more to suggest stockpiling. He was echoed by Sabin, who joined the defectors. Sabin believed that the vaccine could be stockpiled in fire stations and other public places, and, in an emergency, volunteers could immunize the entire population of America in one or two days. Sencer thought that notion ridiculous. There were other, even more vocal, critics. Dr. Sidney Wolfe of Ralph Nader's Public Citizen Health Research Group began a drumbeat of criticism against the swine flu initiative as soon as President Ford announced it.

A second set of field trials for children pushed back the campaign schedule and raised inevitable doubts in the public mind. When the results of the second trials were in, recommendations for vaccine doses were made in nine different categories for four different vaccines—monovalent and bivalent, whole and split viruses—greatly complicating the program's logistics. One of these recommendations was for children under three. They should not take it at all.

While the field trials were under way, the swine virus disappeared. There were no cases of swine flu anywhere, either in the United States or in South America, where, if a pandemic were imminent, they should have appeared. But no one would say that there was no threat. In CDC's laboratory, Dowdle, Allen Kendall, and the staff worked diligently sending reagents to all the laboratories and running down every clue. It was Kendall who discovered the flaw in the Parke-Davis vaccine.

As Sencer said, "We did our best to prove that everything was not swine flu." When word came from the Philippines that the swine flu virus had been isolated from a taxi driver and that a number of schoolchildren had serologic evidence of exposure, Gary Noble went to investigate. He found a laboratory error. There were also two reports of swine flu isolates in the United States, but again both were laboratory errors. Even though any flu virus disappears in the summer, people began to wonder if the virus had gone away.[18]

The Bureau of Epidemiology got ready for the worst—an epidemic of swine flu. As always, surveillance was the key to control, but this time, the staff in "Epi" had unsurpassed equipment for tracking cases: computers. Dr. Philip Brachman, who became Epidemiology chief in 1971 when Langmuir retired, had no philosophical objection to computers, and Dr. Michael Hattwick, chief of the bureau's Respiratory and Special Pathogens Branch, was enthusiastic about them. He organized a staff of people who shared his convictions, including a statistician right out of graduate school who knew the latest techniques. Together they put together the most sophisticated surveillance system the public health system had ever seen. It was manned around the clock, ever alert to outbreaks or to consequences from immunization itself. There would be some adverse reactions; there always were.

It was the possibility of bad side effects from the vaccine that nearly brought the immunization campaign to a halt before it began. Only four days after problems with the vaccine were revealed, the American Insurance Association informed health officials, including Sencer, that the manufacturers of swine flu vaccine would not get liability insurance.

The hazards of vaccines were well known. The Cutter incident dramatically demonstrated that a vaccine can cause harm. So did cases of paralysis associated with the Sabin oral polio vaccine and rheumatoid manifestations traced to rubella vaccine. It had been only a few years since CDC had led the way in stopping smallpox vaccinations in the United States because of adverse reactions to one in a million vaccinees. Whenever vaccine usage went from 10,000 or 50,000 to millions of doses, a few severe reactions would follow. In January 1976, a month before swine flu appeared at Fort Dix, Bruce Dull, CDC's assistant director for programs, sent a memo to HEW Secretary Mathews recommending that the department request authority to establish a program to reimburse individuals who were damaged as a result of participation in immunization programs done for the community's benefit. Since society benefited from an individual's immunization, society had some responsibility for any adverse effects the action might have. The memo was returned to CDC with a note from the assistant secretary's office that the recommendation was not being forwarded to the secretary because there was no evidence that this would become a problem.[19]

The decision of the insurance companies not to provide liability coverage to vaccine manufacturers meant there would be no mass immunization program unless the government assumed responsibility. CDC would provide "informed-consent" forms, but this was not enough for pharmaceutical houses afraid of any program that involved immunization of 200,000,000 people in a litigious age. The congressional hearings took most of the summer. Should the government pay for suits that were baseless or only for those that had some merit? The tort claims bill, which ultimately became law, provided that any claim arising from the swine flu program should be filed against the federal government, but the government reserved the right to sue for compensation from other participants. President Ford pressured Congress to pass the legislation, but the bill might never have become law had not events in Philadelphia intervened.

David Sencer was walking down a hallway at CDC on the morning of Monday, August 2, when Mike Hattwick asked him if he had heard about the three deaths in Pittsburgh from something that sounded like influenza. All the victims had attended a recent convention in Philadelphia. A startled "What!" signaled Sencer's thoughts exactly. Was this swine flu? By nightfall, three EIS officers were in Pittsburgh, Harrisburg, and Philadelphia, where they began extensive "shoe-leather epidemiology." They collected specimens and sent them by courier to Atlanta. Ten more EIS officers joined them the next day, integrating their activities with the existing state and city investigations. Dr. David Fraser directed his team from headquarters in Philadelphia. Over the next three weeks, thirty-two CDC personnel went to Pennsylvania. There were twenty-five epidemiologists (a quarter of the entire force), two industrial hygienists, a specialist in occupational health, three statisticians, and an engineer.

For a few days, the number of acutely ill people mounted steadily, and so did the number of deaths. Patients had chest pains, high fever, and lung congestion. All of them had attended the Philadelphia State Convention of the American Legion held at the Bellevue-Stratford Hotel July 21–24, or had been in close proximity to the hotel. The outbreak fit the definition of an epidemic: an excessive number of cases in a community at a given time. Soon, it had a name, Legionnaires' disease.

Early reports from pathologists in Pennsylvania lent credence to speculation that swine flu had appeared; the fatal pneumonia looked suspiciously like viral pneumonia associated with a severe influenza infection. Before the epidemic subsided, 221 people became ill—182 Legionnaires and 39 others who had simply been in the vicinity of the Bellevue-Stratford. Twenty-nine Legionnaires and five others died, a mortality rate of 16 percent. The bell-shaped curve plotting the epidemic indicated a common source of infection, but the cause of the disease remained a mystery.

Legionnaires' disease had a profound effect on the National Influenza Immunization Program and on CDC. In Washington, news of the Philadelphia outbreak spurred Congress to pass the Tort Claims Act, and in Atlanta the epidemic set off the most intense search in CDC's history. Everyone was anxious. If the severe epidemic were swine flu, CDC had a major disaster on its hands. The immunization campaign would not begin for weeks. Should the Democratic Convention scheduled for Philadelphia be canceled? The seed virus could be spread all over the country.

Specimens from Legionnaires' disease victims began arriving at CDC laboratories on Monday night, August 2. Hundreds more followed in the weeks ahead. They were inoculated into eggs, tissue culture, and bacterial media. Specimens from autopsies were prepared for electron microscopy and fluorescent antibody staining. On Tuesday, August 3, the labs ruled out Lassa fever, rickettsiae, and some bacteria. By Wednesday, they knew that it was not bubonic plague or typhoid, and that it was unlikely to be swine flu. By Thursday, to everyone's relief, they were certain it was not swine flu, and the search for a toxin began. Dowdle relaxed a bit. Sencer went to Washington to testify on the liability issue before Senator Kennedy's subcommittee. He expressed confidence that the Philadelphia epidemic was not swine flu, but the appearance of such an acute illness highlighted the critical nature of the problem. If swine flu should occur, the nation was in trouble.[20]

Legionnaires' disease was a huge news story, ranked that year second in importance only to the election of Jimmy Carter as president of the United States. The Legionnaires' disease epidemic led the nightly news on television for five nights in a row, and NBC did a live half-hour program from CDC's Clifton Road headquarters. Hundreds of articles appeared in newspapers, and the epidemic was the cover story in *Time*. CDC's public affairs officer, Don Berreth, attributed the newsworthiness of Legionnaires' disease to the fact that it had pictorial qualities making it good for television: marching Legionnaires, coffins being lowered, epidemiologists, laboratorians, and no talking heads. The eight telephone lines in Berreth's office were busy for two weeks, with eight people always on hold. The center got 1,500 calls an hour during those two weeks, double the usual number. Three separate offices were set up to handle them—one for the news media, one for the general public, and one for scientists, engineers, physicians, and other professionals. On Saturday, when only the emergency line was open, the guard was so overwhelmed that Sencer took a turn at the telephone. He prided himself on his accessibility, but when the calls started to come to his home, he got an answering machine. There he often listened to the callers, "well-meaning people, not cranks."

In addition to calls, there were thousands of letters from the public suggesting a possible cause. The majority of these fell into several major categories: contaminated cigarettes or cigars, faulty air-conditioning, insect spray, toxic cleaning agents, drinking water from rusty pipes, homemade liquor, and contaminated food. One person sent a newspaper clipping dated 1905 telling of an immense terrapin pond that lay three stories beneath the Bellevue-Stratford (sic). Could turtles be blamed? Some of the more anxious members of the public, fearful that they might have Legionnaires' disease themselves, sent along specimens. The extraordinary interest in Legionnaires' disease might be attributed to the rarity of devastating epidemics, a measure of how far public health had come.[21]

At first, the publicity cast CDC in a favorable light. The disease detectives had a well-established reputation for solving difficult epidemiological puzzles, and there was every expectation that Legionnaires' disease would be no different. The *New York Times* ran a story on EIS exploits of the past: tracing hepatitis in Michigan high school students to the glaze on doughnuts; pinning the famous salmonella outbreak in Riverside, California, to a single well in the city's water system; identifying the cause of a typhoid outbreak in New York City to dry mix for mashed potatoes. The *Times* also reported the similarities of Legionnaires' disease to the Pontiac outbreak of 1968. "Everyone at the Center knows the Pontiac case by heart. It was one of their very few failures."[22]

As the weeks went by, however, and the cause of the disease was not found, the tone of the stories became strident. Conditioned by Watergate, investigative reporters sharpened their attack. References to past triumphs gave way to full-scale attacks on what they saw as current ineptitude. Legionnaires' disease became an albatross, hung first around the neck of the Bellevue-Stratford, which closed its doors forever in mid November, and then around the neck of CDC, whose very existence also seemed threatened. CDC was accused of ignoring the needs of the medical profession and public, giving too much attention to epidemiology and not enough to the needs of people who were actually sick. It was blamed for looking too hard for an infectious agent and not hard enough for a toxic cause; for collecting too few specimens, which might contain clues to the mystery; and the wrong kinds. The *New York Times* attacked the center editorially. Questioning why toxicologists had played such a small role in the investigation, it concluded, "The Center for Disease Control has not added to the lustre of its record by its performance here."[23]

Critics of CDC concentrated on its alleged failure to search for a toxin, a charge vigorously denied. In the toxicology laboratories at Chamblee, the staff worked sixteen-hour days performing complex tests, using the most advanced equipment—the gas chromatograph and the atomic spectrometer—to look for metals, traces of chlorine, bromine and fluorine compounds, fungicides, pesticides, and herbicides. "Chemistry," Sencer told one reporter, "is sometimes even more complicated than microbiology." Tests that could not be performed at Chamblee were done at the NIOSH laboratories in Cincinnati.

Nickel was most often cited as the culprit. Nickel carbonyl, an odorless, tasteless, colorless gas, was found in some tissue samples of the victims, and a toxin specialist at the University of Connecticut, Dr. F. William Sunderman, Jr., suggested that the gases might have seeped into the upper levels of the hotel from a smoldering fire of multiform invoices nearby. That suggestion brought the press in droves to Dr. Sunderman's university laboratory, and he let them in, cameras and all, to see what he was doing, quite likely skewing the results of his research.

CDC never put much faith in the nickel theory, a lapse for which it came under sharp attack. Lawrence Altman, a former EIS officer who had become a reporter for the *New York Times,* was especially interested in nickel as a possible cause and began to publish his own epidemic curve based on the theory of nickel poisoning. The syndicated columnist Jack Anderson raised the issue of a mad killer on the loose, someone with a bit of knowledge about chemistry who had mixed nickel carbonyl with dry ice and put it in the hotel's air-conditioning system. According to Anderson, CDC had tried to discourage Dr. Sunderman from talking. In Washington, Congressman John Murphy scheduled hearings. He wanted to know why CDC had dwelled so long on the possibility that Legionnaires' disease was swine flu at the cost of delaying or making impossible the pursuit of the real killer, a mysterious toxin. Berreth, speaking for CDC, denied the congressman's charges. "There's just no question but what toxic substances were considered from the outset here," he said.[24]

For weeks medical and scientific consultants trooped to Atlanta to look at the evidence and make suggestions. They could find nothing definite, but if they were certain of anything, it was that the cause of the epidemic was not a bacterium. The CDC staff were increasingly frustrated. Epidemiologist David Fraser kept asking himself what he had overlooked. In the toxicology laboratory at Chamblee, Dr. David D. Bayse, director of clinical chemistry, decided that everything had been done that could be done and that it was time for "review and appraisal." His laboratory contained the world's most advanced equipment for tracking and identifying chemicals in the body, and they had found nothing. "We have other projects which must be given attention," he told a reporter from a Philadelphia paper. "It is a matter of priorities."[25]

Congressional hearings on Legionnaires' disease were held in late November. Sencer reviewed CDC's activities on a day-by-day basis, cited the extensive work done by the health departments of Pennsylvania and Philadelphia, and concluded:

> One must adopt a certain sense of rational objectivity and scientific humility in acknowledging our failure to date to solve the question of etiology. . . . we must admit that there are diseases and conditions of ill health with which we are not familiar and which, as yet, we are unable fully to understand. This is not so much an admission of human failure as a recognition of how medical and biological science and knowledge evolve.

His explanation did not satisfy Congressman Murphy who, after two days of hearings, said that "the job done by the federal people, to be charitable, was botched up." He did not understand how "we could have been awarded three Nobel prizes this year in medicine and at the same time blow the search for the cause of the Philadelphia epidemic."[26]

By the time of these hearings, Legionnaires' disease had long since subsided, disappearing as mysteriously as it came, and the much-delayed campaign to immunize the nation against swine flu was under way. Difficulties with the vaccine itself, the necessity for a second set of field trials, and protracted debate over the liability issue cost the campaign much of its momentum. Millar's staff used the time to prepare and print sixty million consent forms. Before the campaign could get under way, however, Congress attached a proviso to the tort bill requiring that a wholly separate body, the National Commission on Protection of Human Subjects, review and consult on these forms. The commission criticized CDC's efforts and required an additional sheet be attached to the forms already printed. It was another major complication in a program already plagued with problems.

CDC staffers staged a slogan contest for the swine flu campaign. The winner was "No flu! Roll up your sleeve, America." The day finally came when the slogan was appropriate. The campaign began in fits and starts on October 1 because not all areas of the country had adequate supplies of the vaccine. Still, in only ten days, over one million Americans had received their shots, and the campaign was picking up speed. The next day, on October 11, three elderly people dropped dead in Pittsburgh shortly after receiving their immunizations. Although the first news story said there was no connection, later reports linked the deaths to a single batch of vaccine. Other apparently vaccine-related deaths were reported from around the nation. All three Pittsburgh victims had had existing serious heart conditions, and most of the others were not good risks, but this fact got lost in the news.

The deaths posed a dilemma. They were reported immediately, demonstrating the superiority of CDC's surveillance system, but did nothing to inspire confidence in the immunization campaign. It took four days to show that the Pittsburgh deaths were not vaccine-related. To reassure the nation, President Ford paused briefly in his campaign for reelection to get his own flu shot, an event duly aired on national television.

The campaign briefly sputtered after the deaths in Pittsburgh, and then resumed its pace. Immunization centers were set up in armories, shopping centers, and other public buildings, but not in schools as originally planned, because results of the first field trials excluded everyone under the age of eighteen. Results of the second field trials, on which recommendations for young people were based, did not come in until after the campaign got under way, and it was November 15 before the Advisory Committee on Immunization Practices made its report. In spite of this missed opportunity to immunize whole families at once, the campaign still accomplished a major miracle. In ten weeks, nearly fifty million doses of swine flu vaccine were given in the United States, most of it to civilians. There had never been anything like it.

With so many receiving the vaccine, CDC expected some complications, and Hattwick's surveillance unit was on guard. It investigated all reports of serious reactions—more than 2,000—including 181 deaths supposed to be vaccine-related. Many of these occurred within forty-eight hours after immunization and might have been vaccine-related, but when all adjustments for age, sex, and other medical factors were made, the statisticians concluded that the risks posed by the vaccine were slight. Deaths overall were actually fewer than might have been expected had no vaccinations been given.[27]

Nothing prepared Michael Hattwick or anyone else at CDC for the appearance of Guillain-Barré syndrome (GBS) among the vaccinees. The first indication of a problem came during the third week of November, when the surveillance network picked up the case of a Minnesota man who became ill with Guillain-Barré syndrome soon after he received a swine flu shot. The case raised few suspicions, but during the next week, three additional cases were reported from Minnesota, another three from Alabama, and one from New Jersey, all in people recently inoculated. A red flag went up in surveillance.

Guillain-Barré syndrome is a rare neurological disease that afflicts four or five thousand people in the United States every year. It has symptoms like polio, although usually not as severe, and is sometimes called French polio. In fact, is was by that name that Sencer first heard of this newest development in a campaign full of problems. His daughter in Minnesota called him one day and asked, "What's going on with the French polio?"

Nobody had an immediate answer. In early December, Michael Gregg asked Dr. Lawrence Schonberger, deputy chief of the Enteric & Neurotropic Disease Branch, to look into the cluster of Guillain-Barré cases in Minnesota and Alabama. When a case from New Jersey came in, that state was added to the list. Colorado was used as a control.

Schonberger could not determine whether or not Guillain-Barré syndrome was related to swine flu inoculation until he had more information on what the normal incidence was, and he could find only one study that gave reasonably good rates. The results of his initial study bothered him. The cluster of cases appeared the second or third week after the patients received the vaccine, and that was unusual. "If it were a coincidental thing, you might have a clustering during the first week. The patient would make an association. As you got further and further away, it would be less likely that you would make the association."

He reported his concerns to a Friday meeting of Millar's task force. They notified Sencer, who came in over the weekend to see what could be done. Surveillance was extended to eleven states. As the new data came in, Schonberger began to get a feel for it and became increasingly convinced that there was a problem. On Monday, December 13, he went over the data with top CDC officials, who called in outside experts. Among them was Alexander Langmuir. Over a telephone hookup Schonberger presented the data he had analyzed in terms of person-time of risk, a standard epidemiological procedure. He divided the total number of cases by the total number of those vaccinated. He thought the data showed a connection, but Langmuir, the most influential of the outside consultants, convinced Foege that while the data looked suspicious, GBS was not a major problem. CDC issued a press release acknowledging that some cases of GBS had occurred; it was not enough of a problem, however, to stop the national immunization program.

Schonberger left the meeting concerned and came to work the next day dejected. It was difficult to present the data on the telephone, and he thought he must have done something wrong. That day he got a call from Dr. Ronald Altman, an epidemiologist for New Jersey, who had just listened to the tape-recording of the regular Tuesday meeting of EIS officers at which Dr. Michael Hattwick of Epidemiology had announced that an investigation of GBS was being conducted. Hattwick had reported cases in New Jersey among people who had not been vaccinated and seemed to imply that the connection between swine flu inoculation and GBS was a chance occurrence. Altman protested that New Jersey was not being treated fairly. New Jersey had begun its immunization program two weeks after Minnesota; Altman did not think it was fair to count cases that occurred before anyone was inoculated as constituting evidence that there was no association with the vaccine.

Altman had a good point, and it set Schonberger to thinking there was something wrong with what he was doing. How should his analysis take into consideration the fact that Minnesota and New Jersey had not started vaccinating people at the same time?

> At two o'clock in the morning, I woke up. "My God, I've got it. I'm not analyzing this. It's *persons : weeks of risk*. The denominator for the unvaccinated would get bigger and the denominator for the vaccinated would be relatively smaller. I called my boss, John Bryant, and told him we had a problem. We had to do the reviews over again.

Schonberger had recently completed a year's study at Johns Hopkins University in CDC's Career Development Program. In Dr. George Comstock's advanced epidemiology class, he had done an exercise using person-time of risk as the appropriate denominator in certain situations. He pulled out his old lecture notes, and recalculated the numbers on

Guillain-Barré syndrome. When he finished his work, he saw that the risk factor had jumped to seven. A person who received swine flu vaccine had seven times the risk of getting GBS as by chance. In another conference call to the outside consultants on Thursday, December 16, Schonberger once again presented his data, this time using the new calculations. On the basis of fewer than three dozen cases of GBS, epidemiology demonstrated once again its power to predict. The National Influenza Immunization Program was suspended immediately. It was never resumed.[28]

The next day Foege was at a meeting in the office of Assistant secretary for Health Cooper in Washington. Cooper asked how many thought the association of Guillain-Barré syndrome and swine flu immunization was real. Foege was the only person who raised his hand.[29]

A variety of emotions marked the end of the swine flu program. For Schonberger, it was the exhilaration of discovery. For others, there was pride in having set the world's record for immunization and comfort in having found its Achilles' heel themselves. Everyone was relieved that the epidemic never arrived; most defended the correctness of CDC's response. In so doing, they demonstrated an unflinching, but perhaps unwarranted, faith in science and a naiveté about the politics of public health. The swine flu campaign was a painful lesson in the necessity and the difficulty of demonstrating to the public the degree of risk any threat to health poses.

At year's end there was still no answer to Legionnaires' disease, but William Foege was philosophical: the "unnerving [publicity] helped us develop humility about our own limitations." He predicted that "in five, ten, or twenty years from now when our technology is further advanced, we will find out what killed the Legionnaires."[30] He did not have to wait that long.

During the quiet of the Christmas holidays, Dr. Joseph McDade, a young scientist in Dr. Shepard's virus and rickettsia laboratory, had the leisure to clean out his desk. Among the things he found to read was the final report on the Legionnaires' disease epidemic, the Epi-2, which David Fraser with great thoroughness had delivered to all those who worked on the Philadelphia puzzler. Rickettsiae were an unlikely cause of Legionnaires' disease, but McDade had run tests in August and September as part of the CDC's leave-no-stone-unturned approach. He infected guinea pigs with material from dead Legionnaires. Within two days the guinea pigs became ill, and some of them died. He injected samples of spleen from sick guinea pigs into chicken eggs, and the embryos were dead within six days. He tested the eggs and blood samples from the guinea pigs for any rickettsia, and looked especially for *Coxiella burneti,* the organism that causes Q fever. He found nothing, put the slides away in a wooden box on his desk, and went on to other things.

In the Christmas lull, he had time to reflect a bit. Reminded of the Legionnaires' saga by the Epi-2 report, he decided to look at his slides again; he searched for anything that was unfamiliar, not just the usual rickettsiae. He put one slide under the microscope and looked at it for twenty minutes or so, and then at another and another. It was, he said, "like looking for a contact lens on a basketball court by crawling on your hands and knees with your eyes only four inches from the floor." After an hour or so, he saw something he had not noticed before, a small cluster of bright red rods. He pulled out more and more slides, and with increasing excitement, looked at them. Dr. Shepard looked at them, too, and agreed with McDade that something was there. Checking the notes he had made in August, McDade found the reason he had missed the organism earlier: he had concentrated too hard on rickettsia. The bright red rods were bacteria, which all the experts had ruled out.

In September he had tried to grow the organism in eggs treated with antibiotics, a standard procedure for rickettsiae and viruses, which allows them to grow without bacterial competition. The antibiotics killed what he was looking for. After seeing the bright red rods on the slides, McDade decided to try again. It took three days to get eggs from chickens that had not eaten feed laced with antibiotics. On December 30 he injected the eggs with tissue from the guinea-pig spleens. In six days, the embryos started to die. He made slides of the egg material, put them under the microscope and found them strewn with clusters of red rods. It was only then that he told Shepard and one or two colleagues that the material came from the Legionnaires' epidemic. They told no one else until they were more certain of the data.

Shepard got four samples of Legionnaires' blood from the virology lab and mixed it with the organisms McDade had grown. The indirect fluorescent antibody test for two of them was positive. The organism that made the Legionnaires sick was the same one just grown in the laboratory. McDade could not believe what was happening to him, "the rookie on the block" who had been at CDC for less than a year. The most distinguished pathologists in America had agreed that it could not be a bacterium, but he had evidence to the contrary. "You are disbelieving and mistrustful of your own data," he said. In the days that followed, Shepard's lab was alive with activity; dozens of tests on blood samples from CDC's stocks were run. The evidence held up. It was time to report to Sencer.[31]

Dr. Roslyn Q. Robinson, chief of the Bureau of Laboratories, made the appointment for Thursday afternoon, January 13. Dr. Dowdle would be there, and so would Drs. Brachman and Fraser from Epidemiology. Shepard and McDade arrived together at the big corner office on the second floor. McDade was very nervous. He was not sure of his data, and being new to CDC did not know all the people there. It was the first time he and Fraser had ever met. Nobody said much until Dowdle broke the silence, saying, "I guess we have found the organism that causes Legionnaires' disease." It was a startling announcement, the best news Sencer had had in months. Shepard did most of the talking, explaining step by step the work they had done. Over the weekend, he said, he wanted to repeat the work in a clean room where none of this material had been before. He was already "pretty sure."

To Sencer's query as to how sure that was, Shepard replied, "Well, I'm 99.9 percent sure," but for him that left too much margin for error. On the way out of the room, Shepard warned that nothing was to be said until McDade had published in the scientific literature, saying, "I won't have Dr. McDade being made fun of by his peers." Sencer knew this story could not be kept quiet. Legionnaires' disease had been front-page news for months; CDC would have to go back to Pennsylvania for more blood samples; the story was certain to leak. So Sencer and Shepard reached a compromise. A special edition of MMWR would be published on Tuesday, putting the work in the scientific literature.

Everything went well. Tests done over the weekend confirmed the earlier data, and MMWR went to press. About ten o'clock Tuesday morning, Shepard literally "came running" into Sencer's office. He had just run the serum from the unsolved St. Elizabeths epidemic of 1965, and it was caused by the same organism as Legionnaires' disease. They stopped the presses in the basement of CDC, the new information was inserted, and the deadline met.[32]

At the Tuesday afternoon conference, 300 CDC employees crowded into the auditorium. Don Berreth orchestrated the event so that the press was kept waiting outside until the CDC family heard the news. Although Sencer qualified his remarks—a bacterium had been found that was "quite definitely associated with the disease"—everybody knew what he meant. CDC had found the cause of Legionnaires' disease. The news boosted everybody's morale at a time of trauma. It was a big day, one to be savored.

CHAPTER 19

Aftermath

The euphoria at 1600 Clifton Road was short-lived. CDC had to atone for its failings in what came to be known as the swine flu affair. Just twenty days after the breakthrough in Legionnaires' disease, as national television cameras bored in, David Sencer was fired. At least, that was the way it appeared. The ostensible reason was that Joseph Califano, President Carter's newly appointed secretary of health, education and welfare, wanted to name his own staff. To Sencer's colleagues at CDC, however, he was the sacrificial lamb.

The Carter administration was but two weeks old when Sencer was called to Washington for a conference with Hale Champion, undersecretary of HEW, who told him he would be replaced as director of the Center for Disease Control. There would be no immediate announcement, but Sencer reminded Champion, "This place leaks like a sieve." The word was certain to get out by Monday, when the secretary had scheduled a conference of outside experts to consider resuming use of A/Victoria vaccine to halt an outbreak of flu in nursing homes. That was a mere three days away. It did not take that long for the news of Sencer's dismissal to get out. By the time he got back to Atlanta, a colleague had a verbatim account of what had taken place in Champion's office.

Sencer wanted to break the news to his top staff before they read it in the newspaper. He tracked down Champion to get permission, and called them one by one. He did not cancel the party at his home that evening to which they had already been invited. The party was a "bit wake-ish," but no one was prepared for what happened on Monday.

The conference on resuming use of A/Victoria vaccine (all of which had been combined with the swine strain) was held in the penthouse of the House Office Building. Dr. John Knowles of the Rockefeller Foundation, and Dr. Ivan Bennett, dean of the New York University Medical Center, were in charge. About midday, the press officer entered, motioned to Sencer, told him the press had the story and asked how he wanted to respond. Sencer answered with a one-liner: "The Secretary wants to select his own staff." But, as Sencer recalls, it did not end there.

> A bit later, the Secretary came in and leaned over John Knowles and asked in a stage whisper, "Which one is Sencer?" John pointed to me. The Secretary came over and said, "Come here." The TV cameras followed. The Secretary said, "I want to say something nice about you: 'Even though Dr. Sencer is not going to be with us anymore, we appreciate his contributions.'"

The walk to the back of the room made the nightly news, and Sencer got home in time to see himself fired.[1]

The next day Califano explained that he was looking for "some fresh air . . . some fresh faces" at CDC, where Sencer had been director for eleven years. Sencer's head was not the only one to roll. Califano replaced the directors of all PHS agencies except Dr. Donald Frederickson at NIH. The secretary insisted politics would play no part in choosing Sencer's replacement. "[B]elieve me," he told the press, "if you had just been through what I have been through in the last week in trying to think through this swine flu program, you would be damned sure that there were no politics in the health area and that you had the best minds available in this country to help with those issues."

The staff at CDC were both hurt and angry. Sencer was a popular, effective leader, and one whom many regarded with awe. To them he personified the best in public service and in public health. They sent a petition to the secretary with 349 signatures asking that he be allowed to stay.[2]

Announcement of Sencer's imminent removal was but one of the shocks the Center for Disease Control endured in that gloomy February of 1977. Robert Dubignon and George Flowers, two employees in Building 7, where many of the center's laboratories are located, died of Rocky Mountain spotted fever. One was a janitor, the other a laboratory services employee who delivered glassware and ran the autoclave. Neither had been immunized against *Rickettsia rickettsii*. February was not the right season for tick bites; both had to have been exposed while at work.

At first it was feared that the Legionnaires' bacterium or "dirty" viruses from the "Hot Lab" had somehow escaped and killed the two men, and that others would be stricken. The mobile quarantine facility was put on standby. Karl Johnson, guardian of the "Hot Lab," did not see how it could be Ebola or Marburg or Lassa fever, since he allowed no maintenance help in the building (he and the staff did all the cleanup themselves), but he worried nonetheless and was greatly relieved when his lab was absolved. It was a relief, too, when Legionnaires' disease was ruled out. For two employees to die of a disease on which the CDC had worked for years, however, was a devastating blow. A feeling of gloom pervaded the center. The low point of Walter Dowdle's career was attending the funerals.

More than a week passed after these funerals before the cause of death was definitely determined, and on that day an intensive investigation into laboratory safety began. Some of the blame could be laid on the gap between procedures and practices, to a kind of casual attitude engendered by the center's heretofore unblemished safety record. Some blame could be attached to the numerous changes made in Building 7 since it had first been occupied in 1960. Laboratories that were supposed to have negative air pressure no longer had it. The investigation also zeroed in on the buildings at Chamblee, still in use seventeen years after they were supposed to have been replaced. They had glaring flaws. Viral research, particulary, needed much more secure facilities. Karl Johnson thought that CDC's "we can do it" spirit had pushed such difficult investigations as hemorrhagic fevers without the proper facilities. The need for a new building could be ignored no longer, and the long process of lobbying for it got under way.[3]

For the rest of 1977, CDC picked up the pieces left in the wake of year-long trauma and savored overlooked triumphs. The public fascination with swine flu and Legionnaires' disease distracted attention from CDC's work on Ebola fever. CDC had stopped an epidemic that had killed hundreds in Africa in its tracks and identified the cause. The final chapter in the global eradication of smallpox was written that year as well.

Still, the swine flu affair could not be forgotten. Legal claims from victims of Guillain-Barré syndrome kept it alive. Dr. Martin Goldfield of the New Jersey State Health Department, the most vocal critic of the influenza immunization program, turned his attention to Lawrence Schonberger, who had linked GBS to the swine flue vaccine. Goldfield said the risk of getting GBS continued for twenty-six weeks after getting a swine flu shot; Schonberger insisted the risk was greatest during the first five weeks and disappeared after ten weeks. This disparity was of obvious interest to victims of GBS claiming compensation from the government. Schonberger had to deal with one lawyer after another, who even searched his trash baskets for evidence. The Justice Department asked a group of experts, led by Alexander Langmuir, to analyze the data again. One of them, the distinguised epidemiologist Dr. Leonard T. Kurland, saw no association at all between swine flu vaccine and Guillain-Barré syndrome. Kurland's reputation was too great for CDC to ignore his challenge, so the investigation was reopened. The scientific dispute continued for ten years, with Schonberger being first vindicated, then repudiated, then once more vindicated.[4]

Except for this controversy, the swine flu affair was finished, but publication of a report made it impossible to forget. Secretary Califano asked Richard Neustadt, a political scientist at Harvard, to study and analyze the national immunization program. Neustadt in turn recruited Harvey Fineberg, Harvard colleague, physician, and leader in the field of medical decision analysis. *The Swine Flu Affair: Decision-Making on a Slippery Disease* was published as a government report in November 1978. It detailed the swine flu story from the outbreak at Fort Dix to Sencer's dismissal. The authors found no villains among the government's officials and advisors: "[A]nyone (ourselves included) might have done as they did—but we hope not twice." If Sencer was no villian, the authors nonetheless described him as "an able, wily autocrat" and pictured him as manipulative.[5]

Neustadt's indictment of CDC in general and of Sencer in particular was perceived as harsh, but accurate, by at least one reviewer of the book, Robert D. Bahn, of Duke University, who called the "swine flu caper" a "classic fiasco, replete with premature commitment, personal agendas, incomplete analysis, unspecified uncertainties, unstated assumptions, the neglect of implementation, and the failure to reconsider prior decisions." Bahn found CDC's efforts indefensible and asked how the president or the secretary of HEW could protect himself and the public "from scientific expertise gone, not mad, but conscientiously and collectively amuck?"[6]

Dr. D. A. Henderson, the dean of the School of Public Health at Johns Hopkins University, who had such long ties to CDC, was irate about the Neustadt book. Sencer was irritated, not so much with what was said about him as with the implication that CDC was Machiavellian. Don Millar felt betrayed. He likened Neustadt's and Fineberg's "attack" to a scene from the movie *Bonnie and Clyde.*

> There is a big shoot-out. Clyde's brother is killed and his girlfriend is blinded. Bonnie and Clyde escape. The girl is sitting in a cell bandaged all over. This guy whose life purpose is to run down Bonnie and Clyde comes in behind her and sweet-talks her about how good he is going to make

everything. He gets her to open up and she starts revealing information, and he gets the piece that he wants and walks out the door. She thinks in her blindness that he is a friend trying to help. . . .

Neustadt sat here and said, "I know you people are emotionally upset; it is a big blow for you; you have been an outfit with great prestige; you know people are saying things about you that are not true. Tell us about it."[7]

There was comfort to be found in work, and at CDC the work of unraveling the mystery of Legionnaires' disease had barely begun. Within days after McDade and Shepard linked the St. Elizabeths outbreak to Legionnaires' disease, they retrieved serum of Pontiac fever victims from CDC's deep freeze. Analysis showed that Pontiac fever and Legionnaires' disease were caused by the same organism, even though Pontiac fever was a much milder disease. Strangely, that discovery, resolving one of the center's few epidemiological failures, set off new waves of criticism. Why had not the organism been discovered in 1968? Why had CDC abandoned the search after only two years? It should have been more diligent. Critics questioned if McDade had really found the cause of Legionnaires' disease. Had CDC given the toxin theory short shrift?

An atmosphere of doubt permeated the meeting of the American Society of Microbiology in New Orleans in the spring of 1977. McDade and Shepard were there to give a preliminary report of their data. Hundreds of scientists along with some reporters crowded into the large ballroom. Afterwards, there were questions. Some in the audience were skeptical; some wanted clarification; some hinted at sinister plots; some were congratulatory. Shepherd fielded the questions while McDade stood by "pretty much overwhelmed by it." Shepard, a world-renowned man in his sixties, distinguished for his work in leprosy, was calm and cool. For a bit McDade thought it would have been nice to be answering the questions himself and wondered why Shepard was doing this. After all, Shepard's role had been mostly advisory. But as McDade listened, he realized he would not be doing very well and was glad Shepard was there. They did not talk about it then, but a year or so later, when the relationship between the two had grown easy, the subject came up. McDade said he had come to realize that Shepard was protecting him that day in New Orleans. Shepard looked at the younger man and said, "That's exactly why I did it." He did not need the limelight. "He was clearly protecting me," McDade said, "making sure that I was not turned around and made to look foolish."[8]

McDade's discovery of the casuative organism was just the starting point for the laboratory work on Legionnaires' disease. The nature and life cycle of the bacterium had to be ferreted out, its habits discovered. This could not be done until the bacteria were grown in quantity, which was difficult to do. McDade asked a CDC bacteriologist, Dr. Bob Weaver, to help. Weaver, described by his boss Dr. Albert Balows as a "bread and butter bacteriologist," put the organism in several different mediums, including a "chocolate" one containing virtually everything self-respecting bacteria would want nutritionally. After three or four days, something appeared to be growing, even though under the microscope it did not look like much. When Shepard and McDade mixed it with serum from the Legionnaires' patients, however, they got a reaction that indicated infection. "It was 'Eureka!' if there ever was one," said Balows.

The fact that the same bacterium caused the highly fatal outbreaks in Philadelphia and St. Elizabeths and the relatively mild Pontiac fever meant that it had a wide spectrum. Scientists had seen both ends of it, but not the gradations in between. Using the guinea pig as a model, they got to work. Gradually, the Legionnaires' bacterium released its secrets. It was fastidious and difficult to propagate. Its growth characteristics were quite unlike those of any other bacteria. It grew best on solid nutrient media plates rich in hemoglobin and the amino acid cysteine. It liked a temperature close to that of the human body and a carbon dioxide–laden atmosphere. It was slow growing but exceptionally hardy. It was gram negative. Almost a year after McDade saw the first red rods in his microscope, information was still too sketchy for the bacterium to be named. Only when its characteristics became better known was it called *Legionella pneumophilia.*[9]

For the epidemiologists, identification of the Legionnaires' bacterium opened up exciting possibilities. There were probably other Legionnaires' victims out there. With a positive means of identifying them available, David Fraser was ready to search the country. He looked especially at the thousands of cases of pneumonia caused each year by unknown organisms. He arranged for six health officers from Connecticut to Florida to send serum from these patients. Within weeks it began to arrive, not only from Fraser's sources, but from physicians all over the country who were suspicious of any pneumonia not quickly diagnosed.

The volume of work quickly overwhelmed McDade's and Shepard's small laboratory. The indirect fluorescent antibody test was too complicated and time-consuming for the amount of work that poured in on them. They looked for a simpler, quicker test that could be taught to other laboratories. The number of sporadic cases of Legionnaires' disease postively identified quickly mounted. By November 1977, there were eighty-eight in twenty-seven states, the District of Columbia, and several foreign countries. Among them were three Scottish tourists who had died while on holiday in Spain in 1973. Scottish health officials, who had saved the serum for four years, sent it to CDC for analysis.

The numerous leads on Legionnaires' disease created an air of excitement on Clifton Road. McDade outlined the scope of the problem for a reporter:

> If it [the unnamed bacterium] is in the air, you have to find out how it gets in the air. If it's in the soil, you have to find out how it's replenished in the soil. . . . [I]f an animal excreted something in the soil in a certain spot, does this make this one little spot full of organisms? And if they're stirred up, do they infect people? It's more complicated than the average person realizes, and it takes a lot of time.[10]

In November 1977, the Senate Health Subcommittee held a hearing on Legionnaires' disease at CDC. Senators Jacob Javits, Edward Kennedy, and Richard Schweiker were there, as well as the subcommittee's counsel. Representing CDC were David Fraser, Walter Dowdle, and William Foege, CDC's new director. Foege, the lead-off witness, testified that CDC had devoted 73,000 man-hours and $1.5 million to solving the mystery of Legionnaires' disease, that the discovery of the causative organism was accomplished in the face of overwhelming odds, and that science was only in the infancy of understanding it. What they did know was that the bacterium had been around for a long time, that its likely mode of transmission was through the air, that its natural home was most likely somewhere in nature rather than in the human population, and that the bacterium caused both outbreaks of disease and isolated cases. In the latter, the fatality rate was high. No more than 1.5 percent of unexplained pneumonias, however, could be blamed on it.[11]

Dr. Leonard Bachman, the secretary of public health for Pennsylvania, was also at the hearing. He voiced two complaints: Legionnaires' disease had become a media event, and CDC had given too much help during the epidemic in Philadelphia. "I believe the public health power is clearly a right reserved for states under the Constitution," said Bachman. "On some things I would rather they not relieve us, and let us fight our own battles." Senator Kennedy was amazed that Bachman had raised the states' rights issue. He thought CDC had taken "the rap [for] Pennsylvania," which the State Health Department could not have done. "Everybody here deserves a Nobel prize," Kennedy said. The statement fell pleasantly on the ears of those at CDC, but Dowdle noticed that as soon as it was made, the camera lights went off, and the newsmen left. Press accounts of the hearings made no mention of the senator's praise.[12]

Criticisms of CDC's handling of Legionnaires' disease continued for months. A New York physician ridiculed the agency's pursuit of what he called "their bug" to the neglect of such a promising target as phosphene gas. Lawrence Altman of the *New York Times* asked if it was not the "embarrassment of failing to find an immediate solution in a widely publicized epidemic [that] gave the crucial extra impetus for the search?" The *National Enquirer* chimed in with the charge that CDC's claim to have found the cause was "a great hoax . . . a desperate bid to save their reputations" in the wake of public outrage over the swine flu fiasco. But there was praise, too, and sweet it was. It appeared as an editorial in the prestigious *New England Journal of Medicine*, which called the work done by the Center for Disease Control "a brilliant example of scientific achievement. . . . This is a saga of medical science at its best, and the public have been the beneficiaries." Secretary Califano sent Christmas greetings to CDC staff congratulating them on the "fine job you have done in Legionnaires' Disease. I am proud of you."[13]

Gradually, information about Legionnnaires' disease accumulated, not only at CDC but in laboratories around the world. Hundreds of scientists began to probe its secrets. CDC speeded the process by training health officials in lab techniques. In December 1977, 120 of them came for the first course. The following May, CDC published the first edition of *Legionnaires': The Disease, the Bacterium and Methodology*, a manual intended for worldwide distribution. By the time four hundred scientists from thirty nations met in Atlanta in November 1978 for a symposium on Legionnaires' disease, more of its mystery had been stripped away. Rarely in the history of microbiology had knowledge developed so quickly about a new organism. In welcoming the delegates to the international symposium, CDC Director Foege praised this "restless passion to understand."[14]

CHAPTER 20

The Lengthened
Shadow of a Man (3)

Appointment of Dr. William Foege as director of CDC in the spring of 1977 was good news. For two months after David Sencer was summarily fired, CDC was rife with rumors that the new director would be chosen for political reasons. HEW Secretary Joseph Califano came to Atlanta to make the announcement personally. He said Foege's appointment was a "clear signal . . . that the health programs of this Department will be headed by the finest professionals in the nation."[1] There was a palpable sense of relief.

Foege had a long association with CDC, and he was immensely popular. For two years he had been Sencer's assistant and protégé. He had not sought the job of director, but he was the only person Sencer recommended. That recommendation may have influenced Foege's appointment; it was essential to his acceptance. Like Sencer, Foege wanted to broaden CDC's mission, to apply the principles of prevention to environmental and lifestyle issues that had worked so well with infectious diseases. His plan was similar to that of the Under 42 Committee, and it accorded with a general shift of emphasis in public health towards chronic diseases.

The new director had grown up in a family of six children, his father a minister, his mother a proud woman who even in the depression did not want anyone to know they were poor. She believed that if you instilled in children a sense of curiosity, they would educate themselves. She taught them that the world is governed by cause and effect, not by an irrational fate. It was good training for a future scientist.

Foege graduated from the University of Washington Medical School, and after an internship at the Public Health Hospital on Staten Island, he joined the EIS and was assigned to the State Health Department of Colorado. While there, he got orders to go to New Mexico to examine a child suspected of having smallpox. He knew nothing about smallpox, but found out from colleagues in Atlanta which book he should read en route. He had time only to learn the difference between smallpox and chicken pox, but to those who met him at the airport, he was the out-of-town expert. His interest in smallpox began that day and never waned.

Medical missions with the Lutheran Church were Foege's destiny, and as soon as he received his Master of Public Health degree at Harvard, he went to Nigeria. But for the Nigerian Civil War, he probably would have spent the rest of his life there. As it was, the war drove him out of the country, and he found a home at CDC in the smallpox program. Millar recruited him and Langmuir encouraged him. This was missionary work with a different twist; it was done under auspices other than those of the church.[2]

The CDC staff knew Foege as the architect of the E^2 plan for smallpox eradication, as an overseer in the swine flu program, and as a dedicated scientist with almost no ego. They knew him, too, as a practical joker, Sencer being his favorite target. When EIS celebrated its silver anniversary in 1976, Sencer could not be there to see Alexander Langmuir receive the Creation Award, edging out God and Zeus, nor to accept for himself the Foresight Award, presented to him for having made the most ridiculous prediction during the past year: the eradication of measles in the United States. Foege accepted the "Silver Alex" (a shoe with a hole in it) for Sencer and began to plot. He would even the score with his boss, who had once had the whole Foege family detained by quarantine officials in Honolulu on the grounds that their vaccination certificates were bogus.

Sencer wondered how the shoe would be presented. Would it be at WHO headquarters in Geneva? At a staff meeting in Washington? Foege would do nothing so mundane; he had it presented in church. Sencer muttered Foege's name as he slipped out of the pew and went to the front. The minister presented the shoe and read the citation Foege had written. The congregation applauded enthusiastically; Sencer shifted from one foot to the other. Just for a moment, Foege thought he should not have done it.[3]

The first picture of Foege as director of the Center for Disease Control is one with eight inches of shirtsleeve showing. Califano told him of the appointment the day before the public announcement but cautioned him to tell no one but his wife. Don Berreth, ordered to get a photograph of the new director, decided for the sake of security to take it himself. He asked Foege to come to his office in his usual shirtsleeves, lest the staff get suspicious. Berreth lent him a jacket. From the shoulders up, it did not matter, but Berreth could not resist taking shots with inches of shirtsleeve showing. Although he assured Foege the pictures would never see the light of day, he immediately had twelve copies made and distributed throughout the building.[4]

The photo session was a light-hearted moment preceding the assumption of a very tough job. CDC was still in turmoil. It had been under intense public scrutiny for a year, and the spotlight was unlikely to go away. As one science reporter for a TV network told Richard Neustadt, CDC "lost its innocence" in the swine flu affair. After Watergate and Vietnam, it was "almost the last Federal agency widely regarded by reporters and producers as a *good thing,* responsible, respectable, scientific, and above suspicion."[5] Unfairly or not, the perception of CDC had changed, with devastating results for staff morale and confidence. The old fear that CDC would be dismembered returned. Foege's first job, like that of Ted Bauer a quarter of a century earlier, was to keep that from happening.

Sencer had groomed Foege for a year and a half for the directorship of CDC, and he continued to offer guidance from nearby Emory University, where he had a short-term appointment. But the new director was left pretty much on his own insofar as relations with those in Washington were concerned. A new administration brought an entirely new contingent to the PHS and HEW. Obviously, Foege had won Califano's confidence, but the new HEW secretary was not an easy man to please. Foege found him both very demanding and very supportive. When Califano, the architect of many of Lyndon Johnson's Great Society programs, decided to back a program, as he did with immunization (see chapter 21), that support was total. Still, he was exacting in his demands. Foege's trips to Washington increased geometrically. In his determination to manage the behemoth that was HEW, Califano demanded an instant response from all who worked for him. Foege was no exception, even though Atlanta was six hundred miles away. If Califano notified Foege in the morning to be at a conference in Washington in the afternoon, he expected him to be there. On one occasion, as

Foege was returning home, he was paged at the Atlanta airport. Califano ordered him back to Washington; Foege caught the next plane.

Most of Califano's staff were as hard-driving as he was, but in Dr. Julius Richmond, who held a joint appointment as assistant secretary of health and surgeon general, Foege found genuine support. A pediatrician and founder of the Head Start program, Dr. Richmond was dedicated to the idea of child health. He also believed that the American people should take more responsibility for their health by practicing healthier lifestyles. Along these lines, his thinking paralleled Foege's.

A long-time staff member said that Foege's main trouble as director was that "he assumed that everybody at CDC and in Washington was as good as he was, and he was wrong." Sencer tried unsuccessfully to convince him otherwise. When funds were short, and they often were, Foege was left pretty much on his own to fight the battles on Capitol Hill. He knocked on doors and shook hands. Simply showing up to talk to people helped, and he wished later that he had done more of that; he thought he was far too slow in understanding how Congress worked. CDC was a good team player and never went behind the backs of its PHS bosses, but Foege learned that much is expected on the Hill. What frustrated him most was navigating through the different layers of government. Each level cut out things, mostly for the cutting's sake.

The real competition for funds in the late 1970s came not from other agencies of the PHS but from the huge demands of Medicare and Medicaid. During the Califano years, the increase in the budget for those two programs alone was more than the total budget for all of the PHS. Foege learned that whatever party was in power, the odds were stacked against funding for public health. It never competed well. He had to show that public health was not only safe and efficacious but that it had a positive benefit-cost ratio, and he had to do it over again every year. Usually, the Senate was more sympathetic to his pleas than the House, but no other field of medicine had to run such a gauntlet.[6]

Foege's particular genius in bolstering the fortunes of CDC in a difficult time was in reaching out to the medical profession and the lay public for advice on shaping the agency's future. Sencer's Under 42 Committee came entirely from within the institution. Foege sought advice from hundreds of people outside CDC, the first time in more than two decades the agency had actively sought outside guidance. He benefited from this collective wisdom, and, more important, he developed a national mandate for an institution that had been under attack.

The replies were varied, but many voiced a common theme: CDC should not forget its original mission of service to the states as advisor and educator. Neither should it forget its historical long suit—the control of infectious disease—but its horizons should expand to include health issues of the past decade that seemed to have passed CDC by: environmentalism, consumerism, ecology, occupational health, and medical-care evaluation. It should do more in international health, building on the solid foundation laid in the Smallpox-Eradication Program. There was but one caution. In expanding its scope, CDC should lose neither its humanity nor its informality.[7]

From the respondents, Foege chose sixteen health professionals and laymen to study CDC's programs and policies.[8] This "Red Book Committee," as it came to be known, was chartered in December 1977, met three times during the next six months, and submitted its report in July 1978. None of the members had a formal connection with CDC, although there were several alumni: D. A. Henderson and George I. Lythcott of the Smallpox-Eradication Program, and James O. Mason, once CDC's deputy director and destined to become its next director. The committee's best-known non-scientist was Betty Bumpers, wife of Senator Dale Bumpers, the former governor of Arkansas. She was intensely interested in immunization programs. Foege appointed a CDC insider as chairman of the committee, J. Donald Millar, the man who had recruited him and had directed so many of CDC's major efforts.

The committee's charge was to study the morbidity and mortality statistics and point out what had to be done to prevent illness and premature death. Millar designed a three-stage process: identifying the leading diseases and health problems in the country; determining how to work in those areas; and defining CDC's role in the process. The work of the Red Book Committee was a first step towards a complete reorganization of CDC (see chapter 23).

After lively debate, the committee drew up a list of the twelve most important health problems in the United States. Initially, hernia made the cut, and it might have stayed on the list had it not been for D. A. Henderson's objections. As it was about to be approved, Henderson, the leader of the global smallpox-eradication effort, jumped up. It was too much for CDC to recommend that hernia be considered one of the principal health problems of the United States. Henderson won the day. The final list had a broad scope: alcohol and its consequences; cancers (when detected early); cardiovascular diseases; contamination of drinking water; dental diseases; hazardous health exposures in the work place; infant mortality; motor vehicle accidents; newly recognized diseases and unexpected epidemics; nosocomial infections; smoking; and vaccine-preventable diseases in children. After much discussion, three others were added for special consideration: mental illness, social disorders, and stress.[9]

The committee agreed that *primary* prevention was the best means of reducing morbidity and mortality, and pointed to the undeniable fact that there was no agency in the United States responsible for advocating primary prevention activities. It recommended that CDC become that agency. The technical knowledge to prevent much unnecessary morbidity and mortality was available; what was needed was a national commitment to apply that knowledge in a rational, efficient manner. CDC's close relationship with the states, its long experience in epidemiological investigations and surveillance, and its excellent laboratories made it ideally suited to become the nation's premier institution dedicated to prevention. As the nation's "conscience for prevention," CDC should champion the cause loudly, continuously, relentlessly.[10]

Foege became the chief advocate of prevention. During the next two years, he sold the idea both within CDC and in Washinton. The CDC staff met twice at Berry College in Rome, Georgia, to voice any objections to the Red Book report, and decide what, if anything, should be added. The principal change was the addition of environmental health as a major issue. Also added to the list were violence and unwanted pregnancy. This brought the number of top priority items to fifteen. Of all the areas, violence was the most controversial and the one the public health community found hardest to accept. Foege needed all the persuasive powers at his command to convince others that murders and suicides were health problems. He believed that the basics of infectious-disease control—epidemiology and surveillance—could be used to control violence just as they had been used to provide relief in famines. Gradually, as the scope of a broader program for prevention emerged, it became obvious that CDC was not structured to handle it. The institution would have to be reorganized. The first discussions on changing the organizational pattern, little altered since the institution was founded, took place at the second Rome conference, but more than two years passed before reorganization became a reality.

Planning for reorganization went on simultaneously with the more pressing task of producing a broad-scale national prevention strategy. The United States had never had a national health plan, but Canada had recently detailed such a policy in *A New Perspective on the Health of*

Canadians. The conceptual framework of Canada's program was that lifestyle made a difference. At Foege's behest, the CDC staff drew up a prevention strategy for the United States and set goals for 1990. Foege took the report to Washington, showed it to Surgeon General Richmond, and asked permission to publish it as a CDC document. Richmond was so impressed that he proposed giving the study a broader base by publishing it under the aegis of the Public Health Service. He appointed a task force to make it readable and persuasive and give it popular appeal.

Dr. James Michael McGinnis, the assistant surgeon general, and two members of CDC's staff, Martha Katz and Dennis Tolsma, were the principal architects of the popularized report, although many people worked on it in both Atlanta and Washington. They drew on a general sense that something was not quite right in the world of public health, that medicine did wonderful things but at enormous cost, that some people were kept alive with no marginal gain in the quality of life. One day Richmond asked those working on the report what it would be called. Tolsma pulled out the thesaurus. They played around with "Advanced Health" and the "Notion of Wellness." Then Tolsma asked what the goal of the project was. The answer: healthy people. Why not call it that? Tolsma asked. *Healthy People: The Surgeon General's Report on Health Promotion and Disease Prevention*, published in 1979, was widely distributed. It came to be synonymous with the concept of health objectives and with the idea that lifestyle is important in promoting health.[11]

In an introduction to *Healthy People*, Secretary Califano wrote that the aim was "to encourage a second public health revolution in the history of the United States." The first revolution, which occurred in the late nineteenth and early twentieth centuries, was against infectious diseases. The second revolution, aimed at the killers and cripplers, could be achieved more by prevention than by cure.

> We are killing ourselves by our own careless habits.
> We are killing ourselves by carelessly polluting the environment.
> We are killing ourselves by permitting harmful social conditions to persist—conditions like poverty, hunger and ignorance—which destroy health, especially for infants and children. . . .
> You, the individual, can do more for your own health and well-being than any doctor, any hospital, any drug, any exotic medical device.

He cited the goals for 1990: a reduction in the mortality rate for everyone under sixty-four and a major improvement in health, mobility, and independence for older people.[12]

Healthy People contained commonsense advice. Do not smoke; cut down on alcohol; reduce the intake of calories, fat, salt, and sugar; exercise; get a periodic screening for high blood pressure and certain cancers; obey the speed laws, and fasten your seat belt. Foege saw it as not unlike the advice your grandmother might have given you. In that sense, the second revolution in public health was not a revolution at all.

Distribution of *Healthy People* had far-reaching effects. The 1990 objectives became a policy statement and were taught in the schools of public health. The National Institutes of Health stepped up its research for prevention; health education became increasingly important. The report also set the stage for publication a year later of *Promoting Health / Preventing Disease: Objectives for the Nation,* which listed 226 specific goals. Progress towards reaching them was regularly reported in *Public Health Reports.*[13]

Paradoxically, as CDC began its broad-scale prevention emphasis, it lost its Clearinghouse on Smoking and Health. CDC was accused of giving the program less than its full attention, and Secretary Califano, a militant ex-smoker, decided arbitrarily to move Smoking and Health back to Washington, where it would be under his own watchful eye. Like a reformed sinner, the secretary often gave personal witness to the evils of tobacco and recounted how in 1975 his eleven-year-old son had asked him to stop smoking as a birthday present. From his life in public work, Califano knew that "cigarette smoking is Public Health Enemy Number One in the United States." From his private experience, he knew how difficult it was to stop. In what one medical journal described as "demonic fashion," Califano set off on a crusade against tobacco. Even though he never got the funding he needed, he exploited his connections with the press and "stirred up more anti-smoking fervor than had ever been seen in the government since the Surgeon General's 1964 report, *Smoking and Health.*"[14] This fervor may have contributed to his dismissal by President Carter when the 1980 presidential campaign began. Although the president repeatedly expressed his approval of prevention as a priority in public health, he needed the political support of the tobacco-producing states.

While CDC (temporarily) lost the Smoking and Health program, Foege pushed ahead in other important, and sometimes controversial, areas of prevention. When the Supreme Court ruled that states had the option to restrict public funds for abortion, CDC monitored the impact of the decision. It found that while women did not generally take the route of illegally induced abortions, they did wait longer, thus increasing the danger to their lives. In 1977, the number of abortion-related deaths rose for the first time since 1972. CDC also moved ahead on injury control, and by late 1979 had a system in place using epidemiological principles to help state and local governments reduce unintentional injuries.[15]

At the same time, CDC added diabetes to its list of concerns. The National Commission on Diabetes recommended in 1975 that a program in diabetes education and control be established at CDC, and it was funded for the first time in 1977. The purpose of the program was to make knowledge about advances in diabetes control better known so that the complications of the disease might be reduced. CDC did a ten-state study to collect data and select priorities. Senator Richard Schweiker of Pennsylvania was a chief supporter of the program in Congress and worked hard to get the million-dollar funding. When Pennsylvania did not make the cut for the study, Foege went personally to explain why. It was the beginning of a warm relationship. When Schweiker became secretary of the Department of Health and Human Services (successor to HEW) in the Reagan administration, Foege was the only PHS agency head to be retained.[16]

Expanded prevention was one dimension of Foege's program for CDC. International health was the other. He saw the world as a "global village," where everything affects everything else from the birth rate, to the price of oil, to health. Especially health. Unlike many of his colleagues, Foege saw the smallpox crusade as just the beginning of his career, not its high point. For him the greatest satisfaction came in the continued improvement of health in the Third World.[17]

International health is a twentieth-century idea, and both the World Health Organization and CDC were established after World War II. In its early years, CDC's contributions to international health were primarily in malaria control and in training health workers from overseas, but expansion of CDC's activities in the 1960s brought it an international reputation. By the mid 1970s, CDC had a credibility overseas that even WHO did not have.

Soon after leaving the smallpox program, Foege was assigned the job of mapping CDC's future in international health. He was chairman of a committee that pinpointed the major problems: a misplaced emphasis on cures rather than prevention, an insufficient data base, and inappropriate training. These were the areas of CDC's expertise where it could play a significant role in improving world health. The Smallpox-Eradication Program served as an example. The committee concluded that the SEP's chief benefit "may, in fact, be the demonstration that global programs are workable and that global health objectives are attainable rather than simply idealistic projections." CDC could become a fulcrum in the effort by training people in international health administration to be assigned to the relatively few offices where decisions on international health were made: the World Health Organization, World Bank, Agency for International Development, Food and Agriculture Organization, and certain regional health groups.[18]

When Foege became director of CDC, his ideas on international health were echoed at the highest levels in Washington. President Carter included as part of his emphasis on human rights the right of every human being to be free from unnecessary disease. Secretary Califano embraced the World Health Organization's commitment to the idea of "health for all by the year 2000." This was no utopian notion, even though there were sizable obstacles to be overcome. Foege was a persuasive spokesman for a "managed" approach to international health. Testifying before a congressional committee on aid to Africa, he spoke of the huge gaps in "what is known and what is actually applied." He said that vaccination against disease and safe water supplies would do more to improve the health of many nations than elaborate national health-care systems. In disasters, managers were more important than doctors; reestablishing housing and food and water supplies was more important than setting up medical facilities.[19]

CDC had accomplished much overseas with a marginal mandate and wanted to capitalize on its growing international reputation, but it had neither the legislative authority nor the funding for foreign expansion. One conduit to the international health arena was through Public Law 480. This statute authorizes expenditure of local currency not usable elsewhere for special projects. If the United States sold wheat to India and was paid in rupees, those rupees could pay for a demonstration in malaria control. By 1979 CDC had dozens of projects under way in India, Yugoslavia, Egypt, and Poland.

The ultimate goal in international health was to help countries help themselves. David Sencer had wanted to export CDC's expertise and, in his last months as the agency's director, suggested the creation of a global epidemic intelligence service. CDC often sent epidemiologists overseas in an emergency and brought people from other countries to Atlanta for training, but Sencer felt that the best training for foreign epidemiologists was on their home ground. A plan was worked out with the World Health Organization, and the first global EIS program got under way in Thailand in 1980. It was funded by WHO and the government of Thailand, but CDC provided an epidemiologist and paid his salary. Similar EIS programs were established in Indonesia, Mexico, Taiwan, and Saudi Arabia. Each worked towards self-sufficiency. After five years, CDC's epidemiologist was moved out and the country was on its own.[20]

The burgeoning refugee population in Aisa underscored the urgency of problems in international health. By 1979 there were 200,000 Indochinese refugees in the United States, and the worsening situation in Cambodia meant there would be many more. In June, President Carter raised to 14,000 the number allowed to enter the United States each month, doubling the previous quota. In so doing, he doubled the responsibilities of those charged with guarding the public health.

A CDC team, which Foege headed, went to the West Coast and on to Asia to visit refugee centers in seven countries. Malaria and diarrheal diseases were the most common illnesses in the camps, but there were also cases of tuberculosis and other quarantinable diseases. All the camps were overcrowded; water and sanitation facilities were inadequate, and medical facilities limited or nonexistent. To handle the immediate emergency and to provide for follow-up health care after the refugees arrived in the United States, more public health personnel would be needed. Califano duly requested 112 positions and $101 million.[21]

When the Thai government agreed to accept Kampuchean refugees in designated camps in the autumn of 1979, Foege returned to Thailand with First Lady Rosalyn Carter and Surgeon General Richmond. They found a virtual absence of children aged one to four in the camps, mute testimony to the suffering of the people in the wake of the rise to power of the Khmer Rouge and the subsequent invasion by the Vietnamese. There is no better yardstick for measuring the overall health of a population than infant mortality. To Foege it seemed ironic that in the World Health Organization's Year of the Child, so many children were suffering. Mrs. Carter, much affected by the misery she saw, called a meeting at the White House to discuss what government officals and voluntary agencies could do.

An international effort was launched to help the Kampuchean refugees. CDC had epidemiologists at the Sakaeo camp shortly after it opened. Surveillance was the first priority. Using techniques developed over three decades, a young team from Atlanta identified the principal causes of death and severe illness and initiated appropriate treatment and preventive measures. They studied the mortality figures, weighed and measured all the children under ten, tested every fourth person for malaria, and monitored laboratory logbooks. Within seven weeks they brought down a sky-high death rate to normal levels.

When a second camp opened at Khao I-Dang, CDC was on hand from the first day to set up an orderly arrival and screening system and begin surveillance. There were immediate results. The death rate at Khao I-Dang was never as high as at Sakaeo. This was the second time that epidemiologic techniques had been used in the planning process for dealing with a disaster. About two dozen people from CDC had successfully used these techniques to plan famine relief in Nigeria in the late 1960s. The Kampuchean operation, important in itself, demonstrated to health officials from around the world what surveillance could do. For several years after the CDC staff came home, Khmer health officials kept the original surveillance system functioning efficiently.[22]

The Kampuchean experience was followed by a similar undertaking with refugees in Somalia. From 1980 to 1983, CDC used surveillance to make humanitarian efforts effective. In asking for CDC's help, an official of Somalia's Refugee Health Unit wrote, "In the past and even now CDC has been the one to help us solve our problems. Again we request CDC to make the big difference."[23]

Making the big difference was what CDC hoped to do at home as well as abroad. The first challenge CDC faced at home after Foege became director was a piece of unfinished business. Once again it would try to eliminate measles.

Immunization: The Third Crusade

The national campaign against measles and other childhood diseases was a casualty of swine flu. Weakened by budget cuts (federal funding for immunization dropped 75 percent in five years), the crusade against measles almost expired in 1976 when so many immunization specialists became, as Lyle Conrad put it, "swine-fluologists." Just a week before that effort was abruptly terminated in mid December, Conrad lamented the diversion of attention, time, personnel, and money from the fight against other diseases. The number of cases of measles was up 64 percent over the previous year, and 1977 might be even worse. Conrad looked forward to spring, when the limited number of people who could conduct immunization compaigns would be through with swine flu and could go on to other things.[1]

A move to restore life to the fight against childhood diseases was already under way. A national conference on immunization, held in Washington under PHS auspices in November 1976, established six committees to make recommendations on everything from policymaking to consent forms; they were to report at another conference in April. The need was urgent. Immunization levels were dangerously low, and so was the vaccine supply. Several pharmaceutical manufacturing houses refused to produce vaccines for measles, rubella, and polio without assurance of protection from law suits. At Senate hearings inquiring into the shortage, Senator Kennedy made a vitriolic attack on David Sencer, and he became the scapegoat.[2]

There was no clue in the fall of 1976 that childhood immunization was on the eve of success, but the juxtaposition of the abrupt end of the swine flu campaign and a change of administrations in Washington made it possible to start anew. In the national arena there were different players with different priorities. Among them was Betty Bumpers, who had championed childhood immunization in Arkansas when her husband, Dale Bumpers, was governor of the state. The new Carter administration gave her an opportunity to push her pet project at the national level. She mentioned the nation's low levels of immunization to First Lady Rosalyn Carter, who passed it along to the president, who in turn mentioned it to HEW Secretary Califano. The secretary, recognizing both an order from his boss and a good issue, proceeded in his usual vigorous fashion to make immunization a national priority.[3] When Califano came to Atlanta in early April 1977 to announce Foege's appointment as CDC director, he stated publicly that the swine flu effort had set back the ordinary, but highly important, efforts to immunize children against polio and measles, but acknowledged that important lessons had come from the abortive campaign: disease-reporting techniques were much improved, and there was much more knowledge about development and control of new vaccines.[4] Privately, Califano asked the CDC staff what the chances were of getting 90 percent of the nation's children immunized. "I would hate to see that in my job description!" Don Millar replied. The only times CDC had ever achieved more than 80 percent coverage was with special programs like the Sabin Sundays.

The next day the second national conference on immunization convened at NIH. Without prior warning, Califano announced a national Childhood Immunization Initiative. By October 1, 1979, he said, two targets would be met: immunization levels of the nation's children would be raised to 90 percent, and a permanent system would be in place to maintain these levels. The deadline was only two and a half years away.[5]

The Childhood Immunization Initiative required both tremendous effort and a lot of money. Califano assumed responsibility for persuading Congress to make the necessary appropriations: $23 million for grants to the states, about equally divided between vaccine purchases and personnel.[6] The program made a visible impact on CDC's Immunization Division. Five public health advisors were paired with five medical officers to work directly with the PHS regional offices and with the states. Dr. Alan Hinman, a former EIS officer, returned to CDC to serve as division director.

The program went well. Funding was adequate, public and private sectors worked together, and many volunteer agencies participated. At HEW, the Office of Education pushed it and so did the Human Development Program, overseer of Head Start. Califano regularly asked each of his subordinates what they were doing on immunization. He gave specific marching orders to Hinman and the Immunization Division, but he also gave them all the money they needed. The speed with which the program moved ahead pointed to something more powerful at work than the will of a few people. Foege believed it was a change in the social norm. Before 1977, the Office of Management and Budget looked at immunization facts and figures and asked how much it would cost to squeeze out the last 5 to 10 percent of coverage, deciding always that the cost was too high. In 1977, OMB decided it was worth the effort.

In a matter of months, a national program emerged. Califano's goal of immunizing 90 percent of the nation's children against the major childhood diseases—diphtheria, pertussis, tetanus, polio, measles, rubella, and mumps—turned out to be unrealistically low, so the program aimed still higher. The second part of the program—maintaining full coverage by making sure that newborn infants got into the immunization pipeline—was more difficult. It required a new kind of record-keeping on a national scale.

There was nothing uniform about the way immunization records were maintained. In the late 1970s, everybody put them out: the Academy of Pediatrics, the Academy of Family Practitioners, all manufacturers of vaccines, insurance companies, and even dairies, which printed them on milk cartons. None of them looked the same, and nobody had a record that included everything. Hinman convened a meeting of all those who put out these forms, added the Red Cross, and got everybody to agree that only state health departments would print immunization records. CDC developed the basic format, and within a year and a half, the multiplicity of records was replaced by a standard form presented to parents along with the child's birth certificate. The states began to enforce laws already on the books making regular vaccinations for a requirement for school entry. Standardized forms made checking easy.[7]

Participation by the schools was vital to the success of the program. Alaska was the first state to require immunization for first graders. Los Angeles County, California, was the next major area to do so. By the end of 1978, well before the deadline set for 90 percent protection, forty-seven states had laws requiring immunization as a condition of school entry, and thirty-one states vigorously enforced them. By 1980, all fifty states had fallen into line. Fewer than 1 percent of parents objected. Certainly the program was cost-effective. A few million dollars spent for vaccines saved many times that amount in reduced medical costs. Califano saw the immunization crusade as proof that government can work, that human compassion can be translated into effective programs.[8]

Success was measured by that most sensitive of indicators, the incidence of measles. The number of cases dropped dramatically in 1978 — so much, in fact, that once again there was talk of eradication within five years. The Immunization Division, fearing this would seem an impossibly long time to the public, scaled it down to four, which might just be possible. Foege mentioned this idea to Califano, who thought it so marvelous that he called a news conference and announced that by October 1, 1982, indigenous measles would be eliminated from the United States.[9]

To some it seemed an impossible goal, and no one thought it would be easy. Lyle Conrad, a staunch advocate of measles control, remembered the on-again, off-again support the program had received, and thought it would fail once more if the necessary resources were not provided. Michael Lane, a veteran of the Smallpox-Eradication Program, knew that the campaign against measles, unlike that against smallpox, might never end. High immunization levels and the ability to deal with imported cases would have to be maintained indefinitely. Requiring a second dose of vaccine at school entry, just to make sure of protection, might undermine credibility of the program with the public.

Experience in West Africa showed two approaches to the successful interruption of measles transmission: an annual cycle of mass vaccinations that reached 90 percent of susceptibles, or a continuing effort in which a minimum of 75 percent of all susceptibles were vaccinated. Either method required knowing where the susceptibles were and tracking each outbreak. Surveillance and epidemiology were vital.[10]

The model of measles had changed since the 1960s. The level of immunity that had to be sustained to prevent spread was generally thought to be 95 percent, although some set the figure as low as 93 percent and some as high as 97 or 98 percent. The number of cases of measles in the United States had been reduced by 90 percent from the time the vaccine was introduced in the mid 1960s to 1978. Within four years, it was reduced by another 90 percent—about 1,300 cases a year.

Surveillance indicated there would continue to be about 500 cases a year, stemming from 100 imported cases, each of which would probably spread to four others.

Squeezing out the last few susceptibles was one of the most difficult parts of the campaign, and was never completely achieved. The vaccine does not always work, and some people, typically about 4 or 5 percent, remain susceptible even after vaccination. Hinman did the arithmetic. If you immunize 95 percent of the population with a vaccine that is 95 percent effective, you have reached 91 percent coverage, which, with measles, may be enough to allow transmission. A second dose would raise coverage a few percentage points but at twice the cost.[11]

Some adverse reactions are inevitable with any vaccine. The first large system for tracing these was in the swine flu program, and a similar system was established for vaccines given in the Childhood Immunization Initiative. The most troublesome of the vaccines was the one for pertussis, a problem brought dramatically to light by the unexplained sudden deaths of seventy-four infants in Tennessee during a five-month period from November 1978 to March 1979. Eight babies died within a week of receiving DPT vaccine. As a precaution, CDC and FDA requested Wyeth Laboratory to withdraw the vaccine lot used in Tennessee. The data did not indicate a definite cause-and-effect relationship, making the decision difficult. There were strong arguments against withdrawing the vaccine, not the least of which was undermining confidence in the national immunization crusade, but the decision was made to take the safest course. The company called in 100,000 doses. From the perspective of a decade, Foege thought that decision had been correct, although he was convinced that the relationship between the deaths and the vaccines was a statistical aberration.[12]

The Childhood Immunization Initiative and the campaign to eradicate measles went forward without a solution to the knotty problem of liability. Assistant Secretary for Health Dr. Theodore Cooper outlined some of the difficulties. There would always be a small number of deaths whenever vaccines were administered to millions of people, but setting an acceptable number of deaths was impossible. "Is it all right to have twelve deaths? If twelve is acceptable, how about thirteen?" Cooper did not have an answer, but he believed that in any program where people take a risk for their own protection and as a perceived benefit to society, the community must have a policy to deal with the problem. In 1984 six countries provided compensation for those who were injured as a result of vaccination, but not the United States. Americans had to sue.[13]

The crusade to immunize the nation's children achieved remarkable success. The incidence of all the childhood diseases steadily declined, although measles was not eradicated.[14] The uniform method of maintaining immunization records was firmly in place by 1980; Mrs. Bumpers was chairman of the newly organized National Immunization Records Work Group. New parents in all states got information about immunization along with birth certificates.

Gains made in the third immunization campaign were maintained, whereas earlier gains had often been lost. There was a change in what society deemed to be the norm. The difference between 1962, when Congress first passed the Vaccination Assistance Act, and 1977, when the Childhood Immunization Initiative began, was a difference in social will. Foege was convinced that the battle for immunization would never have to be fought again.

Immunizing children in the rest of the world would take much longer. The United States became committed to WHO's Expanded Program on Immunization in 1974, and the program actually began three years later, with CDC playing a major role. The goal was to provide immunization for all the world's children by 1990. CDC assigned people to long-term duty overseas, and one of its staff, Dr. Ralph Henderson, was put in charge of the world program. Only 10 percent of children in the developing countries had been immunized when the program began. A decade later, about 40 percent were receiving the DPT shot. Enormous difficulties had to be overcome. Vaccines are fragile and must be kept cold, even frozen. CDC developed a "cold chain," which kept vaccines cold all the way from the manufacturer to the recipient. Both kerosene refrigerators and solar power were tried before small cold boxes were developed that kept vaccine cold for a week without any power at all.

The program is expensive. To attract increased resources and commitment, the World Bank and the Rockefeller Foundation joined with two UN organizations—the United Nations Development Programme (UNDP) and the United Nations International Children's Emergency Fund (UNICEF)—to organize a Task Force for Child Survival. WHO and various governments provide vaccines and equipment. Among those committed to the project are the members of Rotary International. Dr. Albert Sabin persuaded Rotary to provide any country in the world with the polio vaccine it needed for five years. Rotary originally intended to raise $180 million for the cause by 2005, when it celebrates its centennial, but its drive was so successful that in less than four years it raised $240 million, a tremendous catalyst towards the global eradication of polio.

As always, the eradication of measles proved to be the most difficult job. Every fifteen seconds a child dies somewhere in the world from measles. Global eradication of measles, Foege wrote in 1982, probably would not come for a long time. Failure would be measured by each case; success required a major test of will.[15] Success at home and abroad in immunizing children also depended on educating the public, a job not always helped by the media. During the controversy that followed the deaths of the babies in Tennessee who had received DPT vaccine, a Washington television station produced a one-hour documentary entitled "DPT: Vaccine Roulette." The program purported to be a balanced view, but Foege considered it "distorted." It focused on reactions known, suspected, or alleged to be owing to pertussis vaccine and gave very little emphasis to the benefits of vaccination and the risks of whooping cough. It attempted to produce a major controversy where one did not exist.[16] In the information age, presenting the degree of risk clearly entwined public health with public relations.

CHAPTER 22

Maintaining Credibility

Public perception of government and its institutions changed markedly in the 1970s, and inevitably CDC was affected. For three decades such public attention as it received was nearly all laudatory. That changed in 1976. While attention was still paid to CDC's successes, reporters schooled in Watergate searched for flaws as well. Scientists were also bureaucrats who could be blamed for any perceived wrong. The change in attitude was most obvious whenever economic or environmental issues were involved.

The liquid protein diet was a case in point. *The Last Chance Diet* by Dr. Robert Linn, an osteopath, spawned a new generation of over-the-counter diet products, predigested liquid protein supplements. Composed mostly of animal hides, tendons, and bones, the product was supposed to supply just enough protein to keep the body going without breaking up lean tissue. It became a fad overnight. As many as four million people consumed it, and some lost up to ten pounds a week.[1] Within a few months, however, there was trouble: thirty-nine deaths among the diet's overzealous, but otherwise healthy, adherents.

CDC investigated. The deaths were caused by irregularities of heart rhythm associated with starvation. In testimony before Congress, Foege blamed neither the doctors who cared for the patients nor the product's manufacturers. Subsisting for a long period on 300 calories a day (less than was given people in Nazi concentration camps during World War II), no matter what the source, could lead to death from starvation, a condition with which few doctors were familiar. Nothing in general medical knowledge suggested that patients on a low-calorie diet should have their hearts monitored regularly. When the Food and Drug Administration moved to take the product off the market, at least one columnist, reflecting the new combative attitude of the press, rushed to judgment. Jack Anderson wrote: "The government that brought you the swine flu vaccine is now threatening to take away liquid protein."[2] The implication of a blunderbuss bureaucracy at work was clear.

The swine flu campaign and the warning against liquid protein diets were unrelated, but the revelation that Reye's syndrome was more likely to occur in those who took aspirin came as a direct result of the swine flu effort. Reye's syndrome is a rare, but serious, disease of children that sometimes follows flu or chicken pox. It kills about 40 percent of its victims and leaves many others brain-damaged. During the fall of 1976, as swine flu shots by the millions were given, epidemiologists fanned out over Ohio identifying cases and asking a lot of questions. Their main purpose was to get blood samples so that what appeared to be cases of flu could be linked to a particular virus, but at the same time they took medical histories and asked patients how they treated their symptoms. Although the survey confirmed the well-known statistical connection between Reye's syndrome and cases of flu and chicken pox, no one assumed at the time that aspirin put children at greater risk. Nor did anyone have an inkling of the enormous political pressure that would be brought to bear on CDC when that relationship was published.

Dr. Karen Starko, an EIS officer assigned to the Arizona Health Department, first suggested a connection between the two. About a year after the swine flu campaign, she called Lawrence Schonberger to tell him about a flu outbreak. Among the victims were seven children who had developed Reye's syndrome. She compared them with sixteen controls and found that Reye's syndrome patients had taken aspirin more frequently. She did not quite know what to make of it. Schonberger suggested that more data might be available in the Ohio study.

Many of the Reye's syndrome patients in Ohio had also taken aspirin, but it was not known just when they had taken it. To verify Starko's idea that there was a connection between aspirin and the onset of Reye's syndrome, the Ohio study was changed to get exact information. Meanwhile, a similar study was begun in Michigan. Within a year there was no doubt that a child who took aspirin in any amount for the symptoms of flu and chicken pox was more likely to get Reye's syndrome than one who did not. The first report that something was going wrong with salicylates appeared in *MMWR* in the summer of 1980, and a few months later, details from the Ohio and Michigan studies were published there also. Because the aspirin industry was certain to be upset, the second article was accompanied by an extensive editorial note pointing out weaknesses in the study, but nevertheless concluding that the "association between Reye's syndrome and salicylates may indeed be real." The article created a sensation. Critics assailed it because it preceded publication of the detailed data in the medical literature. The first of these, giving the results of the small Arizona study, was published a month later in *Pediatrics*. Some critics concluded incorrectly that CDC's warning was based on only seven cases.[3]

The aspirin industry immediately went on the attack. Company officials went to Foege and then to the Food and Drug Administration. Their argument was rather clever: "It would be a shame to have the credibility of CDC built up over the decades destroyed by one wrong decision—to put out information that would later turn out not to be true." Foege, convinced of the scientific validity of the studies, listened but went ahead with plans to publish a more definitive report of the Ohio and Michigan studies. Just before the December 1981 publication date, spokesmen for the aspirin industry pleaded for time to present additional information. The proposed *MMWR* article was duly delayed, but when the industry came up with nothing new, publication of the data was rescheduled. It was to be accompanied by a joint statement by CDC and FDA warning against giving aspirin to children with flu or chicken pox. The night before this article was to appear in *MMWR*, FDA pleaded for more time. The aspirin industry had brand-new information, and FDA had to listen. "It seemed to me a clear pattern," Foege recalled, "that we would just delay this thing forever." With FDA's concurrence, he decided the article would be published without FDA's endorsement.

It summarized the number of cases of Reye's syndrome in the nation for 1981 and used stronger language than before. It cited the opinion of eight outside consultants who had reviewed the data from the studies in Arizona, Ohio, and Michigan and concluded that "until the nature of the association between salicylates and Reye syndrome is clarified, the use of salicylates should be avoided, when possible, for children with varicella infections and during presumed influenza outbreaks." The warning was quite clear, but it came in February when the flu season was well advanced. The surgeon general's advisory against the use of salicylates for children with influenza or chicken pox was published in *MMWR* four months later.[4]

Foege thought the ethics of public health demanded that the public be warned against a health hazard even if the warning was based on studies not yet published in the medical literature. The American Academy of Pediatrics' Committee on Infectious Diseases concurred, but when pressured by the aspirin industry, backed down from its strong endorsement. Having failed to influence Foege, who wanted a warning about Reye's syndrome put on aspirin bottles, industry officials turned next to the assistant secretary of health, Dr. Edward Brandt, and to Health and Human Services Secretary Schweiker, both of whom held firm. The industry then appealed to the Reagan White House, and an order came down to make yet another study. This would take several years, delaying the warning on bottles. Dr. Walter Dowdle headed the committee that oversaw the new study, and Dr. Eugene Hurwitz, who did the first study in Ohio, set a new task force to work. The Institute of Medicine, in constant touch with the aspirin industry, monitored everything. A pilot project worked out procedures for the definitive study, but even this modest effort showed the problem to be worse than had been supposed.

Nothing, not even the swine flu campaign, prepared CDC for the pressure, both political and economic, of the controversy over Reye's syndrome. Dowdle said simply, "It was something we had not experienced before." In 1986 when warning labels finally appeared on aspirin bottles, the aspirin industry was congratulated on its public-spiritedness. "In fact," Foege said, "they avoided letting parents know for more than a year that there was a problem with aspirin. It shows how strong the profit motive . . . can be in trying to make good health decisions." As the word filtered down that aspirin should not be given to children with flu and chicken pox, the number of cases of Reye's syndrome plummeted. CDC took much pride in saving lives and making a big scare go away.[5]

It was a really big scare, the accident at the nuclear plant at Three Mile Island outside Harrisburg, Pennsylvania, on March 28, 1979, that thrust CDC into the role of environmental watchdog. At about 7:45 A.M., a series of events stemming from a minor plumbing problem in the cooling system led to the shutdown of the plant's number 2 reactor. Thousands of gallons of radioactive water spilled within the plant and the reactor core dangerously overheated. Within hours, CDC's offer of help with epidemiology and surveillance was accepted by the Pennnsylvania Bureau for Radiological Health and by FDA, the principal federal health agency involved. The next four days were tense; radiation was measured and plans were made to evacuate the area if necessary. Rumors made the pursuit of truth difficult, but within twenty-four hours

Foege began to think that the problem was probably not as great as the news media portrayed it. Dr. Tony Robbins, director of NIOSH, and Dr. Clark Heath, director of CDC's Division of Chronic Diseases, went to the scene immediately and were soon joined by two epidemiologists, Mark Stein and Gary Nelson. Fifty public health advisors were available to be moved in on short notice.

The evacuation never took place, and within a week the crisis passed. Radiation exposure was quite small. A person standing unprotectecd along the border of the plant site for ten days would receive no more radiation than from three to five chest X-rays; one living five miles away would receive no more than a passenger in a jet plane on two round trips across the United States. Nor was there much danger to future generations. No more than two excess deaths would occur among those living near Three Mile Island on the day of the accident and their descendants. Much of an apprehensive public remained unconvinced, partly because of the association of radiation with cancer, and partly because of an innate suspicion of government experts. It was, after all, government experts who had assured them that nuclear power itself was perfectly safe. Why should anyone believe those who came along later and told them the danger was not great? To allay fears, CDC began a health census of all those living within five miles of the reactor. Additional surveys made at five-year intervals would pinpoint any problems. At Three Mile Island, the real threat was not radiation but psychological stress.[6]

It was after the accident at Three Mile Island that CDC was designated to coordinate the PHS response to envirnomental emergencies: disposal sites, transportation accidents, explosions, fires, chemical spills, and clusters of cases apparently of toxic origin. Threats to health long in the making often proved more difficult to handle than sudden emergencies.

One of these involved high concentrations of DDT in the little town of Triana, Alabama. In 1978 the Tennessee Valley Authority released information that fish from the Indian Creek Embayment of the Tennessee River contained up to forty times the level of DDT cleared by FDA. The mayor asked CDC if the health of Triana citizens was endangered. From 1947 to 1971, DDT had been manufactured at the Redstone Arsenal plant, ten miles from Triana, and waste from the plant had been emptied into the creek that ran through the town. Fish from that creek were a major source of food for the poor, mostly black, community.

A team went to Triana from Atlanta, and the mayor selected for the study a dozen lifelong residents of the area who ate a lot of fish. Nearly all Americans have measurable levels of DDE, a metabolite of DDT, in their blood, but nothing comparable to the amount found at Triana. Eleven of the twelve people in the study had 225 parts per billion of DDE, about fourteen times that of most Americans and equal to that of industrial workers once engaged in the long-banned manufacture of DDT. The twelfth had a concentration of 3,256 parts per billion, four times higher than any value previously reported. It could only have come from eating the creek's fish, which showed a high concentration of DDE. The CDC team could not prove, however, that DDT posed a definite health hazard, just as those who had worked on the problem of exposure to DDT since the 1940s had never been able to prove a deleterious effect. The point was probably irrelevant. The revelation of the massive exposure to DDT affected the way people in Triana thought. One resident worried that the experience would kill ambition in his sons. "The mind will create whatever is planted in the body, and we have DDT planted in our bodies," he told a reporter. "A lot of [the young people] don't do their best because they have a crutch now."[7]

CDC's most difficult environmental assignment was at Love Canal, New York. A problem years in the making came to light in April 1978, when evidence of toxic chemicals was found in several homes built in an area once used as a chemical dump. There were miscarriages and more birth defects than usual. The state health commissioner pronounced the area a health hazard, and Governor Hugh L. Carey announced that the state would purchase the 235 homes nearest the landfill, evacuate the families, and find them new homes. President Carter declared Love Canal a disaster area, the first such proclamation for chemical pollution.

The problem had its roots in the nineteenth century, when the visionary William T. Love sought to build a model industrial community at Niagara Falls to take advantage of the area's cheap electric power. The key to the project was a navigable canal connecting the Niagara River above and below the falls. Discovery of a way to transmit electric power cheaply ruined Love's plan, and the canal was never finished. In the 1920s, the Hooker Chemical Corporation and the city of Niagara Falls used the abandoned canal as a dump for chemical wastes. In 1953 the canal was covered over, an elementary school built on top of it, and hundreds of residences built near by. A quarter century later, chemicals were found in those homes.[8]

CDC did not get involved in the Love Canal investigation until two years after the first residents were evacuated, the houses boarded up, and a chain-link fence put around the contaminated area. By then a climate of fear developed in the community, making any effort to help extremely difficult. Investigations conducted by both the state of New York and the federal Environmental Protection Agecy (EPA) left residents either dissatisfied or furious. Two years of uncertainty left many people feeling they had lost control over their lives.

The EPA report revealed the possibility of damaged chromosomes, but offered no help. The study was not done for strict scientific purposes, but to help the agency in its multimillion dollar lawsuit against the company that had dumped the chemical wastes. A panel from the Department of Health and Human Services found the EPA study scientifically flawed, but its opinion did nothing to allay the community's fears. Indeed, Love Canal residents accused the HHS panel of trying to "whitewash some very scary data"; they felt betrayed by all levels of government.[9]

President Carter declared a state of emergency, clearing the way for relocation of an additional 2,500 residents, and two weeks later, on June 3, 1980, CDC assumed responsibility for providing physical examinations and health studies of the residents. Foege saw the "extraordinary public concern" as one of the most important elements in the problem, and he knew that the existing health structure, both federal and local, was ill equipped to handle it. He noted the schism that existed between concern for the environment per se (the concern of EPA) and responsibility for human health aspects of environmental exposure, CDC's new assignment.[10]

He made $500,000 available for the project and engaged a team from the nearby State University of New York at Buffalo to do much of the on-site work. The first meeting with residents of Love Canal was tense. The "nearly physically violent, certainly verbally violent" meeting was one Dr. Arthur D. Bloom would not forget. The advisor from Columbia University's Pediatrics Department had gone to explain the new science of chromosome-testing. He explained that chromosome breakage could be caused by many things other than exposure to toxic chemicals; radiation from dental X-rays, illnesses like measles or influenza, drugs used to treat cancer, even caffeine. He spoke in an atmosphere of palpable fear and anxiety, which in itself constituted a serious medical crisis. The residents, believing they had been lied to repeatedly, distrusted both the state and federal government, and "erupted in vituperation."

[T]he residents made it clear that the priority issue for them is relocation. . . . Without some action, and soon, there will almost certainly be overt violence. They again threatened . . . to torch their houses. And there is a barely concealed threat against those residents who might be inclined to cooperate with the Government in the proposed studies. . . . [Only after a] satisfactory resolution of this issue . . . will the CDC be able to do the health studies to which it is committed and in which the residents will then cooperate.[11]

Dr. Philip Taylor, CDC's medical officer assigned to Love Canal, was even more explicit. Love Canal residents considered all government agencies as one, and health studies had to take second place to the government's purchase of their homes. "The EPA's problematic chromosome tests are our problem. The Justice Department's lawsuit against Hooker is our lawsuit. The White House's failure to purchase homes is our failure. Separation of responsibility by agency does not exist for them. Our relationship is clearly an adversarial one." In such an atmosphere, Taylor doubted that CDC could provide any service to the people or "shed *any* light on the scientific issues involved."[12]

The extensive studies CDC originally planned included an analysis of chromosomal abnormalities in a selected group, but these plans gave way in a few months to something much simpler. Congress refused a request to allocate unused funds from the swine flu campaign for the project, and a panel of scientists meeting in Atlanta concluded that although Love Canal was a "political reality," it did not rank high on the national agenda of health priorities. The scaled-down study concentrated on the effect of exposure to chemicals on children. By the end of 1980, as funds allocated by CDC petered out, Foege recommended that the project be abandoned.

CDC was never able to show that the citizens of Love Canal suffered any damage to their health from exposure to toxic chemicals, much to the latter's consternation, but the staff learned a great deal about the importance of public relations in handling an environmental crisis. You had to get on the scene early, involve the citizens in the decision-making process, and speak a language people could understand. The film on chromosome damage was too technical for the lay public and only made them angry. Dr. Vernon Houk, director of CDC's environmental studies, who understood their frustration, observed:

Scientists tend to be so scientifically precise that no one knows what in hell they are talking about. . . . We have learned to be there early in the process, have a reasonable plan worked out, involve the community in the plan and get them to understand what you are trying to do. . . . [O]nce the community becomes polarized, as [at] Love Canal, . . . it becomes virtually impossible to turn that around, because there are so many suspicions in that community that they don't believe anybody.[13]

The principal threat to health at Love Canal was dioxin, the contaminant found in the Times Beach, Missouri, community in 1982 and used as a defoliant in Vietnam, where it was called Agent Orange. CDC investigated both. At Times Beach the situation was not more dangerous than at Love Canal, but when flood waters covered much of the community, the problem took on a special urgency. The state, the EPA, and CDC were all involved at Times Beach, just as they were at Love Canal, and the communication among the three, while better than in the New York community, left much to be desired. The contamination in Times Beach came from streets and roads that had been sprayed with the unwanted by-product from the manufacture of herbicides. It was believed that flood waters might have spread the contamination to yards and homes. Just before Christmas 1982, as the waters subsided, CDC was called to investigate. A preliminary check showed much higher concentrations of dioxin than had been suspected, so Dr. Henry Falk, the CDC epidemiologist dispatched to Times Beach, advised citizens returning to their homes to leave again and wait for the final report of EPA. Most people ignored him.[14] They cleaned up their property and, as tempers rose, waited for the promised report, which did not come out until spring. Ultimately, the social problems in Times Beach, like those at Love Canal, proved more difficult to resolve than the scientific ones. The final report showed that the flood had not spread dioxin from the roadways and ditches, but the community was polarized by uncertainty long before that information got to residents.

The investigation of Agent Orange paralleled that of Love Canal and Times Beach. When many veterans of the Vietnam War blamed a variety of illnesses, including cancer and birth defects, on exposure to Agent Orange, Congress ordered an inquiry and established a budget of $70,000,000. At a time when many agency budgets, including that of CDC, were being cut, this huge amount was an indication of the political sensitivity of the issue. Elaborate plans were drawn up. In 1982 CDC began the search for enough veterans exposed to Agent Orange to do a scientifically valid study. The military records were so inexact, however, that these veterans were never found. Houk thought this indicated there was not as much exposure to Agent Orange as was generally thought to have occurred. Research done in the next half dozen years showed that Agent Orange does not pose as much risk as was originally supposed. The news did not make the veterans happy, and emotions got ahead of the scientific data. Some veterans wanted to shoot the messenger. They railed at CDC, which absorbed the blows rather than sacrifice scientific credibility. It is better to appear stupid by remaining silent, Houk said, than to make public pronouncements without facts. "Credibility once lost is never recovered."[15]

CDC's credibility was enhanced by its continued ability to solve medical mysteries. There was the case of three infants in Memphis, Tennessee, who had renal problems and did not thrive. Three epidemiologists from CDC—David Erickson, Jose F. Cordero, and Frank Greenberg—went to investigate and found that all three children were taking the same soy-based formula. When they called a national sample of physicians treating infants with renal problems, their suspicions that the formula might be at fault were confirmed. All the babies were being fed Neo-Mull-Soy, which probably did not contain enough chlorides to meet an infant's nutritional requirements. One of the investigators flew to California, presented the information to the company, and the product was taken off the market that afternoon. The whole investigaton took but five days.[16]

Equally dramatic was the tracking down of the source of a polio outbreak in a Pennsylvania Amish community and preventing its spread. News of a single case of Type I polio in the community in January 1979 raised immediate questions at CDC. Was it vaccine-related or was it a wild virus? If the latter, the threat to health was serious, since the wild virus spreads, whereas the weakened vaccine virus does not; one case attributable to a wild virus constitutes an epidemic. CDC suspected that the virus was wild, since vaccine-related polio is nearly always Type II or Type III. Laboratory tests, steadily refined over the years, confirmed these suspicions. An immediate effort was made to immunize people in the Amish community and the surrounding area. When a second case appeared, health officials in the nineteen states with Amish communities were alerted to the danger.

Quite early it was clear that the spread was within the Amish community itself and not in the general population, but it was almost as difficult to control the panic in the general population as it was to persuade the Amish to be vaccinated. For the most part, the Amish had not received the standard immunizations and were wary of anything that smacked of governmental regulation. The state epidemiologist of Pennsylvania met with elders of the Amish community to persuade them to do something about the polio problem, and while the Amish were eventually responsive, it was a slow, tedious process. The breakthrough came when the elders finally permitted an article on the need for immunization to appear in the national Amish newsletter.

Because there was little chance that the virus would spread to the general population, with but one exception, no mass vaccination campaigns were planned. The exception was in Lancaster, Pennsylvania, where the Amish community attracted many tourists. If polio was going to spread to the general populace anywhere, it would be there. Everybody in Lancaster was asked to participate in a reprise of Sabin Sunday, and the residents responded well. Most of them, however, had already been vaccinated and did not need it. Only a few of those who really needed protection showed up.

The epidemiology of the polio outbreak among the Amish in the United States indicated that it had its origin in similar religious communities in Canada and the Netherlands. Serologic tests pointed to the same conclusion, but the association was definitely confirmed by a new test performed in the CDC laboratory in June 1979. A technique called oligonucleotide mapping "fingerprinted" the virus exactly. It was the first time specific differentiation between wild polio viruses had ever been done.[17]

The most dramatic instance of medical sleuthing was the quick association of toxic shock syndrome (TSS) with the use of tampons by menstruating women. In January 1980, the health departments in Minnesota and Wisconsin reported nine cases of TSS in adult women. The disease, first described in 1978 by Dr. James Todd of the University of Colorado School of Medicine, is characterized by high fever; low blood pressure; a diffuse rash, with subsequent peeling; vomiting; diarrhea; and multiple abnormalities in laboratory findings. Unlike the victims in Wisconsin and Minnesota, Todd's seven patients were children and young people, aged eight to seventeen. When *Staphylococcus aureus* was isolated, Todd suggested that a toxin was elaborated from it.

In response to reports of TSS in women, Dr. Kathryn Shands began CDC's informal surveillance. Todd's hypothesis that *S. aureus* was involved had not been proved, so a case definition that included the consistent features of Todd's cases and those in Wisconsisn and Minnesota had to be made. Fifty-five cases were reported nationwide by late May, and *MMWR* summarized the findings. The mean age of the patients was 24.8 years, and all but three of them were women.[18] Association of the onset of illness with the menstrual period was so striking that a case-control study began the following month.

One hypothesis to be tested was pursued by Dr. Jeffrey Davis, state epidemiologist for Wisconsin: that the use of tampons might be important in the pathogenesis of the disease. Results of the study, involving fifty-two women and fifty-two controls, showed a definite association. *MMWR* published the first warning on June 27, 1980.[19] It was picked up immediately by the news media. Senator Kennedy read about it in the *Washington Post* and wanted it to get quick public notice. He asked Foege, who was already scheduled to testify at an environmental hearing on toxic dumps, to be prepared to answer questions about TSS. Foege took Kathryn Shands to the hearings, and on the way to Washington they discussed how long it might take to come up with an answer. When Senator Kennedy asked that question specifically, Foege replied that he thought CDC would have the answer by the end of the year. "We had to revive Kathy Shands, who was on the floor, because she thought there was little chance that we could do that," said Foege. "I worded it in a way that did not say we would have solved the toxic shock problem, but correctly put it in terms that we would have an answer."[20]

They did have the answer before the end of the year. As soon as the association of TSS with tampons was made, the question arose of why the illness had not been noticed earlier. What was different about tampon use in 1980 from all the years before? When the results of CDC's study were announced, Utah health officials zeroed in on brand names, and found that one product, Rely, had been used by many women with TSS. In early September, CDC did a second study, which verified the association. Women using Rely tampons were 7.7 times more likely to have TSS than if they had used other brands. *MMWR* published the results on September 19. Three days later, the manufacturer voluntarily removed the product from the market. The question of why TSS was associated with the use of tampons, and specifically the Rely brand, still had to be answered, as did the illness's relationship to *S. aureus*, but incidence of the disease dropped immediately.[21]

The toxic shock story got enormous attention. For days it was on national television and in the national press, and Shands was much in demand for interviews. People whose lives had been affected by TSS called CDC and wanted to talk. Among them were the parents and husband of one of the earliest fatalities of TSS, who wanted to give CDC whatever information they could. Another was a man whose bride had become ill on their honeymoon and died within days. He came to Atlanta and talked for hours with an epidemiologist about the research being done. The publicity affected the lives of those doing the research, and appearance on national television became almost routine. Publicity also enhanced the public perception of CDC's disease detectives as wizards. This time the glare of publicity had no adverse effect on CDC itself.[22]

Although TSS was a new phenomenon, it was a disease that fit into CDC's traditional area of expertise. While that investigation was under way, CDC was thrust into another arena in which it had almost no previous experience. On May 18, 1980, the volcano at Mount Saint Helens in Washington State erupted, spewing millions of tons of ash into the air. Three days later, by invitation from the states most involved, CDC staff, including some from NIOSH, were on the scene. They set up hospital-based surveillance of acute repiratory disorders. While particularly concerned with the danger of silicosis in lumber workers, highway crews, police, and others most exposed to the ash, they also laid the groundwork for long-term follow-up studies in the general population. Except for comparing the effects of the Mount Saint Helens eruption with the 1979 eruption of the Soufrière volcano on the island of St. Vincent in the West Indies, they worked in uncharted territory. They monitored the air from the Dakotas to Utah and for months issued the Mount Saint Helens Volcano Report. The lack of specific data made it impossible to do much more than recommend that people wear masks. The whole approach to the problem of pollution at Mount Saint Helens was different. As Dr. Robert Bernstein, a NIOSH officer, explained, "In industry you can diagnose the problem . . . and clean it up. But a 'scrubber' on St. Helens?"[23]

The work at Mount Saint Helens enhanced CDC's credibility at home. Its credibility abroad, nurtured over many years and bolstered by the success of the smallpox-erediction campaign, was never in doubt. In 1981, when the Agency for International Development began a new project in Africa to protect children against communicable disease, it invited CDC to participate. The program—Combatting Childhood Communicable Disease (CCCD)—is designed to reduce sickness and death in children in virtually all of sub-Saharan Africa. It involves malaria control, immunization, and oral rehydration, the almost-miraculous cure for infantile diarrheas in Third World countries. CDC provides the majority of the technical expertise and support for the program.

Further evidence of its international credibility came when CDC was invited to assess the health risks after the chemical accident at Bhopal,

India, in December 1984. The accident took the lives of thousands of people and made many more thousands desperately ill. The request for help came from the U.S. embassy in New Delhi and a team of four, led by Dr. Jeffrey Koplan, CDC's assistant director for public health practice, left for India. The team included Dr. Henry Falk, an epidemiologist who had been at Times Beach and Mount Saint Helens; Dr. Jim Melium of NIOSH, and Professor Garreth Green, an environmental toxicologist. Their experiences proved how much CDC had learned about the psychology of emergencies since the difficult days at Love Canal.

Koplan's three team members arrived in New Delhi eight to ten hours before he did. As they stepped off the plane, microphones were shoved at them and they were asked which one was Mr. Belli. (Melvin Belli, the famous American attorney, was said to be going to represent the people of Bhopal in their suit against Union Carbide.) When they identified themselves as doctors, the microphones vanished. They spent the rest of the day at the U.S. embassy and at the AID mission, where they learned that their chances of getting into Bhopal were slight to none. The U.S. embassy had pushed for the CDC team to be invited, but Indian bureaucrats had not approved and did not want them.

When Koplan arrived, he found his colleagues depressed. Instead of getting information, they had to win the support and trust of officials from India's Ministry of Environment and Ministry of Health. The environmentalists wanted to assess the effects of the accident on the environment; the health officials wanted to assess blame. The next day, at a meeting of a government commission convened to review the situation, the four Americans were very careful to listen to everything and say little. Above all, they did not want to represent themselves as experts. They suggested only that they had some experience that might prove useful.

Koplan, who had worked in Bangladesh during the smallpox campaign, knew it was important to determine the rhythm and pace of the place, and even more important not to appear pushy. By the second day, they had established cordial relations with the minister of the environment, who was a botanist and Shakespeare scholar. During an afternoon meeting at which all the foreigners who had come to help were asked to give their opinions, Koplan realized that the Indians intended to let the foreigners speak their piece, then bid them good-bye. As spokesman for the American team, he decided to say as little as possible. He watched his colleagues "getting antsy" when all he said was: "Sounds like you have put it together pretty well. We have nothing to add."

As the meeting was about to end, he asked to make a couple of points. He congratulated the Indian officials on a splendid response to a very difficult situation, on dealing well with tens of thousands of ill people in the middle of the night in a provincial city. He then asked to hear from the Bhopal representative at the meeting, who had not spoken. The man from Bhopal warmed to the recognition. When the meeting ended, the other foreigners left for home; the Americans returned to their hotel.

The next day, thanks to the intervention of the minister of the environment, the Americans were off to Bhopal, where they stayed for several days. They visited patients, looked over hospital records, and wrote a report with a few practical suggestions. Chief among these was the need to reconstruct as nearly as possible the environment and the neighborhoods as they were on the day of the accident. This meant taking a census of those living in the area. From the smallpox crusade, Koplan knew that boys aged twelve to fifteen were the best source for that kind of information. That fact went into the report, although Indian officials seemed reluctant to use untrained personnel.

"Again, we could have pushed," Koplan recalled, "but I did not think this was appropriate. . . . [O]ur role was to give a set of recommendations. If they wanted them, fine, if not, then they might have good reasons. . . . They cordially accepted our reports, and we were gone. We did what we set out to do. We established the framework for measuring health effects."[24] The lessons of Love Canal and Times Beach had been learned well: in a psychologically charged atmosphere, science does not advance.

Toward the Twenty-first Century

Expansion of CDC's activities into areas far-removed from infectious diseases made reorganization necessary. The structure of CDC had been minimally adjusted numerous times over the years to accommodate change, but in the late 1970s the basic framework—laboratory, epidemiology, and training—was still in place. William Foege had been in his new job for only a short while when he advanced the notion of something entirely new.

The reasons were compelling. As the national advocate of prevention, charged with the responsibility of working towards the 1990 goals, CDC needed a more efficient organizational structure. Room had to be made for environmental and lifestyle issues and for the study of chronic diseases. Also, it was time to phase out some existing units. The Smallpox-Eradication Program certainly had to go before it won the Golden Fleece Award, the dubious honor Senator William Proxmire bestowed from time to time on government projects he considered utterly useless. Every time Michael Lane, who had worked in the smallpox campaign from its beginning, went to a congressional hearing on nutritional issues—nutrition still being located within CDC's smallpox unit—he had to explain why that program still existed.

Canada provided a model for CDC's new structure. Canada's health program was divided into four areas—biological, environmental, lifestyle, and medical care. Foege liked the concept; it was not unlike Joseph Mountin's old blueprint for the Public Health Service, with a center for infectious diseases and one for environmental health. It seemed natural to reshape CDC along those lines. In Washington, Assistant Secretary for Health Julius Richmond thought so, too.[1]

For weeks Foege explored the idea with his staff individually. In 1978, at a staff conference held in Rome, he sought a consensus. There were two schools of thought. One favored the classical functional approach, which had worked well at CDC for three decades. The other considered the end product: teams would work together towards a particular outcome, whether it was to control disease, prevent accidents, or lower the level of violence.

Reorganization should make CDC's work more efficient, and it might foster goodwill. The historic rift between the Laboratory and Epidemiology branches of CDC was still there, although not so apparent as when Ralph Hogan headed the Laboratory Branch and Alexander Langmuir directed Epidemiology. Dr. Roslyn Q. Robinson, director of the Bureau of Laboratories in the 1970s, tried manfully to close the gap and heal the wounds, but was never completely successful. Resentment simmered about slights real or imagined. Abstracts of papers at the annual EIS conference named only the presenter of the paper, not the laboratory staff who had contributed to it. "I was not aware that the personnel in the Bureau of Laboratories have evidently for a long time felt that this 'practice is unethical and demeaning,'" Philip Brachman, director of Epidemiology, wrote in late summer 1980. He promised a change.[2]

To a remarkable degree, the staff put aside personnel problems as they discussed reorganization and concentrated on what was best for the nation's health. Foege knew, however, that some staff members were sending out their resumes. With morale at the center already low as a result of the swine flu affair and the firing of Sencer, it was not an ideal time to shake up the organizational structure. No one liked giving up the old familiar identities. Even Michael Lane, one of the most vigorous supporters of reorganization, was a bit daunted by the massive change. He attributed its ultimate acceptance to "the tremendous . . . respect and affection that everyone had for Bill Foege. We felt that there was no evil intent, no malign thing. He was not out to get any of us. It was not some ploy to jump on somebody's turf."[3]

After the Rome conference, the staff settled on four general areas of concern. There were two old ones, infectious diseases and occupational health, and two new ones, environmental health and self-induced risks. Most public health issues could be lumped in one of those four categories, which provided the basis for the new organizational structure.

Those with the most passionate—and negative—feelings about reorganization were the laboratory scientists and the epidemiologists. Their large fiefs were cut up and redistributed to other bureaus, and there was concern about loss of identity and esprit de corps. In the reorganized CDC, EIS officers would be together only in training. After that they would go to different units and march to different drummers. The lab scientists would lose their central focus, too. The Bureau of Laboratories was, as Robinson put it, "a unique resource," which depended on a critical mass of committed and creative scientists with freedom to pursue promising leads. He saw reorganization as a threat to both critical mass and freedom.[4]

Combining the Laboratory and Epidemiology bureaus into the Center for Infectious Diseases (CID) was the most difficult step in the reorganization process, and Foege was afraid that in putting these two competitive units together he would lose key people. He decided it would work only if a laboratory person, well respected by the epidemiologists, headed it. He asked Walter Dowdle, an eminent virologist, to take the job. Dowdle was conversant with epidemiologic principles and had the right temperament. He was less than eager to take on the assignment; he enjoyed being a scientist and was not interested in becoming an administrator. He met with Foege several times before he finally agreed.

There was precedent within CDC itself for combining Laboratory and Epidemiology in a single unit. For years Laboratory and Epidemiology staffs had worked together at the field stations in Kansas City and Phoenix, and the staff at Phoenix liked to think the harmony they enjoyed set an example for Atlanta to follow. Foege hoped that the new structure would reduce the need for negotiating what the Laboratory branch would do every time CDC investigated an epidemic. It was time to stop reinventing the wheel.[5]

The rest of reorganization was easy by comparison. NIOSH was already a part of CDC; the other areas of emphasis were too new to have built-in allegiances. Some feared that a center concerned specifically with the environment might be taken away from CDC, but Foege decided to take the risk. CDC was already heavily involved in environmental issues at Triana, Love Canal, Three Mile Island, and Mount Saint Helens, but it had not yet tackled the hard-to-sell issues of controlling violence and injuries.

Among those most pleased with emphasis on the environment was Mark Hollis, CDC's first director. He had always wanted CDC to be involved in environmental issues and had tried without success to interest Alexander Langmuir in them. "Just envision what would have happened if you had put a few people on the environmental field earlier," he said to Langmuir when the problems of the environment became too great to be ignored. "If we had worked on this and had done what we did in infection, what would have happened?"[6]

The difference that lifestyle could make in preventing disease was the raison d'être of the new Center for Health Promotion and Education. Its object was to apply the flexible principles of epidemiology to behavior. Since smoking was the lifestyle choice that posed the greatest single threat to health, the implication was clear that the Office of Smoking and Health should be moved back to Atlanta from Washington.

The rest of CDC was easier to rearrange within the new structure. The traditional service functions would be carried out by the Center for Prevention Services and the Center for Professional Development and Training. Three program offices—one in epidemiology, another in international health, and the third in laboratory improvement, cut across all lines to provide a focus for external relationships in these areas.

The staff's doubts about reorganization were echoed in Washington. Ellen Wormser, director of Health Budget Analysis, suggested that CDC was undergoing an identity crisis. "In the past, the agency has been very successful in achieving its primary, historical mandate of controlling and preventing communicable diseases. Because of this nationally acclaimed success, CDC's role in this area has shrunk to the unglamorous one of maintaining the nation's high resistance to outbreaks of these diseases." Some members of Congress opposed what they called CDC's "recapture" of the smoking program, which, as they perceived it, had been "liberated" by the creation of the Office of Smoking and Health. They also objected to putting the health education–health promotion function within CDC when Congress had only recently mandated an office of Health Information and Health Promotion in the office of the assistant secretary for health.[7]

There was a difference of opinion, too, about what to call the agency when and if reorganization were approved. The name had to reflect its enlarged scope. Dr. Richmond very much wanted *Prevention* in the title, reflecting an emphasis Justin Andrews had advocated thirty years earlier. "Centers for Disease Control and Prevention" was his choice, even though it was unwieldy and changed the well-established initials. The staff were adamant that the initials be retained, and Foege thought they could be sacrificed only for a title that rolled easily off the tongue. When wordsmiths proved unequal to that task, the initials were kept and *Center* was simply changed to *Centers*.

Foege hoped that the reorganized CDC would become to preventive health what the National Institutes of Health was to health research: it would make possible the delivery of "well conceived and exceedingly effective prevention/control services to the American people."[8] Reorganization was linked to the prevention initiative; they moved forward together. In spite of the Carter administration's commitment to "healthy people" and the enthusiastic support of Assistant Secretary of Health Richmond for an emphasis on prevention, reorganization of CDC was in limbo for more than two years after the ideas were first hammered out. It was not until October 1, 1980, that the reorganization became official.

The change made an immediate difference in the area of health promotion and education. EIS officers were available for the first time for this different kind of epidemiological work. They were mostly young, lifestyle-oriented, nonsmoking exercise buffs; one was a marathon runner. They chose surveillance and research on exercise as their first project. The work was important, nobody else was doing it, and it had a certain "pizzazz," not an insignificant factor in a health field just coming to prominence. Although new, it met the religious test of CDC: that epidemiology is a science.[9]

From the dismantled smallpox program, the Center for Health Promotion and Education inherited nutrition studies, and from Epidemiology, work in family planning. From modest beginnings, family planning had leapfrogged to national and international prominence. Private foundations contributed liberally to support the work, which brought up issues related to legal abortion and contraceptive safety. The center's investigations of the relation of contraceptives to spontaneous abortion and cancer were classified as "landmarks."[10] Its work on the logistics of contraceptive distribution affected family-planning programs around the world.

The combination of lifestyle studies, nutrition, and family planning gave the Center for Health Promotion and Education an undeniable solidity, even though the Office of Smoking and Health, the original centerpiece of health-education activities at CDC, remained in Washington for several more years. When this important program was eventually moved back to Atlanta, most of the major areas in which education could make a real difference in promoting health were in a single place.[11]

The Center for Environmental Health, the second "new" program created in the reorganization, was actually not new at all. It was put together from what was left of the rat-control, lead, and dental-disease studies, plus the work started years before by Dr. Clark Heath on cancer clusters and by Dr. Godfrey Oakley on birth defects. The clinical labs from the Bureau of Laboratories were added to give this center a critical mass. It was not long before these labs measured dioxin in parts per trillion and did other equally sophisticated tests, moving CDC into a leading role in environmental investigations.

The task of combining these varied activities into a workable whole was assigned to CDC verteran J. Donald Millar. At the time of reorganization, Millar was assistant director for public health practice and complaining that he had nobody to lead. As chief of the Center for Environmental Health, he would be in charge in investigations covering a broad scope, from a proper response to earthquakes to disposal of nerve-gas weapons. Although exposure to toxic chemicals had achieved much prominence in the investigations at Love Canal and Times Beach, such exposure proved to be the least important of environmental hazards, well behind injuries and accidents. The public supported the study of toxic wastes, but it was almost impossible to get funding for injury control. Every year Foege put it in the budget, and every year it was cut out. The Center for Environmental Health was a half dozen years old and under the leadership of another director, Dr. Vernon Houk, before it was possible to move in any significant way into the fields of injury and violence.

Of all the prevention studies, the one on birth defects turned out to be the most controversial. CDC's data source on birth defects is the best in the world, but the ability to diagnose in fetuses conditions for which there is no therapy continually raises the touchy issue of abortion. A relatively simple blood test to measure the level of alpha fetoprotein in the blood of an expectant mother can indicate if a child will be born with spina bifida. But if the test is positive, science can offer no help beyond abortion, a solution unacceptable to many. In the conservative 1980s, funds for the study of birth defects were cut and a significant reduction in birth defects was removed from the 1990 objectives. On this issue, as in some others, science was too far ahead of social acceptance.[12]

In reorganizing CDC, the National Institute for Occupational Health and Safety (NIOSH), created by law, was left alone. Yet it soon became obvious that something had to be done about NIOSH. Although occupational safety and health had started as part of the public health movement, it had gradually become something of an orphan. When state health departments abandoned their work in the field, politicians filled the vacuum. Foege was concerned not only about the influence of politics on NIOSH but about the credibility of the institute's science. NIOSH's report on beryllium, for example, made it seem that exposure to beryllium was very dangerous to workers, but an expert panel reviewing the findings disagreed. To many people it seemed that NIOSH was pro-labor, more influenced by politics than by the impartial pursuit of science. Foege found the situation intolerable. He thought that much of the problem lay in the fact that NIOSH, while organizationally a part of CDC, was entirely removed from it physically. It did its scientific work in laboratories in Cincinnati, Ohio, and Morgantown, West Virginia, and had its headquarters in Rockville, Maryland. Foege began a campaign to convince the new administration in Washington to move the headquarters to Atlanta.

With the inauguration of President Reagan, all the personnel in the Department of Health and Human Services changed. Senator Richard Schweiker of Pennsylvania became HHS secretary, and Dr. Edward N. Brandt, Jr., became the assistant secretary for health. On Brandt's first visit to Atlanta, Foege discussed the need to move NIOSH headquarters. It would improve scientific credibility, reduce political influence, and effect economy in management. Brandt was persuaded and Secretary Schweiker was supportive also. In June 1981 the top-secret decision was made to move NIOSH headquarters.

It fell to Bill Watson, who had been through nine such transfers, to go to Rockville to break the news. The employees were surprised, unhappy, and upset, and one of them asked Watson, "How can we stop this?" He said they had asked the wrong person. Times had changed since 1957, when Watson, as a public health advisor in the Venereal Disease Division, had been on the receiving end of a transfer to Atlanta. "When the surgeon general made [that] decision, we were unhappy, just as the NIOSH people were unhappy, but in effect, we saluted and went on and did it," he says. In 1981, people were more inclined to bring their union in and fight for their rights.

Announcement of the move was made simultaneously with Foege's selection of Don Millar as NIOSH director, replacing Dr. Tony Robbins, whose pro-labor stance made him unacceptable in the Reagan administration. Millar was not interested in the job so long as the headquarters was away from Atlanta and "political games" took precedence over science. He was well aware of the fate of the first three directors of NIOSH. The first, Dr. Mark Key, had resigned after four years in office; the second, Dr. John Finklea (whom Millar himself had recruited) was fired after three years; the third, Dr. Robbins, had lasted a bit longer than two years. As any good epidemiologist would do, Millar produced a little chart showing the length of service and the success of incumbents in the post of NIOSH director. The curve went straight down. Millar figured that he might last a year.

If his first encounter with the NIOSH staff had foreshadowed the future, he would not have lasted even that long. On July 13, 1981 (he remembered the date clearly), Millar and Foege went to Rockville to talk to the staff about the things CDC was interested in doing. In the midst of the meeting, Darlene Christian, the leader of union opposition to the move, walked into the room dressed entirely in black, carrying an elaborate black wreath emblazoned with a banner reading "Death of NIOSH."[13]

In opposing Millar's appointment, the local union of the American Federation of Government Employees referred to him as the head of the "infamous Tuskegee Study" and the swine flu program "when 38 people died within 48 hours after receiving the vaccine." His appointment demonstrated "a profound moral bankruptcy which is unworthy of public trust. We will not stand idly by and allow Dr. Millar to look after American workers the way he looked after the Tuskegee subjects."[14] For Millar it was a hard time. TV cameramen camped out in his front yard and filmed him driving his daughter to school. It was shown on a Washington station. The next night four tires on his car were slashed.[15]

NIOSH personnel claimed that it was Millar's refusal to leave Atlanta that made the headquarters move necessary. Congress lent a sympathetic ear. Congressman David Obey of Wisconsin, a member of the House Appropriations Committee, proposed that NIOSH be transferred to the National Institutes of Health. That move failed, but Obey attached a rider to the appropriations bill prohibiting the move to Atlanta. More than a year passed before CDC had an opportunity to do something about it. The prohibition was not included in the continuing resolution in 1982, and Foege was told by a sympathetic senator that when that resolution came up, there would be a "small window of opportunity" where funds could be spent for a couple of weeks. A last-minute attempt to defeat the maneuver was unsuccessful, and NIOSH was moved to Atlanta over one weekend.

The long delay in moving NIOSH from Rockville may have been

salutary. While the move was pending, all those who did not really want to be part of CDC went elsewhere, repeating a historical pattern established when the Venereal Disease Division was moved to CDC in 1957. When NIOSH finally moved, only a handful of the original Rockville staff remained, and they were committed to CDC. A "no-nonsense" scientist, Dr. Elliott Harris, who had once run NIOSH's behavioral and biomedical sciences program at Cincinnati, was named Millar's deputy. The two men made certain that the work done was "good science" with no political overtones. An outside peer-review process was mandated and a Board of Scientific Counselors established to scrutinize the institute's work.

In an echo of the Red Book process that had identified the nation's leading diseases and health problems, Millar got his staff to identify the ten leading work-related diseases and injuries in the United States. The results were published in *MMWR*,[16] and a national debate ensued. Some issues, like occupational cardiovascular disease, stress, and psychological disorders, were controversial, but generally, there was broad acceptance of the list. Millar and Harris also involved the states more closely and thrust NIOSH into a health-promotion campaign. *Health promotion* had once been "a bad word" among unions, Millar explained:

> If you said that people ought to stop smoking and start exercising, they said that . . . cleaning up the work place is more important. We agreed with them. There was no sense in telling people to quit smoking when you asked them to breathe toxic fumes, but similarly, there is no sense telling them not to breathe toxic fumes if they are going to keep on smoking.

NIOSH also began surveillance of occupational health, and it dispatched investigators to look at health problems in the work place, just as EIS officers had for years investigated epidemics. Millar calls them "the cavalry . . . [always ready] to ride out and look at a problem and figure out how to prevent it."[17]

Moving NIOSH headquarters to Atlanta almost completed the reorganization of CDC. There was one other step. The Phoenix laboratory where all the work on hepatitis was done was two thousand miles away. The Phoenix staff were a strong group and would reinforce the Center for Infectious Diseases, so the decision was made to move the laboratory, much to the dismay of everyone in Phoenix. They had thought they were safe. More than two years had passed since the reorganization of CDC had become official, and the Phoenix laboratory was still untouched. The staff had begun to believe they would be able to stay where they were. The laboratory occupied a building owned by a landlord to whom the government paid rent. After twenty years, the building would revert to the government for a dollar, and the twenty years was up in 1983. The land would still have to be purchased at fair market price, but even in the lean budget years of the 1980s, it seemed to make sense to do that. In the end, however, the government bought the building, but CDC moved the laboratory anyway. The move brought the laboratory's valuable chimpanzees to Atlanta, and more important, a distinguished staff to invigorate the work being done on viral diseases.[18]

The massive reorganization caused less trauma than might have been expected, although the epidemiologists continued to worry about the loss of critical mass and a sense of identity. The laboratory staff had similar concerns. Physical facilities posed a problem as well. The laboratory for virology work was hopelessly out of date and much too small even before the Phoenix laboratory was moved. When the buildings on Clifton Road had been constructed, only twenty or so Class III and Class IV viral agents were known. By the 1980s, there were four times that number, and the use of electron microscopy was routine. There was space enough to work safely with only one or two viral agents at a time. For years Foege tried unsuccessfully to get funds for a new virology building. He first asked for $25 million. When this proved to be a hopelessly large amount, he cut the request in half, but even that sum was struck from the budget.

The coming of the Reagan administration made the situation particularly bleak. All health budgets were cut, those for prevention by 25 percent.[19] Foege asked again and again for the new building. When the 1984 budget was being considered, the request for planning money for a virology building made it through the PHS review, but it was removed at the departmental level. So were a number of other items, but Foege was told he could select three for appeal to Secretary Schweiker. Assistant Secretary for Health Brandt warned him specifically, however, not to appeal the decision on the virology building. If any such attempt was made, all appeals would be lost on the grounds that he had violated instructions.

The night before Foege was to appear before the secretary, he returned to his home in Atlanta to find that the house had been robbed. By the time the police finished their investigations, it was 1 A.M. Foege spent about an hour working on budget materials, slept briefly, and caught the early-bird flight to Washington. On the way to the secretary's office, Dr. Brandt warned him again not to mention the virology building. In fact, Foege probably would not be called on to say anything. The Public Health Service would present CDC's three appeals, and Foege could answer questions, if any.

In the course of the presentation, the PHS spokesman got confused on some numbers, so the secretary turned to Foege for clarification. Foege supplied the needed information and went through the three appeals. Then he told the secretary about the robbery at his house the night before and how angry he had been until he realized that those who robbed him were so poor they had a different set of values. He could understand that; he could not understand elected officals who robbed the American people of health by not giving them something that was so obviously needed.

Schweiker directed that CDC should have all three, then asked Foege, "If you had known it was going to be that easy, would you have asked for anything else?" Foege glanced at Brandt, who nodded, so Foege talked about the virology building. Schweiker asked him what priority it should have. "I would have put it Number 1," Foege replied. "If we had a virological Tylenol problem in this country, it would be clear how vulnerable we were. We simply [do] not have the capacity to deal with any more volume or more than one agent at a time."

Schweiker again directed, "Add the building to that." Some weeks later, he called Foege from the White House to tell him that the building would be included in the president's 1984 budget.

As it happened, CDC never had to defend the request before Congress. The virology building was put into a continuing resolution for 1983, and when this made it appear that CDC's budget had actually been cut for 1984, Congress saw a vacuum and increased funding. CDC had asked only for planning money, but it got building money too.[20]

The need for a virology building had become painfully obvious in 1977, when two employees died in a laboratory accident. By the time construction began, CDC was deeply involved in investigating the most frightening epidemic of the century. All its scientific expertise and persuasive skills would be tested.

CHAPTER 24

Discovery of the AIDS Epidemic

In the midst of CDC's reorientation towards lifestyle and environmental issues, a mysterious and devastating disease, subsequently named AIDS, appeared. It was not surprising that the epidemic was discovered at the institution that for more than three decades had been the nation's sentinel for health, but it was ironic that an infectious disease became CDC's center of concern in the decade when so many plans were made for a different thrust.

From her tiny office in Room 161 of Building 6, Sandra Ford answered requests from physicians for rare drugs to treat seldom-seen diseases. On an afternoon in April 1981, she mailed pentamidine to a New York physician who needed it to treat patients with *Pneumocystis carinii* pneumonia, not one of whom had an underlying reason (like a kidney transplant or leukemia) for the unusual disease. It was the fifth request that this particular physician had made for the drug in just three weeks, and Ford was suspicious.[1]

Dispatching rare drugs and vaccines wherever they were needed was a job CDC had done since 1966, and it was the only source in the United States for pentamidine. Until 1974 there were many calls for it, but when a less toxic, more widely available sulfa drug proved effective in treating most *Pneumocystis* patients, demand for pentamidine dropped sharply.[2] CDC got about eighty or ninety requests a year for it. Beginning in February 1981, however, the demand for pentamidine went up. Even more striking was the fact that nine of the orders in a three-month period were for young adult males in New York and California who until recently had been well. When two of these patients did not respond to the first treatment, the doctor made an unusual call for more of the drug. Ford wrote a memo to her boss, Dr. Dennis Juranek, deputy director of the parasitic disease division. That memo started CDC's investigation of AIDS.

The search for more information led to Dr. Michael Gottlieb in Los Angeles, who had recently treated four young men for *Pneumocystis carinii* pneumonia. He and Dr. Wayne Shandera, an EIS officer assigned to the Los Angeles County Department of Health, happened to be friends, and the two of them talked over the unusual circumstances of Gottlieb's patients. All had been healthy until they sought help for candidiasis (yeast infections in the mouth), fever, and pneumonia. They all had cytomegalovirus (CMV) infection, a herpes virus sometimes linked to cancer; all were homosexuals. From Health Department records Shandera knew about a fifth case, a young man who had died of CMV infection the month before. To have five such cases in a single city in a single segment of the population spelled epidemic. Gottlieb wanted to publish in one of the medical journals, but that took months. Shandera suggested the *Morbidity and Mortality Weekly Report*, and he called friends in Atlanta to expedite publication. A short account of less than two pages, entitled simply "*Pneumocystis* Pneumonia—Los Angeles" appeared in the edition of June 5, 1981. Written in *MMWR*'s terse, straightforward style, it appeared on the less important second page, but any knowledgeable person could read between the lines. This was a big story. The appended editorial note, almost as long as the article, clearly suggested the seriousness of the situation: "The occurrence of pneumocystosis in these 5 previously healthy individuals without a clinically apparent underlying immunodeficiency is unusual. The fact that these patients were all homosexuals suggests an association between some aspect of a homosexual life style or disease acquired through sexual contact and *Pneumocystis* pneumonia in this population."[3]

Just a few days before the article appeared, two physicians in CDC's sexually transmitted disease (STD) division (the new name for what was once called the venereal disease branch), Dr. James Curran and Dr. Harold Jaffe, were in San Diego for a conference on sexually transmitted diseases. They knew publication of the *MMWR* article was imminent, so they brought it up at the conference and discussed it at length privately with several gay physicians from San Francisco and New York who had unreported patients with similar symptoms. When Curran and Jaffe got back to Atlanta, they went to their boss, Dr. Paul Weisner, and suggested this was a problem that needed much more study. Had it been going on for a long time unrecognized, or was it a new phenomenon? There were two ways to answer the question, both of them unique to CDC. One was to check pentamidine use over a period of years, a relatively simple task since the records were readily available. The other was to ask EIS officers assigned to cities and states to contact teaching hospitals and find out if such a disease had been seen in the past.

The pentamidine records showed that until 1980 there was only one case like those in New York and Los Angeles that had so puzzled Sandra Ford. From June until December 1980, there were nine. From the EIS officers in the field came a disturbing report that some of the *Pneumocystis* patients also had Kaposi's sarcoma, a form of cancer rarely seen in America and then only in old men. In eighteen months, from January 1980 to July 1981, twenty-six cases of Kaposi's sarcoma were diagnosed in homosexual men in New York City and California. They ranged in age from twenty-six to fifty-one, and eight of them had died. *MMWR* ran a report on the front page and moved the reference to homosexual men from the text to the headline. It had been only a month since the first article appeared.[4]

The discovery of KSOI (Kaposi's Sarcoma and Opportunistic Infections) or GRID (Gay Related Immunodeficiency Disease), as the outbreak was sometimes called, came during the shakedown period of CDC's reorganization. Under the old structure, the Bureau of Epidemiology would certainly have been in charge, soliciting extensive help from the Bureau of Laboratories. In the new organization, the investigation began in the STD division of the Center for Prevention Services. Curran was chief of research for the division; Jaffe and Dr. Mary Guinan worked with him. They knew the strange outbreak was important. The juxtaposition of two unusual diseases would have attracted attention. The addition of a third factor—the appearance of the diseases in a particular segment of the population—was a fire bell in the night. It meant one of two things: there was a very high attack rate in a localized area, or the problem was relatively common and only the tip of the iceberg could be seen. From the very first, they were afraid it was the second possibility.

A couple of days after the first *MMWR* article appeared, Curran, Jaffe, and Guinan went with Weisner to the office of Dr. Michael Lane, director of the Center for Prevention Services. They outlined the bizarre and unusual nature of the disease and asked permission to drop many of their regular activities to study the outbreak in detail. They wanted to determine if it was a bigger problem than the illness of five young men in Los Angeles seemed to indicate. To Lane it sounded "scary and interesting." He told them to go ahead.[5]

The work began with surveillance. To get information quickly by telephone, the small core of investigators developed a rough definition of the disease: a biopsy-proved case of Kaposi's sarcoma or other life-threatening or fatal opportunistic infection in persons under sixty years of age without an underlying reason for immunosuppressive disease. This strict definition made it possible to collect information by telephone, but it also paved the way for later criticism. They solicited cases and asked health departments to report them.[6] By midsummer they had decided to talk to patients themselves in the hope that something they were missing, perhaps something obvious, would pop up. They went in three directions, to Los Angeles, San Francisco, and New York, seeking answers. Jaffe went to San Francisco.

> We were struck by how sick these men really were. Many were obviously dying and were just wasting away. . . . Secondly, we were struck that these men did lead a particular kind of life style. These were not gay men who were in long-term monogamous relationships. These were highly sexually active gay men. Often they were well-to-do, had good jobs, traveled a lot. They tended to have sexual partners in many parts of the country, often anonymously. . . . They tended to use a lot of drugs along with this . . . [in the] fast track life style.[7]

CDC investigators went armed with a long questionnaire. They asked the men dozens of questions about their medical histories, travel, occupations, use of drugs (prescription and nonprescription), and sexual habits. The two- or three-hour interviews were difficult, but the patients cooperated in spite of their illness. When some thirty interviews were completed, the data were tabulated; the most striking thing setting KSOI patients apart was lifestyle.

By midsummer an informal KSOI Task Force had been organized within CDC to study the strange new epidemic. It was a loose coalition of a half dozen or so people from various disciplines—cancer epidemiology, immunology, virology, and parasitic diseases besides the original core from STD.[8] Initially, Curran had been given three months to work on the problem. Within two months, he and his small group were "drowning." He and Jaffe went back to see Weisner. "This is big!" they said. "Bigger than you believe [Weisner believed it was quite big at that time], bigger than Foege believes or the Center for Infectious Diseases [does]. This is a huge problem and we have got to get going on it."

The next day Weisner assigned six or seven epidemiologists from the medical STD division just to work on AIDS. Lane agreed to the new assignments, which meant that the entire STD division would be working on the new disease, dropping everything else, including work on penicillin-resistant gonorrhea.[9]

Weisner made Curran chairman of the beefed-up task force, primarily, Curran insists, because he had a good secretary, Ellen Shapiro, who could take minutes of the daily meetings. Within CDC's new organizational structure, however, there was no obvious place to put Curran's group. For a time it reported to a steering committee, of which Dr. Philip Brachman, head of the Epidemiology Program Office, was chairman. That committee was made up of representatives from each of the centers. As the scope of the task force's job grew, however, better arrangements had to be made, not only to facilitate work on the new disease but to preserve ongoing CDC programs. With "considerable emotion," Michael Lane outlined the problem to Foege: all the research activities in STD were grinding to a halt, and there were not nearly enough resources to cope with the new problem. Everyone assumed that this was an infectious disease as yet unidentified and that laboratory assistance would be needed in identifying and characterizing the etiologic agent.[10] In the spring of 1982, Foege took the task force into his own office, giving it much-needed administrative support, but there was little he could do to wring more money for it out of a recalcitrant government.

Budgetary problems, especially orders for a reduction in force (RIF), were far more troublesome than those of organization. The Omnibus Budget Reconciliation Act (OBRA) of 1981, which closed PHS hospitals, meant a reduction in the size of the commissioned corps.[11] Though unrelated directly to CDC's work, this action inevitably affected it. There were orders from Washington to reduce the staff by 15 percent. Anyone with less than three years' experience was expendable. The only exceptions were those in training positions. The RIF would have taken away Jaffe, an original member of the KSOI Task Force, who had rejoined CDC's staff in 1980 after a three-year infectious disease fellowship at the University of Chicago. The three years he had worked in the venereal disease division in the mid 1970s did not count. As a newcomer, he was on the list of those susceptible to being cut. To keep him, CDC quickly took advantage of the loophole in the RIF order. Jaffe was recruited into the Epidemic Intelligence Service, class of 1981.[12]

The first major job of the enlarged KSOI task force was a case-control study to compare victims of the strange new disease with healthy homosexual males. Again some of the team fanned out to the most likely cities—San Francisco, New York, and Los Angeles—prepared to stay a month or two, while others remained behind to study Atlanta's gay community. For controls, they selected homosexual men from VD clinics and the practices of private physicians, as well as friends (but not the sexual partners) of patients. Of the seventy-five living KSOI patients at the time, they interviewed about fifty.

Harold Jaffe and Mary Guinan went to San Francisco, where they had rooms in a "sleazy motel," all their per diem afforded. The men came to the motel by appointment, were interviewed, and had blood samples drawn. These were packed up and sent to Atlanta, and the next day the process was repeated for another group. When the task was done and the data from all the cities were analyzed, there was little doubt it was a sexually transmitted disease. The lifestyles of the patients and the controls were quite different, the patients being much more sexually active, much more likely to have sex with people they did not know. Reports from the lab showed that cases had much lower T-lymphocyte counts than the controls. While many of the patients were routine users of amyl nitrites or "poppers," no one in the KSOI task force believed the disease was a toxicological problem.[13]

Those who came to the task force from the STD unit had unusually close contacts with the homosexual community. Even in a political climate less conservative than that of the early 1980s, public health people ordinarily did not have formal ties to the gay health movement. For years, however, CDC had sent representatives to national meetings of gay groups. It set up VD clinics at the Marco Polo Hotel in Florida, where the national gay beauty contest was held, and Weisner frequently addressed national gay meetings. To serve people who are at risk for disease, he had to be familiar with their attitudes and behavior. Weisner talked to them about their major health problems, particularly syphilis and hepatitis B, and he was always well received. The cordiality between the STD unit and the gay community made much of CDC's ground-breaking work in hepatitis B possible. In the late 1970s, when a serologic test made it feasible to study the epidemiology of that disease, the STD division secured the cooperation of large numbers of homosexual men to work with the Phoenix laboratory. That study was a prelude to the important hepatitis B vaccine trials that began in 1980, which led to the licensing of the vaccine. Again, the STD division helped the Phoenix staff enroll gay physicians and patients for the trials. These were conducted entirely within the homosexual community in five cities, among which were San Francisco and Los Angeles.[14] Many of the men whom Jaffe and Guinan included in their study in San Francisco had also participated in the hepatitis B vaccine trials. Their blood samples were especially valuable because they could be compared with those drawn much earlier.

Because CDC staff in both Atlanta and Phoenix had worked so closely and so long with homosexuals, they were quick to sense a problem. For those in Atlanta, the immediate awareness that something was terribly wrong came from years of working with sexually transmitted diseases. For Dr. Donald Francis, who directed the hepatitis B vaccine trials from Phoenix, the outbreak looked like something he had seen before in a different species. A veteran of the global smallpox-eradication program, Francis joined the Phoenix staff in 1978 after years of advanced study in virology at Harvard University. Instinctively, he felt the strange disorder was the human equivalent of the subject of his doctoral research, feline leukemia. Both were marked by cancer and immune suppression. He believed that the new disease, like the common killer of cats, was caused by a little-known organism, a retrovirus. It was a prescient hunch.[15]

The first major publication of the task force appeared in the *New England Journal of Medicine* in January 1982. It reported on 159 cases of KSOI found from June to November 1981. The mortality rate was 38.4 percent. The outbreak was "highly unusual," very probably a single epidemic of underlying immunosuppression. "The high mortality rate among young men with these disorders indicates a serious public health problem." The task force also reported that the magnitude of the epidemic was understated by data from biopsy-confirmed cases of Kaposi's sarcoma and *P. carinii* pneumonia since these were often misdiagnosed or underdiagnosed ailments, and that there were numerous reports of nonfatal opportunistic infections among homosexual men.[16]

A few of the 159 patients, including the only woman in the group, claimed they were not homosexuals but admitted to being drug users. This raised the possibility that KSOI was blood-borne as well as sexually transmitted, but for the moment this fact concerned only some members of the task force—not all of them—and hardly anybody else at CDC. The possibility that the use of "poppers" caused the outbreak had to be checked out, so mice were gassed with amyl nitrites to see if any changes developed in their immune systems. A shortage of funds slowed even that investigation. If a case could be made against amyl nitrites, then the task of controlling KSOI would be relatively easy, but it was a faint hope.

There was not enough money to tabulate the results of the case-control study (these were not published until August 1983, almost two years after the information and blood samples were collected), but it did not cost much to send out a lone interviewer to look at the disease from a different angle. Dr. William Darrow, CDC's senior sociologist, went to southern California where KSOI was prevalent. In the spring of 1982, he began a cluster study to find out what he could by talking to the patients themselves. He had nearly twenty years' experience investigating the sociological aspects of sexually transmitted diseases, although for almost a decade he had been restricted in the kinds of questions he could ask. It was assumed that it was not the business of the U.S. government to know what went on in the bedroom. By 1982, however, the combination of the sexual revolution and the coming of the strange lethal disorder among homosexuals opened the way for a straightforward approach. Darrow could ask whatever he wanted.

With Dr. David Auerbach, the EIS officer assigned to the Los Angeles County Health Department, Darrow tracked down eight of the first nineteen KSOI patients from southern California and close friends of seven others who had died. From thirteen of the patients or their friends, he got the names of sexual partners. Nine of them had had sexual contact with one or more KSOI patients within five years before the onset of their symptoms. Four had had sexual contact with the same KSOI patient—not from California—who was the sexual partner of four KSOI patients from New York City. The cluster study linked forty patients in ten cities by sexual contact. The evidence seemed conclusive that the disease was caused by an unknown infectious organism and pointed to a long incubation period. It also pretty much ended any hope that the cause might be something so simple as "poppers."[17]

April is Cancer Control Month, and Curran went to Los Angeles to testify before an unusual away-from-Washington meeting of the House Subcommittee on Health and the Environment, the group most responsible in the House for health concerns. Congressman Henry Waxman engineered the session held at the Gay and Lesbian Community Services Center. Congressman Waxman was known at CDC as a legislator truly interested in health matters. He had held hearings on liquid protein diet and had conducted a hearing on immunizations in Los Angeles. It was quite natural that he would arrange the first congressional probe into the growing new epidemic.

Curran described the work of the task force for the committee and reported that there were then 300 cases of Kaposi's sarcoma or *Pneumocystis* pneumonia, of whom 119 had died. Beyond the human cost, he cited the high cost of treatment, about $60,000 per case, or $18 million for the first 300 cases. He also reported that other unusal cancers had begun to show up in the same population—rare lymphomas, aggressive cancers of the tongue, and autoimmune disorders. He ended his testimony with the warning that "the epidemic may extend much further than currently described and may include other cancers as well as thousands or tens of thousands of persons with immune defects."[18] His statement gave public expression to the task force's growing private concern that KSOI was a disease that could spread beyond the gay community.

Unlike Legionnaires' disease or toxic shock syndrome, KSOI attracted relatively little attention in the press. Congressman Waxman commented on this in his opening remarks at the hearings. He attributed the reluctance of government and much of the medical community to come to grips with the issue to the fact that it affected one of the nation's most stigmatized minorities, saying:

> Legionnaire's disease hit a group of predominantly white, heterosexual middle-aged members of the American Legion. The respectability of the victims brought them a degree of attention and funding for research and treatment far greater than that made available so far to the victims of Kaposi's sarcoma. . . . [T]he more popular Legionnaire's disease affected fewer people and proved less likely to be fatal. What society judged was not the severity of the disease but the social acceptability of the individuals affected with it.

Waxman pledged to fight anyone who tried to base public health policy on their personal prejudices regarding other people's sexual preferences or lifestyles.[19]

In quickly defining the epidemic in terms of lifestyle and linking it to homosexuals, the task force laid the groundwork for an extended debate on the nature of the disease. Without knowing the causative agent, they engaged in what Gerald M. Oppenheimer has called "epidemiological imagination." In so doing, he writes, "[they] may have skewed the choice of models and hypotheses, determined which data were excluded from consideration until later in the epidemic, and offered scientific justification for popular prejudice, particularly against gay men. On the other hand, the epidemiological approach gave the new disease a human face, . . . [and] offered the possibility of primary prevention in the form of health education and follow-up." CDC provided a model that encouraged others, if not CDC itself, to define the disease in terms of "promiscuous" behavior, a term that carries a heavy moral freight. Even after Kaposi's sarcoma and *P. carinii* pneumonia appeared in other segments of the population, Oppenheimer writes, "CDC was unwilling to disengage itself from the 'life-style' hypothesis or to commit itself to a microbe theory alone." Oppenheimer is particularly critical of CDC for its relative lack of attention in the literature to heterosexual patients before 1984.[20]

The first public disclosure that KSOI would spread to other segments of the population appeared in an editorial by Dr. Anthony S. Fauci of NIH in the June 1982 issue of *Annals of Internal Medicine*. He commended CDC for rapidly deploying a task force to investigate the problem and expressed the hope that eventually important information of scientific interest would result from the study of the syndrome, such as a more precise delineation of the relation between immune defects, viral infection, and oncogenesis. But the immediate goal, he wrote, was to solve the mystery behind an extraordinary disease that struck selectively at a particular segment of society. That population deserved the effort, and to assume that the syndrome would remain so restricted was "an assumption without a scientific basis."[21] That same month, the National Institutes of Health made research on KSOI a "high priority," and CDC's Director Foege held one of many meetings with Assistant Secretary of Health Brandt to urge him to get funding for the work.

Disturbing reports began to come to CDC of lymphadenopathy—enlarged lymph nodes—in homosexual men. Victims often had fever, weight loss, fatigue, night sweats, diarrhea, and other symptoms of general malaise. KSOI patients had those symptoms, too, sometimes for months before they developed Kaposi's sarcoma. The profiles of those with lymphadenopathy and Kaposi's sarcoma were disturbingly similar. The age distribution and other factors were virtually indistinguishable. Dr. Tom Spira, the first immunologist to join the task force, expressed his colleagues' fears when he said, "We don't know if the lymphadenopathy is a prodrome [premonitory symptom] or a milder manifestation of the more severe disease, but our concern is that it is related."[22]

Meanwhile, another aspect of the KSOI story was unfolding. In January 1982 Dr. Bruce Evatt, CDC's expert on hemophilia, got a telephone call from a physician in south Florida. A hemophiliac patient had died of *Pneumocystis carinii* pneumonia, and the doctor thought that he must have been given a contaminated batch of Factor VIII, the clotting factor concentrate pooled from hundreds of thousands of blood donors.

The patient was an older married man from New York who wintered in Florida and had been hospitalized for elective knee surgery. He developed pneumonia, was treated for it, and was subsequently discharged. Within a few days he was readmitted and was diagnosed as having *P. carinii* pneumonia. He died two weeks later. The doctor felt certain that the Factor VIII the patient had received must have been contaminated. Evatt assured him this was not possible, but he called FDA and alerted them to the possibility. He searched the literature and CDC's pentamidine records but found nothing.

Since the patient had died some months before, no further tests could be made, but Evatt knew that if Factor VIII was implicated, if the disorder was blood-borne, more hemophiliacs would fall victim. As Foege said, "If it's real, there will be more of them." Evatt flagged pentamidine requests, asking Sandra Ford to notify him if one came in for a hemophiliac. He waited only a few months. In the early summer of 1982, requests for pentamidine came for hemophiliacs in Colorado and Ohio. Evatt sent Dr. Dale Lawrence to investigate. Both patients had the same disorder that had struck homosexual men in California and New York; their only possible exposure came through the blood supply. Three cases of *P. carinii* pneumonia in hemophiliacs meant two things. First, the underlying immunosuppression was blood-borne. If hemophiliacs were affected, anyone getting a blood transfusion was at risk. Second, the agent had to be a virus. The filtering process used in the manufacture of Factor VIII screened out anything larger.[23]

Just weeks later there was a meeting on KSOI at Mt. Sinai Medical Center in New York City sponsored by the National Institute for Environmental Health. Foege was there to give a ten-minute presentation on why his staff believed that KSOI was caused by a virus or infectious agent. Others at the conference were scheduled to present the case for other possible agents: an environmental toxin, nitrites, drugs, immune overload. Foege previewed the *MMWR* article coming out that week on KSOI in the three hemophiliacs. He made a compelling argument. Curran remembers that the other speakers changed their talks to speak about co-factors. "'We think Dr. Foege is right—it is caused by a virus—however, environmental factors might contribute.' That is how dramatic the three cases in hemophiliacs were."[24]

Between papers, Curran was in the hallway busily arranging a far larger meeting of people from the major blood-banking organizations. "We wanted to get the gay community together so that they would be supportive in deterring gay men from donating blood," he later recalled. "We needed to get all the public health people together including many who were skeptical. . . . [T]he Food and Drug Administration and the National Hemophilia Foundation were saying, 'Let's not over[re]act to this problem; there's a blood shortage.'" The problem was urgent. Just one week earlier, *MMWR* had reported that thirty-four Haitian immigrants had KSOI.[25]

The meeting Curran engineered in the hallway was held two weeks later at the Hubert Humphrey Building in Washington. Dr. Jeffrey Koplan, CDC's assistant director, presided. There were twenty-eight people there from fourteen different organizations representing government, blood banks, pharmaceutical manufacturers, the Hemophilia Foundation, and the National Gay Task Force. The KSOI task force believed that arguments the disease was blood-borne were so convincing that everyone would listen; that possible carriers could at least be discouraged from donating blood. They were disappointed. Almost everyone rejected the argument. Hemophiliacs did not want to return to the primitive methods of treatment they had endured before the introduction of Factor VIII; the blood bank people feared the loss of some of their best blood donors; FDA, which had the authority to enforce regulations, was skeptical that the disease CDC described even existed. Was it just a ploy to get money? Only one positive thing came out of the meeting. The disease finally got a name, Acquired Immune Deficiency Syndrome, or AIDS. The name was more inclusive than KSOI, and unlike GRID, it was sexually neutral. Since the disease had spread far beyond the bounds of the gay community, that was important.[26]

The Washington meeting began the "year of denial." AIDS had appeared in homosexuals, in IV drug users, in Haitians, and hemophiliacs, yet hardly anyone outside CDC wanted to hear about it. There was virtually no coverage in the press, certainly no convergence of reporters like those who had bombarded CDC for information about Legionnaires' disease or toxic shock syndrome. Curran thought that denial served a purpose. As long as you deny that something exists, you do not have to deal with it.[27]

The AIDS task force did not have that luxury. Part of their job was to make projections. Where would AIDS strike next? An obvious answer was recipients of blood transfusions. Another was hospital staff who were daily exposed to blood, urine, and semen specimens from AIDS patients. Predictions of the task force came true with depressing regularity. In fact, sometimes the only lift to AIDS investigators came when one of their predictions—inevitably something bad—came true. There was the momentary satisfaction of having been proved right.

The task force did not have to wait long for one of these predictions to materialize. In the fall of 1982, they received word from San Francisco of a child with an AIDS-like illness who had received numerous blood transfusions shortly after his birth in March 1981. Dr. Arthur Ammann reported the case to the San Francisco Health Department, and CDC helped him track down the blood donors in the case. They found that one of them was a man who subsequently died of AIDS. The case strengthened the belief that whatever caused AIDS, it was blood-borne. The report of this child's illness and an update on AIDS in hemophiliacs appeared in the same issue of *MMWR*. All the first hemophilia cases had died, and four more had been found. The very next week, *MMWR* had another disturbing report. Four more young children had unexplained immunodeficiencies. They had been born to intravenous drug–abusing mothers. But just as there was skepticism in July when CDC first pointed to the possible link between the blood supply and AIDS, so there was skepticism in December that these strange disorders in children could be AIDS. A number of very prominent immunologists insisted the cases were not AIDS. The task force wished fervently that these doubters were right, but they did not believe it. As Jaffe put it, "All these things that represented our worst nightmares were actually happening."[28]

Although the July meeting with blood bank representatives had gone miserably, CDC decided to hold another one on January 4, 1983. The task force had some concrete proposals to make. The meeting was larger this time. Forty-two people from twenty organizations gathered at CDC's Clifton Road headquarters. They were mostly from blood banks, but again hemophiliacs and gay groups were represented. It was a meeting CDC staff would never forget. They planned to present their cases of AIDS in children and hemophiliacs and ask what was to be done about it. It was, Jaffe remembered, an "infamous" session.

We presented our cases, and much to our surprise, people did not believe these cases and were not convinced. One of the people from the Hemophilia Foundation said that he believed that hemophiliacs were getting some unusual illness, but "I don't believe it is AIDS." Those representing the blood banks said the same thing. There was this tremendous denial of the problem. We were stunned. It seemed so clear. But yet it was not being ackowledged by the people who would have to make the decisions. . . . [Finally], Dr. Donald Armstrong, chief of infectious diseases at Memorial Sloan-Kettering in New York, . . . said, "I can't believe what I'm hearing. I can't believe that we are arguing about whether or not this is real. I think there is no question that these people are getting AIDS. We should not be arguing about it, but discussing what we are going to do about it." If applause had been allowed, I would have applauded.[29]

The meeting was Jaffe's first encounter with blood bank people, an altruistic group who could not accept the fact that something supposed to be life-saving brought disease and death.[30] He admitted they had a point. The blood supply in the United States is always precarious, and the blood banks were reluctant even to discuss anything that would compromise it. CDC wanted to exclude high-risk groups like homosexuals from the donor pool, but this was unacceptable, if not unthinkable. In some cities much of the blood supply came from gay groups, and in New York, blood drives had even been conducted in gay bath houses. The suggestion to ban homosexuals as blood donors was offensive to representatives from gay and lesbian groups. They equated it with the old taboo against giving blood from a black donor to a white patient. CDC also proposed surrogate testing of blood donors. Since the exact cause of AIDS was unknown, there was no specific test for it, but Tom Spira's lab had come up with surrogate tests the hematologists believed would be effective. Many AIDS victims had hepatitis B antibodies. That test might be useful for screening, and there were several others. But hardly anybody wanted to listen. Bruce Evatt, who was the first to suggest that AIDS might be blood-borne, remembered the January 4 meeting as "an incredible circus, except that it did start changing minds."

> CDC was going alone. We had a terrible time convincing other people [about] things that had to be done quickly. You can't blame people. These interferences should have been the normal response on the part of these agencies. CDC was calling shots on almost no evidence—educated guesses rather than proof. We did not have proof it was blood-borne; we had five hemophiliacs and two or three blood transfusion cases. We did not have proof it was a contagious agent; we had epidemiological evidence suggesting it. FDA makes recommendations that have to stand up in court. They wanted a different level of proof than could be obtained. The CDC was looking at the trends, and believed that by the time you get proof, you are going to have a major mess on your hands. . . . If [FDA] made recommendations on the things CDC wanted them to make recommendations on, they would long since have lost their jobs. Certainly, the gay groups were putting much pressure on Congress [because of] the emphasis . . . on AIDS being a gay disease. They wanted the emphasis put some place else.[31]

Several factors contributed to the widespread denial that AIDS posed a serious medical problem. The disease affected only marginal groups of society—homosexuals, IV drug users, Haitians, and hemophiliacs, in that order—and there was at least some sentiment in the mainstream populace that whatever happened to the first two groups was only their just desserts. Haitians were recent arrivals, and like any new immigrant group, were more likely to arouse animosity than sympathy. Hemophiliacs made up only a tiny fraction of AIDS victims, 0.9 percent, and they did not want to believe that anything could be wrong with the blood component that had given them near-normal lives. The conservative political climate of the 1980s did not foster faith in the ability of federal government agencies to spot and solve problems. Budgets were severly reduced for even such well-established preventive measures as immunization, and there was pressure to move as much of the responsibility for public health to the states as possible. Then, too, deservedly or not, CDC's stature had been reduced by the swine flu episode. After 1976 the press was more aggressive in its coverage of CDC and probed for weaknesses. The staff consequently became more cautious. All of CDC's documents on AIDS were reviewed an incredible number of times before publication. All statements given to the press were hedged. Just a week before the Atlanta conference in which the staff argued, sometimes with fist-pounding forcefulness, that blood banks should exclude high-risk groups for AIDS from the donor pool, Jaffe was quoted in *Newsweek* as saying, "The risk to the general population [from blood transfusions] is quite small and the need to receive blood far outweighs the concern about AIDS."[32] Considering the millions of transfusions given and the relatively small number of AIDS cases, this was undoubtedly true. Jaffe said it in an attempt to avoid public hysteria, but it did nothing to hasten the end of the year of denial.

There was another legacy of the swine flu affair, one Richard Neustadt and Harvey Fineberg had foreseen four years earlier. In analyzing that giant effort, they said that CDC had lost not only its innocence but also its "clout, not for all time . . . but for some years." For any new departure in preventive medicine, "it almost surely will be tagged as crying 'wolf.'" If CDC foresaw correctly the next public health disaster, they wrote, "its loss of status may affect the lives of citizens."[33]

In the case of AIDS, CDC was not crying wolf, but it had to wait for its message to get through. It might not have taken so long if there had been funds enough to do immediately the thorough analysis of the control-study data that science demands, but almost two years into the epidemic, the staff had learned to live with frustration. A slight softening of resistance was evident in March 1983 when NIH and FDA joined

CDC in publishing some guidelines to prevent the transmission of AIDS. By that time more than 1,200 cases of AIDS had been reported from thirty-four states, the District of Columbia, and fifteen other countries. More than 450 had died. For those whose cases had been diagnosed more than a year earlier, the fatality rate was 60 percent. The five commonsense rules published in *MMWR* were based on experience with hepatitis B infection, which closely paralleled AIDS. The first was to avoid sexual contact with persons known or suspected to have AIDS. The second, "a temporary measure," was the recommendation that those at increased risk for AIDS should not donate blood. The last three were measures to protect the blood supply: better screening procedures for blood, encouragement of autologous transfusions, and research on safer blood products for hemophilia patients. In the dry style of *MMWR*, the document sounds noncontroversial, but before publication, it was, as Bruce Evatt put it, "hounded to death by all the agencies and certainly reviewed by Congress."[34]

The surrogate testing CDC wanted was not implemented, and, in spite of increasing evidence, the blood banks continued to resist the idea that AIDS was blood-borne. Meanwhile, the number of cases continued to grow, doubling every six months. In September 1982, CDC learned of two new cases every day. By June 1983, that number was five or six. Most were from the United States, and of those that had been diagnosed at least two years earlier, 81 percent were dead. By then evidence that AIDS was an infectious disease was compelling enough for the task force to lose its ad hoc status and find a permanent home in the newly formed Center for Infectious Diseases.[35]

Epidemiologists discovered the AIDS epidemic and monitored its spread, but unraveling the scientific puzzle was work for the laboratory. CDC's immunology laboratory was in place and ready to begin work as soon as AIDS specimens began to arrive in 1981. Located in the host factors division (concerned with patients) of the Center for Infectious Diseases, it was the only group at CDC set up to work in human immunology. One of its scientists, Tom Spira, was involved from the beginning. The work in molecular virology got off to a slower start. The distinguished staff of the Phoenix hepatitis laboratory boosted the capability of the virology staff to deal with the AIDS epidemic when that laboratory moved to Atlanta in the spring of 1983 (and this may have been why the laboratory was moved), but even then the work did not always go smoothly. Donald Francis's early suspicion that a retrovirus was responsible for the AIDS epidemic was gaining acceptance, and

Francis was put in charge of setting up CDC's first retrovirus laboratory. It was a mammoth undertaking. The facilities were poor (no one
knew this better than Foege, who had been trying for years to get a new
virology building), and Francis had to recruit a staff. Among the early
finds was Dr. V. S. Kalyanaraman, known to all as Kaly, who came to
Atlanta from the National Cancer Institute. Drs. Cy Cabradilla and
Paul Feorino were already on the staff. That quartet made up the initial
virology lab group, and they did some distinguished work.

Early in 1984, CDC received two ounces of virus associated with
AIDS from the Pasteur Institute in Paris. The French scientists had
isolated it from a lymphadenopathy patient, but they did not know
exactly what they had. They knew it was not HTLV–I (human T-cell
leukemia virus), which Dr. Robert Gallo of the National Cancer Institute had proved in 1980 to be the cause of a leukemia common in
Japan, but, like HTLV–I, it was a retrovirus. The French called it LAV
(lymphadenopathy-associated virus) and sent some of it to CDC and to
Gallo's laboratory. Ever since antibodies to HTLV–I had appeared in
Boston hemophiliacs some months earlier, CDC immunologists had
worked on the assumption that a retrovirus was responsible for AIDS.
Donald Francis, of course, did not have to be convinced. When the
precious sample from Paris arrived in Atlanta, work began at once.
Within hours, LAV was growing well in CDC laboratories.

Gallo also got work under way at the National Cancer Institute. A
full year after the French made their discovery, he isolated a virus he
called HTLV–III, because it was the third such virus discovered in his
laboratory. (HTLV–II had been discovered by Kalyanaraman before he
moved to Atlanta.) HTLV–III was identical to the French virus.

The claim that Gallo had discovered the cause of AIDS was announced to the world by Health and Human Services Secretary Margaret Heckler in April 1984, setting off an international dispute that
was not settled until three years later, when an international panel gave
equal credit to the Pasteur Institute and NCI and changed the virus's
nomenclature to HIV (human immunodeficiency virus.) Resolving the
dispute had more to do with politics than science.[36] President Reagan
and French Prime Minister Jacques Chirac signed the settlement in a
White House ceremony.

The "discovery" of AIDS at CDC took place on several levels. In the
area of hard science, the process began with the arrival of the virus from
France. A test for LAV was quickly developed in Francis's laboratory,
confirming the work of the French and offering one of the earliest

proofs that the virus was indeed serologically and immunologically linked to AIDS. Subsequently, Dr. Paul Feorino proved that the serologic test could be used with considerable confidence to protect the blood supply. He isolated the virus from blood samples that tested positive, thus linking it to transmission by transfusion. At the same time he showed that those samples that tested negative did not contain the virus and thus could safely be used. It took, as one colleague said, "an incredible amount of virus isolation," but it was a milestone in the discovery process with enormous benefits to public health.[37]

Hemophiliacs, the group most vulnerable to blood-borne AIDS, were the major concern of CDC's immunologists. They knew that seroconversions were taking place every day, but there was little they could do about it. Then Bruce Evatt had an idea. If heat killed hepatitis B in plasma, might it not kill the AIDS virus as well? While attending the Hemophilia Congress in Brazil in August 1984, Evatt sought out drug manufacturers and suggested they try it. Most hemophiliacs did not use the heat-treated blood components then on the market because they were more expensive, but Evatt believed they would probably accept the extra expense if it could be proved that heat also worked against AIDS. Two of the manufacturers were interested. As soon as Evatt got home, Dr. Steven McDougal spiked some plasmas with the virus and sent them to the manufacturers for heat treatment. When the plasmas came back, it took but four months to develop the assay and prove without doubt that no virus remained. Evatt described the heat treatment as "incredibly effective"; McDougal considered the work a "triumph." It stopped the exposure of hemophiliacs to AIDS in its tracks.[38]

Another dimension to the laboratory discovery of AIDS was understanding the nature of the virus itself. McDougal found the probe exciting.

> Almost every aspect of it makes sense: mechanistically, on the molecular level [and] cellular level. Everything we learn about this virus just falls right into place. The cells that it infects are explained at the molecular level by the binding of the virus and the T-4 molecule. Its replication in those cells, the reasons it kills the cells . . . the reason the immune system reacts the way it does, makes complete sense. . . . [C]ompared to more infectious diseases, we know more about [AIDS] than any other. The kinds of things that we don't know require years of follow-up. . . .
>
> The science of the virus is really quite exciting, [although] I sometimes feel like Frankenstein. You get in an isolated corner in the lab and you get interested in a concrete discrete problem, and it is not too difficult to lose sight of what this is doing to other people. You do not think that while you are doing an experiment that several people have died from AIDS.[39]

To those studying the epidemiology of AIDS, it seemed as if the discovery would never end. There was always something new: the appearance of AIDS in the wife of a hemophiliac, the revelation that the incubation period averaged five and a half years. That startling figure came from studying the length of time that elapsed between exposure to AIDS in a blood transfusion and onset of the disease. The mathematical curve stretched from six months to eleven years, with the mean at five and a half. It was another blow to those who had been thinking the incubation period might be as long as two years. With the new information, they knew they had not yet explored even the tip of the iceberg.[40]

The discovery process had an international angle, too. In 1983 Joseph McCormick learned that AIDS had appeared in Belgium among immigrants from Zaire. Suspicious, he organized a study team from Belgium, CDC, and NIH to check it out. They found so many AIDS cases that McCormick began arrangements for a long-term study. He returned to Atlanta and reported to Foege. In Zaire, McCormick said, there was heterosexual transmission of AIDS, and men and women were affected in about equal numbers. Foege immediately called Assistant Secretary for Health Brandt. McCormick listened to the conversation on the speaker telephone. Brandt did not want to believe it.[41]

The public's and, to an extent, the government's discovery of AIDS came in mid 1983. Public demonstrations protested the government's lack of action in dealing with the epidemic, the dilemma of those with AIDS being compounded by the fear of many others that they would get "it," too. Overnight, apathy became hysteria. It was then that the PHS called AIDS a "serious health problem," gave it a high priority, and set up an AIDS "hotline" at its headquarters in Washington.[42]

There was also the discovery of AIDS patients, not as victims, but as human beings. CDC's epidemiologists made that discovery in 1981. So did Bill Darrow. He talked to men with AIDS, had tea with them, ate meals they prepared. Within a year or so, he had read more than a hundred of their obituaries. In 1983 he reluctantly followed orders to remove from his files the names and pictures and personal identifiers of all those reported as having AIDS lest the information fall into the wrong hands and the people be stigmatized. To Darrow the people in his files were more than T-cell counts. He remembered their faces.

The end of the beginning of the fight against AIDS was reached by 1984. With incredible speed science had unlocked many of its secrets. Yet AIDS defied solution. The public responded in the same way it had responded to epidemics for three hundred years: first with denial, then with a search for someone to blame, and finally with a demand for action.[43] The action proposed by CDC during these years did not often find ready acceptance. By quickly linking AIDS to a particular lifestyle, epidemiologists acted as a lightning rod for critics, but they also performed the task that historically has been theirs. They pointed out a means of prevention.

Epilogue

The Centers for Disease Control is widely recognized as one of the world's premier public health institutions. From modest beginnings concerned with control of a single disease in one section of the United States, it has gradually broadened its mandate to include not only all the communicable diseases, but also many chronic ones, occupational disorders, and such social ills as violence and accidents. Its efforts have made life much better. During the first three decades of its history, CDC played a vital role in diminishing, sometimes to the vanishing point, the threat of communicable diseases in the United States and the world. There was a time when the staff, with tongue only slightly in cheek, wondered if one day there would be no more worlds to conquer. They reveled in their successes: eradication of smallpox, unraveling the secrets of Legionnaires' disease and toxic shock syndrome, immunizing the nation's children. They learned to be philosophic about their relatively few failures.

How did an institution with modest prospects and comparatively modest funding accomplish so much? Certainly, the drive, energy, and vision of Dr. Joseph Mountin played a significant role. His protégés in Atlanta took him seriously when he said, "There's a lot of ignorance here. Let's exploit it!" Mountin never assigned responsibility without granting the necessary authority. He encouraged innovation: murine typhus disappeared when the exterminators forgot the rats and concentrated on the fleas. He knew how to exploit opportunity: the threat of biological warfare put epidemiology to work on a broad scale.

Freedom to try new approaches no doubt enabled CDC to attract outstanding talent, and scientific excellence early became a hallmark of

Centers for Disease Control Organization, 1990

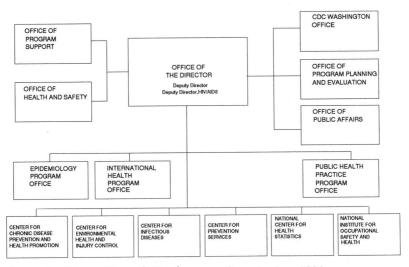

Centers for Disease Control, Headquarters Organization, 1990

the institution. This was most marked at first in the laboratory, where giants in the field established themselves as the world's leading authorities on, among other things, salmonella, shigella, and the toxicity of insecticides. Talent attracts talent, and CDC's roster has always been filled with distinguished laboratory scientists. Although basic research was not CDC's mission, its scientists have been remarkably successful in expanding the frontiers of knowledge. The reasons lie not only in individual excellence but in the availability of a rich lode of material from the nation's epidemics.

The second major pillar on which CDC is built is epidemiology, a science first taught as an academic discipline at Johns Hopkins University in 1919. Exactly three decades later, epidemiology found its institutional base in Atlanta. Both steps were essential before epidemiology could become useful, before it could become the basis of public health practice. The new concept of surveillance, first used for malaria in 1951, ensured that the numbers needed for the practice of epidemiology would be available. The procession of bright young officers in the Epidemic Intelligence Service on two-year assignments ensured a steady supply of fresh ideas. With no personal turf to protect, they could afford to be provocative. Their energy and drive forced a constant reevaluation of what in epidemiology briefly passed as the status quo.

CDC was created to serve the states, to answer any call for help, the routine and the extraordinary. This service mission has tended to attract people with a "Peace Corps mentality." They have a mix of scientific talent and missionary spirit, which makes them believe, often correctly, that they can make the world a better place. The mixture also gives CDC an unusual and heady ferment. It is a place that "allows you to keep your idealism well into middle age," one person put it.

CDC has steadily expanded its domain by acquiring bits and pieces of the PHS, the latest acquisition being the National Office of Health Statistics in 1987. Its current focus is to help people help themselves to become "healthy people." Discovery of the AIDS epidemic was a dramatic warning against complacency about infectious diseases. CDC's encounter with AIDS recapitulated the high and low points of its history. The quick reaction to the five cases of *P. carinii* pneumonia in Los Angeles recalled the Cutter incident, while the difficult public relations problems associated with AIDS were painful echoes of swine flu and battles with the aspirin industry over Reye's syndrome.

In the war against AIDS, violence, occupational hazards, and injurious lifestyles, the art of persuasion may prove to be as formidable a weapon as science. The necessary communication skills for that struggle, however, are still in the dark ages. Assessing risk can be done with considerable confidence, but communicating that risk is at best tentative. Communicating better with all who need to know is among the challenges that lie ahead.

Universal health is a tantalizing dream at least as old as ancient Greece. Appropriately, a bust of Hygeia, the Greek goddess of health, stands close by CDC's front door.

Notes

CHAPTER 1

1. Harry Pratt to the author, January 20, 1988.

2. Justin M. Andrews, "Perspective on Malaria Today," *JAMA* 184 (June 15, 1963): 873; George H. Bradley, "A Review of Malaria Control and Eradication in the United States," *Mosquito News* 26 (December 1966): 463–64; Justin M. Andrews and Jean S. Grant, "Malaria Control History, World War II, Military Malaria Control Experience in the Continental United States" (MS, CDC archives), p. 11.

3. Bess Furman, *A Profile of the United States Public Health Service, 1798–1948* (Washington, D.C.: GPO, n.d.), p. 427; John Duffy, "The Impact of Malaria on the South," in *Disease and Distinctiveness in the American South*, ed. Todd L. Savitt and James Harvey Young (Knoxville: University of Tennessee Press, 1988), pp. 37–45.

4. Paul P. Weinstein, "Parasitology and the United States Public Health Service: A Relation of Science and Government," *Journal of Parasitology* 59 (February 1973): 11.

5. Andrews and Grant, "Malaria Control History," p. 1.

6. Boisfeuillet Jones, author interview, Atlanta, October 1, 1987. Two types of malaria plagued the South, *Plasmodium vivax* and *Plasmodium falciparum*. Vivax malaria is debilitating and subjects its victims to secondary infections, but it is not generally a primary cause of death. Falciparum malaria progresses rapidly and frequently kills its host directly. The vector for both is *Anopheles quadrimaculatus*. Another mosquito, *Anopheles freeborni*, transmits the malaria parasite in the western states. The eastern vector breeds in quiet, sunlit, impounded waters, and would rather feed on animals than man. The western vector requires constantly refreshed water like the seepages from irrigation canals. Control of malaria meant control of the mosquitoes' habitats.

7. Andrews and Grant, "Malaria Control History," pp. 36–37; Joseph W. Mountin, "Adaptation of Public Health Programs to Defense Needs," *American Journal of Public Health and the Nation's Health* 32 (January 1942): 1–2.

8. Andrews and Grant, "Malaria Control History," pp. 36–37.

9. Mark Hollis, CDC Oral History (hereafter CDC-OH), videotape, June 24, 1985. All Oral History interviews are on videotape unless otherwise noted; all are on file at CDC.

10. Melvin Goodwin, CDC-OH, June 1983.

11. Andrews and Grant, "Malaria Control History," p. 41; "History of Malaria Control in War Areas" (MS, CDC archives); Samuel W. Simmons, author interview, October 6, 1987, Atlanta.

12. Andrews and Grant, "Malaria Control History," pp. 43–44; Louis Keenan, "Malaria Control in War Areas: Entomological Warfare during World War II" (Honors thesis, Emory University, 1981), p. 14; Federal Security Agency, PHS, *Malaria Control in War Areas, 1943–44* (Atlanta, 1944), p. 4.

13. PHS, *Malaria Control in War Areas, 1942–43*, p. 31; Furman, *Profile of PHS*, p. 426; Andrews and Grant, "Malaria Control History," pp. 56–57. The Lanham Defense Housing Act paid for ditching. The Lanham Act was concerned primarily with ensuring adequate housing for defense workers, but it also provided funds for day-care nurseries for the children of women employed in defense industries and paid some labor costs essential to maintenance of these industries.

14. PHS, *Malaria Control in War Areas, 1942–43*, p. 66; id., *Malaria Control in War Areas, 1943–44*, p. 20; Keenan, "Malaria Control in War Areas," p. 16.

15. PHS, *Malaria Control in War Areas, 1942–43*, p. 79.

16. Furman, *Profile of PHS*, p. 428.

17. Mark Hollis, CDC-OH, June 24, 1985.

18. Mark Hollis, interview with Harlan Phillips, June 6, 1964 (transcript, George Rosen Oral History Project, History of Medicine Division, NLM), pp. 33–34. Hereafter Hollis transcript, NLM.

19. Samuel W. Simmons, author interview, October 6, 1987.

20. Andrews and Grant, "Malaria Control History," pp. 71–73; Hollis, CDC-OH.

21. Hollis transcript, NLM, pp. 34–35. Dengue was probably introduced to the islands by a pilot returning from Fiji, where an epidemic was in progress.

22. Andrews and Grant, "Malaria Control History," p. 46.

23. Alexander Langmuir, author interview, April 9, 1987, Atlanta.

24. Justin Andrews, "Perspective on Malaria Today," *JAMA* 184 (June 15, 1963); 874; Melvin Goodwin, CDC-OH, June 1983; Mark Hollis, CDC-OH. The Naples epidemic was louse-borne typhus. DDT was to prove equally effective against flea-borne, or murine, typhus found in the southern United States.

25. Carter Memorial Laboratory, "Preliminary Progress Report" (April 1–June 30, 1944, CDC archives).

26. P. F. Russell, "The United States and Malaria: Debits and Credits,"

Bulletin of the New York Academy of Medicine 44 (June 1968): 634; Andrews and Grant, "Malaria Control History," pp. 63–70; Keenan, "Malaria Control in War Areas," p. 25.

27. Minutes, MCWA staff meeting, May 16, 1945, RG 90, 83-0079, Box 1, Federal Records Center, Atlanta. Hereafter, all RG 90 citations, unless otherwise noted, should be understood to be located in the Atlanta FRC.

28. Hollis, CDC-OH; Hollis transcript, NLM, p. 17. Endemic murine flea-borne typhus was found in the southern United States. Like epidemic louse-born typhus, it was effectively controlled by DDT. See John C. Snyder, "Typhus Fever Rickettsiae," in *Viral and Rickettsial Infections of Man,* ed. Frank L. Horsfall, Jr., and Igor Tamm, 4th ed. (Philadelphia: Lippincott, 1965), pp. 1059–94.

29. Minutes, MCWA staff meeting, May 16, 1945. Mountin's ability to move money around was legendary. According to Dr. Norman Topping, associate director, NIH, 1948–52, "Joe used to say, 'You know, if we're not smart enough to move our money around from one pot to another where it's needed more, we shouldn't be in the job we're in.'" See Norman H. Topping, interview, April 24, 1964 (transcript, George Rosen Oral History Project, NLM), p. 56. Hereafter Topping transcript, NLM.

30. Minutes, MCWA staff meeting, May 26, June 2, June 9, 1945, RG 90, 83-0079, Box 1.

31. Minutes, MCWA staff meeting, June 2, 1945; "War and Post-War Tropical Medicine," *Tropical Medicine News* 1 (October 1944): 8–11; Paul P. Weinstein, "Parasitology and the United States Public Health Service: A Relation of a Science and Government," *Journal of Parasitology* 59 (February 1973): 11–12.

32. Marion Brooke, CDC-OH, March 15, 1984.

33. Brooke, CDC-OH; Mae Melvin, CDC-OH, 1985.

34. Minutes, staff meeting, May 16, 1945, RG 90, 83-0079, Box 1.

35. Mountin, "Adaptation of Public Health Programs to Defense Needs," p. 8. The Environmental Health Center was created in 1948 as an outgrowth of work in stream pollution that the PHS had conducted in Cincinnati since 1912. These aging facilities were replaced in 1954 and renamed the Robert A. Taft Sanitary Engineering Center. The Arctic Health Center, established in Anchorage in 1948, was destined to remain quite small.

36. Mark Hollis, CDC-OH.

37. Ibid. Justin Andrews said that it was Surgeon General Parran who gave the Communicable Disease Center its name. See Andrews, interview, July 27, 1964 (transcript, NIH/PHS Oral History Collection, History of Medicine Division, NLM), p. 12.

38. Furman, *Profile of PHS,* pp. 440–41.

39. Topping transcript, NLM, pp. 52–53.

CHAPTER 2

1. In 1931, as an officer in charge of the Office of Studies of Public Health

in the Division of Scientific Research, Mountin conducted health surveys to determine which health protective measures worked and which did not. Four years later, enactment of the Social Security Act gave the PHS authority to make grants to the states for health programs, a powerful new weapon in the war against disease. In 1937, Mountin became chief of the Division of Domestic Quarantine, a forerunner of the Division of States Relations, and served there during World War II. In MCWA, Mountin saw a staff of professionals and a reservoir of experience that could be the source of scientific help the states needed. See Thomas Parran, "A Career in Public Health," *Public Health Reports* 67 (October 1952): 930–43, passim. Hereafter *PHR*.

2. Paul Starr, *The Social Transformation of American Medicine* (New York: Basic Books, 1982), p. 342.

3. Leonard A. Scheele, interview, March 22, 1963 (transcript, George Rosen History Project, NLM), pp. 20–22. Scheele attributes the original idea of building the Clinical Center at NIH to Mountin, but in 1938 (?) the idea was rejected because NIH feared congressional pressure to take pet patients (ibid. p. 23).

4. An anecdote from Andrews's World War II experiences is illustrative. He was in charge of malaria control at Roberts Field, a ferrying airport carved out of the jungle in Liberia. Liaisons inevitably developed between the troops and local women, who met surreptitiously in the bush. Venereal disease and malaria rose alarmingly. Andrews's solution to the malaria problem was to build three houses—Christmas, Valhalla, and Paradise—just beyond the borders of the base and screen them well against mosquitoes. See Martin D. Young, "Fifty Years of American Parasitology: Fulgent Protozoologists," *Journal of Parasitology* 62 (August 1976): 513.

5. Betty Hooper, author interview, May 6, 1987.

6. As president of the American Society of Parasitologists some years after he left CDC, Andrews cut council meetings from two days to a mere five hours, a record for modern times.

7. Young, "Fifty Years of American Protozoology," pp. 513–14; Justin Andrews to Dale R. Lindsay, March 30, 1951, RG 90, 74A1539, Box 2.

8. Surgeon General Parran was not exempt from the pressures of politics. President Truman did not reappoint him to a fourth term in 1948. The ostensible reason was that there should be rotation in that office, and that if Parran stayed on, there would be no room for promotion within the service. He was replaced by Dr. Leonard Scheele, head of the National Cancer Institute, who was not well known in public health circles but had the support of the influential health promoter Mary Lasker. Oscar R. Ewing, administrator of the Federal Security Administration, explained Scheele's appointment as an attempt to balance the factor of morale against the factor of "keeping on a wonderful man." His appointment signaled a shift of emphasis in the PHS away from public health practice, Parran's forte, towards research, particularly into chronic diseases. News of Parran's replacement came as a complete surprise to Mountin, who was visiting the CDC's technology laboratory in Savannah when the announcement was made. "He didn't say a word," S. W. Simmons recalled.

"His mouth dropped." *New York Times,* February 13, 1948, p. 3; February 14, 1948, p. 17; Fitzhugh Mullan, *Plagues and Politics: The Story of the United States Public Health Service* (New York: Basic Books, 1989), p. 128; S. W. Simmons, author interview, October 6, 1987, Atlanta.

9. William Watson, author interview, May 5, 1987, Atlanta; William B. Cherry, CDC-OH, 1982; Ellis Tisdale, CDC-OH, audiotape, February 10, 1982; Sidney Olansky, CDC-OH, June 5, 1985.

10. Justin M. Andrews, "The United States Public Health Service Communicable Disease Center," *PHR* 61 (August 16, 1946): 1203.

11. Andrews to chief, BSS, July 23, 1952, CDC archives.

12. *Atlanta Journal,* December 2, 1947.

13. Justin Andrews, "The Eradication Program in the U.S.A.," *Journal of the National Malaria Society* 10 (June 1951): 102–5; Geoffrey M. Jeffery, "Contributions of the U.S. Public Health Service in Tropical Medicine: Part II," *Bulletin of New York Academy of Medicine* 44 (June 1968): 743; Federal Security Agency, CDC, *CDC Activities, 1946–47* (Atlanta: n.p., 1947), p. 2; id., *CDC Activities, 1947–48,* p. ii; *Atlanta Constitution,* September 20, 1949.

14. Minutes, staff meeting, December 2, 1946, RG 90, 83-0079, Box 1. From Oatland Island, too, CDC acquired the handsome grandfather clock that stands in the director's office in Atlanta, which originally belonged to the Brotherhood of Railway Conductors. Dr. Johannes Stuart of the PHS Venereal Disease Division, which used the Oatland Island facility in the interim between its occupancy by the Railway Conductors and the CDC, did not want CDC to get the clock. He thought the conductors should have it, but with their members scattered, there was no one to take it.

15. Theodore Bauer, CDC-OH, 1985; Seward E. Miller, "Over-All Functions and Objectives of the Laboratory Division," *CDC Bulletin,* April–June 1949, pp. 1–2; Andrews to chief, BSS, July 23, 1952.

16. "Condensed History of Environmental Health Training Conducted by the Communicable Disease Center"(MS, n.d.), RG 90, 75A1154, Box 1; Ellis Tisdale, CDC-OH, audiotape, February 10, 1982; minutes, staff meeting, July 17, 1950, RG 90, 83-0079, Box 1.

17. *Atlanta Constitution,* November 6, 1949.

18. James Steele, CDC-OH, audiotape, May 29, 1981.

19. Minutes, staff meeting, August 5, 1946, RG 90, 83-0079, Box 1; *The Word* 3 (May–June 1971): 6; *Atlanta Journal,* January 22, 1951; David Sencer, author interview, December 27, 1988, Atlanta.

20. *Atlanta Journal,* October 1, 1947; November 30, 1949; *Atlanta Constitution,* July 28, 1948; November 30, 1949; Mark Hollis, CDC-OH, June 24, 1985; Boisfeuillet Jones, author interview, October 1, 1987, Atlanta; Eugene Stead, Jr., to the author, October 16, 1987.

21. The possibility that the fly might be the vector for polio was noted as early as 1911, and the polio virus was isolated from feces-eating flies in 1941 by investigators at the Yale Poliomyelitis Unit, Children's Research Foundation in Cincinnati, and the Department of Pediatrics at Cleveland Municipal Hospital. The Yale Poliomyelitis Unit, working with two PHS entomologists, attempted

without success to stem polio epidemics by fly control in Paterson, New Jersey, and Rockford, Illinois, in 1945. See John R. Paul, *A History of Poliomyelitis* (New Haven: Yale University Press, 1971), pp. 291–99.

22. James Steele, CDC-OH, audiotape, May 29, 1981.

23. Samuel Simmons, author interview, October 6, 1987, Atlanta.

24. Minutes, CDC staff meeting, April 28, 1947, RG 90, 83-0079, Box 1; Frank R. Shaw, "Epidemic and Disaster Aid," *CDC Bulletin,* November 1950, p. 32.

25. James Crabtree, acting surgeon general, to medical director, CDC, October 2, 1947, RG 90, 74A1539, Box 3; Wesley E. Gilbertson to surgeon general, March 2, 1949, ibid., Box 4; Justin Andrews to surgeon general, March 1, 1949, ibid., Box 6.

26. Roger E. Heering to F. V. Meriwether, March 12, 1947; W. H. Wright to Rolla Dyer, March 20, 1947; J. W. Mountin to R. A. Vonderlehr, March 28, 1947; Vernon Link to Mountin, April 1, 1947; Link to Heering, April 16, 1947, in personal file of Marian M. Brooke, Atlanta.

27. E. R. Coffee to Vernon Link, January 6, 1947, RG 90, 74A1539, Box 4; Vonderlehr to Mountin, July 9, 1947, ibid.

28. Minutes, staff meeting, June 7, 1948, June 6, 1949, RG 90, 83-0079, Box 1; Hollis transcript, NLM, pp. 21–22. NIH emphasized basic research from the time of the Steelman Report of 1947. See John R. Steelman, *Science and Public Policy: A Report to the President,* 5 vols. (Washington, D.C.: GPO, 1947).

29. Minutes, staff meeting, February 23, 1948, RG 90, 83-0079, Box 1.

30. Minutes, staff meeting, May 23, 1949, ibid.

31. Alexander Langmuir, videotaped interview in the "Leaders in American Medicine" series, National Library of Medicine and National Audio-Visual Center, March 1979.

32. Association of State and Territorial Health Officers, CDC Conference, October 17–18, 1949, *Report,* RG 90, 74A1539, Box 5; Federal Security Agency, CDC, *CDC Activities, 1950–1951* (Atlanta, 1953), pp. 2–3; Langmuir, author interview, April 9, 1987, Atlanta.

33. Langmuir, author interview.

34. Ibid.

35. Ibid.; Langmuir interview, "Leaders in American Medicine," NLM; minutes, staff meeting, January 30, 1950, RG 90, 83-0079, Box 1.

36. Justin Andrews, Griffith Quinby, and Alexander Langmuir, "Malaria Eradication in the United States," *American Journal of Public Health* 40 (November 1950): 1407–10; Alexander Langmuir, "The Surveillance of Communicable Diseases of National Importance," *New England Journal of Medicine* 268 (January 24, 1961): 183–84.

37. Andrews, Quinby, and Langmuir divided the period 1932 to 1949, when the systematic attack on malaria was under way, into four periods, some of which overlap. From 1932 to 1940, the number of cases of malaria, although high, was grossly underreported; from 1938 to 1943, there was a sharp decline; from 1943 to 1947, there was a slight increase owing to importation of malaria

by troops returning from overseas; after 1947 there was a sharp decline, explained primarily by a change in the method of reporting morbidity statistics. See "Malaria Eradication," p. 1408. After 1942, blood surveys were more useful in determining the virtual absence of malaria than in measuring its endemicity. Andrews told the CDC staff in 1952 that the country was free of malaria, and that it was CDC's job to keep it that way. No one knew why malaria had decreased so quickly, he said, but he thought it was because of "some unknown influences not connected with malaria control programs." See minutes, advisory committee, Malaria Control Field Station, January 8, 1952, RG 90, 74A1539, Box 7.

38. Langmuir, author interview; minutes, staff meeting, January 30, 1950.

39. Alexander D. Langmuir, "William Farr: Founder of Modern Concepts of Surveillance," *International Journal of Epidemiology* 5 (1976): 13.

CHAPTER 3

1. *Atlanta Journal,* October 17, 1949.

2. National Security Resources Board, "Civil Defense Planning Advisory Bulletin" (Doc. 121/1, December 1, 1949).

3. G. H. Bradley, "Miscellaneous Environmental Sanitation Problems: Insect Vector Control following Wartime Disaster" (December 1949); Carl O. Mohr, "Report" (December 19, 1949); "Diagnostic Laboratory Services following Wartime Disaster," all in RG 90, 74A1539, Box 8; *Atlanta Constitution,* December 4, 1949.

4. V. G. McKenzie to [Vonderlehr], February 9, 1950; Langmuir to Vonderlehr, March 2, 1950, RG 90, 74A1539, Box 6; Alexander D. Langmuir, "The Epidemic Intelligence Service of the Center for Disease Control," *PHR* 95 (September–October 1980): 471.

5. Minutes, special staff meeting, August 9, 1950, RG 90, 83-0079, Box 1.

6. Vonderlehr to C. L. Williams, August 14, 1950; Mountin to [Vonderlehr], August 9, 1950; Williams to [Vonderlehr], August 21, 1950, RG 90, 74A1539, Box 7.

7. Langmuir, "Epidemic Intelligence Service of the Center for Disease Control," p. 472.

8. Major General C. A. McAuliffe to Surgeon General Leonard A. Scheele, October 10, 1950, RG 90, 74A1539, Box 2.

9. Alexander Langmuir and Justin Andrews, "Biological Warfare Defense," *American Journal of Public Health* 42 (March 1952): 235; Langmuir, "The Potentialities of Biological Warfare against Man: An Epidemiological Appraisal," *PHR* 66 (March 30, 1951): 393–97.

10. *Hornell* [N.Y.] *Tribune,* May 9, 1951.

11. Members of the committee were Alexander Langmuir (chair), S. W. Simmons, Donald Schliessmann, Larry Hall, and Ralph B. Hogan.

12. "Airborne Disease Studies" (MS [1951?]), RG 90, 74A1539, Box 2.

13. Theodore A. Bauer, CDC-OH, 1985.

14. Dr. Irving Langmuir had a profound effect on Langmuir's life. While the young Alexander Langmuir was in high school, he worked one summer at the General Electric Company, where his Uncle Irving was a distinguished scientist. Alexander worked on the problem of evaporation from the tungsten filament in a vacuum, and "did not have the vaguest idea" what he was doing. "But I was in the laboratory and . . . got a great wealth of . . . general knowledge, of what research process was and, more particularly [over the next fifteen years], . . . a sense of science at its very best . . . the organization of theories and interpretation of laws, making new observations and then drawing interpretation" (Langmuir, interview with Harlan Phillips, March 25, 1964 [transcript, George Rosen Oral History Project, History of Medicine Division, NLM], p. 11; hereafter Langmuir, George Rosen transcript).

15. Langmuir interview, "Leaders in American Medicine," NLM.

16. Elizabeth Fee, *Disease and Discovery: A History of the Johns Hopkins School of Hygiene and Public Health: 1916–1939* (Baltimore: Johns Hopkins University Press, 1987), p. 139.

17. Langmuir interview, "Leaders in American Medicine," NLM.

18. Langmuir to [CDC] Executive Office, July 21, 1950, RG 90, 74A1539, Box 2.

19. Ibid.

20. Minutes, staff meeting, September 25, 1950, RG 90, 83-0079.

21. *Dayton Daily News,* October 3, 1950; *Cleveland Plain Dealer,* October 4, 1950; *Paulding Progress,* October 5, 1950; *Life* 29 (October 23, 1950): 40–41.

22. Langmuir to Thomas Francis, Jr., November 30, 1950, RG 90, 74A1539, Box 2.

23. Langmuir to Ernest L. Stebbins, March 27, 1951, RG 90, 74A1539, Box 4.

24. Langmuir, "Epidemic Intelligence Service of the Center for Disease Control," p. 472; Bruce Dull, author interview, September 28, 1987, Atlanta.

25. A brief outline of the course of epidemiologic history is found in Abraham M. Lilienfeld and David E. Lilienfeld, *Foundations of Epidemiology,* 2d ed. (New York: Oxford University Press, 1980), pp. 23–45; and Abraham Lilienfeld, "Epidemiology and Health Policy: Some Historical Highlights," *PHR* 99 (May–June 1984): 237–41. The statistical approach to disease in America is traced by James H. Cassedy in two books, *Demography in Early America: Beginnings of the Statistical Mind, 1600–1800* and *American Medicine and Statistical Thinking, 1800–1860* (Cambridge, Mass: Harvard University Press, 1969, 1984).

26. Frost's work at Johns Hopkins is recounted in Fee, *Disease and Discovery,* pp. 68–70, 132–36.

27. William Foege, director of CDC from 1977 to 1983, has compared Langmuir's appointment at CDC to Frost's appointment at Johns Hopkins; he sees both as landmarks in the history of public health. Johns Hopkins gave epidemiology its academic base; CDC gave epidemiology an institutional base. William Foege, author interview, October 12, 1987, Atlanta.

28. Farr quoted in Abraham M. Lilienfeld and David E. Lilienfeld, "Epidemiology and the Public Health Movement: A Historical Perspective," *Journal of Public Health Policy* 3 (June 1982): 144; Alexander Langmuir, "The Territory of Epidemiology: Pentimento," *Journal of Infectious Diseases* 155 (March 1987): 349.

29. Richard Prindle, CDC-OH, audiotape, April 23, 1981; 30th Anniversary Dinner, EIS, April 1981, CDC-OH.

30. Langmuir, "Epidemic Intelligence Service of the Center for Disease Control," p. 471. Results of the investigation were reported in "Epi 2."

31. Ibid., p. 473; Epidemiology Branch, quarterly report, second quarter, FY 1952, RG 90, 74A1539, Box 8.

32. Ruth and Edward Brecher, "Disease Detectives," *Saturday Evening Post,* May 30, 1953, pp. 25–26. Dramatic accounts of CDC's work with rabies and histoplasmosis by Berton Roueché are in the "Annals of Medicine" series, *New Yorker* 33 (April 6, 1957) and 36 (September 17, 1960).

33. Langmuir, George Rosen transcript, pp. 20, 45–46.

34. Philip Brachman, author interview, May 7, 1987, Atlanta; James Mason, author interview, October 16, 1987, Atlanta.

CHAPTER 4

1. Andrews to chief, BSS, July 23, 1952, CDC archives.

2. Morris Schaeffer, CDC-OH, 1984.

3. William B. Cherry, CDC-OH, 1982; Marion Brooke, CDC-OH, 1984; Mae Melvin, CDC-OH, 1985; Jim Paine to author, March 24, 1987; David Sencer, author interview, December 27, 1988, Atlanta.

4. Edward K. Kline and Sidney W. Bohls, "Program Review, Laboratory Services, Communicable Disease Center" (MS, January 1951), RG 90, 74A1539, Box 7.

5. Earl Arnold, CDC-OH, 1984; Jim Paine to author, March 24, 1987.

6. Ralph Hogan, CDC-OH, July 12, 1985.

7. Stanley Music, quoted in Hogan, CDC-OH.

8. Hogan, CDC-OH; Langmuir, author interview.

9. William Watson, author interview, May 5, 1987, Atlanta.

10. Hogan, CDC-OH.

11. "A Mosquito's Eye View of CDC" ([1951?] CDC archives). The Laboratory and Epidemiology branches were represented by the mosquito's front two legs; the Vector Control and Investigations, Training, Audio-Visual, and Technical Development branches were represented by the back four. State health departments and the regional offices of the Federal Security Administration were the wings, and the various aspects of administration made up the head and thorax. See chart 3.

12. Chris Hansen to S. W. Simmons, January 13, 1950, RG 90, 74A1539, Box 3. Langmuir hoped that Hansen would be appointed chief of the Vector Analysis Branch, but George Bradley was chosen instead. Hansen later moved to NIH.

13. Simmons, author interview, October 6, 1987; Simmons, CDC-OH, audiotape, August 10, 1979; Theodore Bauer, CDC-OH, 1985; minutes, staff meeting, July 3, 1950, RG 90, 83-0079. Dr. Theodore Bauer, director of CDC after October 1952, took the disloyalty issue in his stride. He had been there before. When he was on the Venereal Disease Commission, he testified before the McCarthy Committee. After Bauer left the room, a member of the committee staff said, "He came clean, but I know that something is wrong with him."

14. Ellis Tisdale to Vonderlehr, March 28, 1951, 74A1539, Box 7. In 1953, CDC had training centers for state health officers in Amherst, Mass.; Columbus, Georgia; Denver, Colorado; Pittsburgh, Pennsylvania; Topeka, Kansas; and Yonkers, New York.

15. Minutes, advisory committee, Malaria Control Field Station, January 8, 1952; M. H. Goodwin, Jr., to R. Hugh Wood, report, November 20, 1952; "New Field Station Section" (unidentified MS), all RG 90, 74A1539, Box 7.

16. Langmuir, author interview; *Atlanta Constitution*, November 30, 1949; "Phoenix Field Station" (MS, n.d.), RG 90, 75A1154, Box 1.

17. Langmuir, author interview.

18. Simmons, author interview; David Sencer, Joseph Mountin Lecture, October 1980, CDC-OH, audiotape.

19. Minutes, executive staff meeting, January 7, 1952, RG 90, 74A1539, Box 9. The experience of CDC in the Midwest may serve as an example of friction with the regional health officers. Dr. Aaron Christensen, director of the Denver Region of PHS, viewed CDC activities with misgiving. He thought his own staff were competent to handle activities carried on by CDC, including epidemiology, and he objected to the practice of the Atlanta office in planning new activities that would take place in the Denver region without informing the Denver office of such plans. LeGrand B. Byington to medical director in charge, CDC, August 13, 1951, RG 90, 74A1539, Box 8.

20. Theodore Bauer to chief, BSS, June 4, 1953, RG 90, 74A1539, Box 3.

21. *Atlanta Constitution*, January 23, 1951; Bauer, CDC-OH.

22. Theodore Bauer, CDC-OH; William Watson, author interview, May 5, 1987, Atlanta. While CDC's budget was cut, other units of the PHS had increased funds during the 1950s, when appropriations for the PHS quadrupled to $840 million. Much of this increase went to NIH, whose budget grew from $37 to $100 million. See Mullan, *Plagues and Politics*, pp. 128–31.

23. Herbert Yahraes, "The Villain Still Pursues Us," *Collier's*, August 21, 1953; "Has the Fly Got Us Licked?" *Popular Science Monthly*, June 1952, clippings, CDC Scrapbook 1.

24. S. W. Simmons, "Insecticides and World Health," *PHR* 67 (May 1952): 454.

25. S. W. Simmons to Wesley Gilbertson, February 1, 1951, RG 90, 74A1539, Box 7.

26. Vernon Link to acting officer in charge, CDC, October 30, 1952; RG 90, 74A1539, Box 2; *Newsweek*, September 29, 1952; *Greensboro Daily News*, October 20, 1952; Thomas R. Dunlap, *DDT: Scientists, Citizens, and*

Public Policy (Princeton, N.J.: Princeton University Press, 1981), pp. 66, 69–70.

27. Simmons, author interview, October 6, 1987.

28. *Atlanta Journal,* October 15, 1952; *Pittsburgh Press,* May 20, 1952.

29. Ralph B. Hogan, "First Quarterly Progress Report of Research at Camp Detrick," July 1–September 30, 1952, RG 90, 74A1539, Box 2; CDC news release, January 27, 1953, ibid.; S. W. Simmons to Chris A. Hansen, March 10, 1953, ibid., Box 7; *Savannah Morning News,* October 22, 1952.

30. Morris Schaeffer, a native of Russia, came to the United States at the age of five, and grew up in New York. After earning both M.D. and Ph.D. degrees from New York University, he taught microbiology at Case Western Reserve and ran a contagious disease unit at the City Hospital in Cleveland before moving to Montgomery. He described the decade he spent at the Montgomery laboratory as "the most exciting, productive, happiest years of [his] career" (Schaeffer, CDC-OH, 1984).

31. CDC, "Western Equine Encephalitis in the Missouri River Basin States, 1950," RG 90, 74A1539, Box 8; *Greeley Journal,* May 21, 1950; *Greeley Daily Tribune,* May 21, 1951.

32. Ralph Hogan to Executive Office, March 9, 1951, RG 90, 74A1539, Box 8; Thomas A. Cockburn to Langmuir, January 4, 1952; Cockburn to Andrews, February 15, 1952, ibid., Box 6; Vernon B. Link, "Notes on Encephalitis Program," April 6, 1953, ibid., Box 2. Cockburn, a native of Great Britain, had a varied career as doctor, author, scientist, soldier, and world traveler. Just before he came to CDC in 1948, he was in charge of animals at the London Zoo. The article over which he and Schaeffer clashed was not published jointly, but they were co-authors, with others, of an article published later. Cockburn left CDC in 1953.

33. Langmuir continued to fret about the complexities at Greeley, where doctors, biologists, immunologists, entomologists, and veterinarians all competed for position. He wondered how to hold them together long enough so that their individual contributions would multiply and not merely add up. (A psychologist told him they must all be equally able or they would fight and break apart.) By the 1960s, Langmuir established a pattern for EIS assignments: either a single investigator or a team of two who complemented each other, one a second-year man, the other a first-year man (Langmuir, George Rosen transcript, pp. 40–41).

34. John Foster, "In the Manchac Swamp Scientists Stalk the Carrier of Sleeping Sickness," *Dixie* [New Orleans], *Times-Picayune States Roto Magazine,* June 17, 1956, pp. 7–9.

35. Schaeffer, CDC-OH; Arnold, CDC-OH.

36. Lillian DeLoach, Montgomery Laboratory Series, #6, *Montgomery Advertiser,* May 17, 1957.

37. Bauer, CDC-OH; Steele, CDC-OH, audiotape, May 29, 1981; unidentified clipping, CDC Scrapbook 1.

38. Steele, CDC-OH; Bauer, CDC-OH.

39. CDC news release, September 18, 1961, RG 90, 64A809, Box 2.

40. Langmuir, memo, December 15, 1950, RG 90, 74A1539, Box 2; Langmuir to Andrews, December 28, 1951, ibid.

41. Tom D. Y. Chin, CDC-OH, 1984; *Wichita Beacon Sunday Magazine,* August 24, 1958; Berton Roueché, "The Liberace Room," *New Yorker* 36 (September 17, 1960): 147–48, 168.

42. Mullan, *Plagues and Politics,* p. 128.

CHAPTER 5

1. Starr, *Social Transformation of American Medicine,* p. 346.

2. The polio virus was isolated in 1948 at Harvard University by Drs. John Enders, Thomas Weller, and Frederic Robbins, who showed that it could be cultivated in non-nervous tissue and that multiplication of the virus in tissue culture caused specific injury, which could be readily recognized with a high-powered microscope. They won the Nobel Prize for their work. Typing hundreds of strains of polio virus was done in university laboratories from Maryland to California and was completed in 1953. It resulted in the classification of multiple strains of polio virus, with Type I accounting for more than 82 percent of all cases. One of the major accomplishments financed by NFIP, the typing project opened the way to all subsequent developments. Dr. David Bodian and Dr. Isabel Morgan of Johns Hopkins University successfully immunized monkeys with *intramuscular* injections of virus over a period of months, and at Yale University, Dr. Dorothy M. Horstmann showed that the polio virus entered the bloodstream during the incubation period. This meant the virus could be blocked from entering the central nervous system by relatively small amounts of circulating antibody. See Paul, *History of Poliomyelitis,* pp. 373–78, 234–35, 389.

3. The value of these fly-control studies was questioned within CDC. Vernon Link suggested that airborne disease studies should be given higher priority than polio, and Budget Officer Abbey said that the work was hard to explain in terms of accomplishment: "We spend $800,000 to $1,000,000 on epidemic work, and they inquire as to whether we are accomplishing anything." Langmuir responded: "Anything accomplished in the field of polio would have to be sensational." Minutes, Epidemiology Section, executive staff meeting, January 7, 1952, RG 90, 74A1539, Box 9.

4. W. McD. Hammon, L. L. Coreill, and J. Stokes, Jr., "Evaluation of Red Cross Gamma Globulin as a Prophylactic Agent for Poliomyelitis. I. Plan of Controlled Field Tests and Results of 1951 Pilot Study in Utah"; "II. Conduct and Early Follow Up of 1952 Texas and Iowa-Nebraska Studies"; "III. Preliminary Report of Results Based on Clinical Diagnosis," *JAMA* 150 (October 25, 1952): 739, 750, 757. The summer after he graduated from medical school, and before he began his internship, Langmuir worked with Hammon on a Rockefeller Foundation Summer Fellowship project. They investigated malaria in Maryland, Tennessee, and Florida.

5. Alexander Langmuir to author, February 2, 1989.

6. States with the highest incidence of polio would get the largest allotment. The formula called for 57 percent of the available gamma globulin to be allotted to the states on this basis: 33 percent for mass community prophylaxis, and 10 percent reserved for national emergencies. Office of Defense Mobilization, "Plan for Allocation of Gamma Globulin" (April 15, 1953), RG 90, 55-0614. Langmuir did not think the formula was epidemiologically sound. He questioned whether predictions could be made accurately on a statewide basis, much less at the county level, where they would be "practically meaningless. Polio in small communities certainly does not behave with the regularity assumed by the plan. . . . There is nothing sacrosanct about a county as far as poliomyelitis epidemics are concerned" (Langmuir to Ralph S. Paffenbarger, June 29, 1953, RG 90, 55-0614).

7. Langmuir to the author, February 5, 1989. Dr. Tom Rivers, chairman of the NFIP's scientific research committee, could not understand how Langmuir had talked O'Connor into testing gamma globulin as a public health measure by giving it to household contacts, nor could he understand how Langmuir, "a pretty smart apple," would want to do such a thing. Rivers told O'Connor he thought the new test would be a waste of time, money, and effort. See Saul Benison, *Tom Rivers: Reflections on a Life in Medicine and Science* (Cambridge, Mass.: MIT Press), pp. 485–86.

8. Basil O'Connor to Mildred Elson, APTA, July 17, 1953, RG 90, 55-0614; Langmuir to author, February 5, 1989.

9. Morris Greenberg to Abraham Lilienfeld, September 2, 1953, RG 90, 55-0614; *Atlanta Journal,* July 23, 1953; August 26, 1953.

10. Langmuir, telephone interview, February 3, 1989; NFIP news release, February 23, 1954, RG 90, 55-0614. A summary of the study, "Evaluation of Gamma Globulin in Prophylaxis of Paralytic Poliomyelitis in 1953," was published in *JAMA* 154 (March 27, 1954): 1086–90. Rivers never bothered to read the report. "You read it," he said to Saul Benison, "and if it proved anything I'll eat it for lunch tomorrow" (Benison, *Tom Rivers,* p. 487).

11. The other laboratories were at the University of Pennsylvania, where Dr. Hilary Koprowski worked at the Wistar Institute, and at the University of Cincinnati Children's Hospital, where Dr. Albert Sabin labored.

12. Morris Schaeffer, CDC-OH. Li was head of the bacteriology department at the Chinese Army Medical College in Nanking until 1947. He fled China and came to the United States when the Communists overran Nanking in 1949. Tom Rivers said Li and Schaeffer "demonstrated a great deal of patience and ingenuity in adapting the Mahoney strain to grow in mice. It had never been done before, and I doubt that before they did their trick anybody ever suspected that it could be done. I don't know why they tried to do this— perhaps it was to get a cheap laboratory animal for diagnostic purposes. If that was their purpose, they got that and more, because the strain they finally developed turned out to be mutant that was avirulent for both mice and monkeys by all routes and later proved very useful to Sabin" (Benison, *Tom Rivers,* p. 565).

13. As the trials got under way that spring, Dr. W. H. Sebrell, director of

NIH, wrote the Dallas County Medical Society that the PHS neither approved nor disapproved of the vaccine. Only when a manufacturer applied for a license would any action be taken, and at that time the government "would consider the safety, purity, and potency of the product and license it only if satisfactory evidence was available on all points" (Sebrell to Millard J. Heath, March 12, 1954, RG 88, 74-8, Box 1, WNRC).

14. Langmuir, telephone interview with the author, February 3, 1989.

15. Just three days later, Dr. Albert Sabin sent a worried note to the director of the Laboratory of Biologics Control. He noted that an appendix between pages 42 and 43 of the report describing thirteen cases of paralytic polio in children up to four weeks after inoculation presented a problem that needs "further scrutiny and consideration." In those cases there was a low incidence of virus isolation, and he wondered whether this "might have been due to the inoculation of a minute amount of virus intramuscularly rather than to natural infection." He suggested that the PHS would perform a useful function by checking reported cases of paralytic polio in children within a few weeks after vaccination. (Sabin to William Workman, April 15, 1955, RG 88, 74-8, Box 1, WNRC.) Sebrell says that the NFIP pushed NIH to approve the Salk vaccine, "but only because of the favorable results of the extensive studies. To refuse the license meant condemning many children to paralytic polio. All of the experts agreed to go ahead" (Sebrell, interview, December 8–9, 1970, NIH/NLM Oral History Project, NLM, p. 110).

16. Aaron E. Klein, *Trial by Fury: The Polio Vaccine Controversy* (New York: Charles Scribner's Sons, 1972), pp. 104–13; William E. Leuchtenburg, *A Troubled Feast: American Society since 1945* (Boston: Little, Brown, 1973), p. 40.

17. Allan M. Brandt, "Polio, Politics, Publicity and Duplicity: Ethical Aspects in the Development of the Salk Vaccine," *International Journal of Health Services* 8 (1978): 265.

18. Langmuir, "The Surveillance of Communicable Diseases of National Importance," *New England Journal of Medicine* 268 (January 24, 1963): 184–85. Langmuir expected that there would be a hundred cases during the next two weeks and possibly more. His epidemiological "diagnosis" proved to be correct, his "prognosis" somewhat high. There were seventy-nine vaccine-related cases.

19. Victor M. Haas to W. H. Sebrell, April 28, 1955, RG 90, 60A-560, Box 44, WNRC. This long letter is marked "Confidential." Access to this material was made possible by the Freedom of Information Act. Sebrell was out of town when news came of the vaccine-associated cases. Although he returned before the all-night meeting, he was not informed of it until the next morning and was miffed that he had not been asked to participate. Sebrell, NIH/NLM Oral History Project, p. 108.

20. Haas to Sebrell, April 28, 1955.

21. "Proceedings, Representatives of National Organizations with Department of Health, Education and Welfare on Availability and Distribution of Poliomyelitis Vaccine" (April 27, 1955), pp. 65–67, RG 90, 60-527, Box 2, WNRC.

22. Langmuir to the author, January 8, 1989.

23. *New York Times,* April 29, 1955, p. 21. Dr. Neal Nathanson headed the surveillance unit; Dr. William J. Hall was the statistician.

24. Those present at the meeting at the National Microbiological Institute were Drs. Sebrell, Workman, Langmuir, Hottle, Hammon, Shaughnessey, Eddy, Murray, Salk, Bodian, Enders, Sabin, Lennette, McGinness, Paul, Haas, and Shannon. The group decided not to release the names of those attending the meeting to the press, which by this time was keeping watch at airports and railway stations to see which authorities on polio came into town.

25. Transcript of Proceedings, NIH, Ad Hoc Committee on Poliomyelitis Vaccine, April 29, 1955, pp. 37, 111, 114–15, 125, 207–8, RG 90, 64A-875, Box 1, WNRC. The Biologics Control laboratory had advance warning that something was wrong with the Cutter vaccine. Dr. Bernice Eddy, a staff microbiologist who tested vaccines for safety, reported in 1954 that the Cutter product paralyzed monkeys. She informed Sebrell, but the vaccine was released anyway; evidence from the paralyzed monkeys was disregarded. See Edward Shorter, *The Health Century* (New York: Doubleday, 1987), pp. 68–69.

26. Poliomyelitis Surveillance Unit, Epidemiology Branch, CDC, *Poliomyelitis Surveillance Report,* No. 1, May 1, 1955. Fifty-five reports were issued in 1955.

27. Langmuir, telephone interview, February 3, 1989.

28. Benison, *Tom Rivers,* p. 554.

29. The committee was a reduced version of the one that had met at NIH on April 29. It included Dr. Salk and Dr. Hammon, University of Pittsburgh; Dr. Francis, University of Michigan; Dr. John Enders, Harvard; Dr. David Bodian, Johns Hopkins; Dr. Albert Sabin, University of Cincinnati; Dr. Edward Lennette, California Department of Public Health; Dr. Joseph Smadel, Walter Reed Army Medical Center; Dr. John R. Paul, Yale; Dr. Foard McGinness, NFIP; and Dr. H. J. Shaughnessey, Illinois Department of Public Health (chairman).

30. *New York Times,* May 8, 1955, p. 1; May 9, p. 14. Those present at this meeting included Drs. Bodian, Enders, Francis, Salk, Smadel, and Shaughnessy.

31. Neal Nathanson and Alexander Langmuir, "The Cutter Incident," *American Journal of Hygiene* 78 (July 1963): 22–23; *New York Times,* November 19, 1955, p. 21.

32. Mrs. Hobby quoted in Klein, *Trial by Fury,* p. 123.

33. Hill quoted in Virginia Van der Veer Hamilton, *Lister Hill: Statesman from the South* (Chapel Hill: University of North Carolina Press, 1987), p. 202.

34. Leonard Engel, "The Salk Vaccine: What Caused the Mess?" *Harper's* 211 (August 1955): 32; *New York Times,* May 12, 1955, p. 1, and July 13, 1955, p. 28; Sebrell, NIH/NLM Oral History Project, p. 103. Dr. Ruth Kirschstein of the NIH staff gives a different picture of the changes in staff that followed in the wake of the Cutter incident. "[It] resulted in everybody up the line who had anything to do with it . . . being dismissed because of it." The director of the Microbiology Institute lost his post, as did the equivalent of the assistant secretary for health. See Shorter, *Health Century,* p. 70.

35. Langmuir, Nathanson, and Hall, "Surveillance of Poliomyelitis in the United States in 1955," pp. 82–83.

36. *New York Times,* November 16, 1955, p. 37; November 20, 1955, pt. 4, p. 8.

37. *New York Times,* September 29, 1956, p. 1.

38. CDC, *Report of Activities, July 1, 1955–June 30, 1956* [Atlanta, 1956], p. 17; *Atlanta Journal-Constitution,* September 16, 1956; *Greenville* [S.C.] *News,* July 4, 1956; *Scope Weekly,* April 11, 1956. Dr. F. Duran-Reynals of Yale University called these viruses "orphan" because they were in search of a disease. They produce changes in tissue culture, and there are hundreds of them. Not all are harmful, but some of them produce diseases like aseptic meningitis (an inflamation of the covering of the brain and spinal cord) that look suspiciously like polio. A high proportion of virus isolated from nonparalytic and aseptic meningitis cases in Montgomery and elsewhere turned out not to be polio at all. There were 3,200 cases of aseptic meningitis in Marshalltown, Iowa, in the summer of 1955. ECHO IV virus was the etiologic agent.

39. CDC, *Report . . . July 1, 1955–June 30, 1956,* p. 17.

40. Ralph Hogan, CDC-OH. Morris Schaeffer said in 1984: "We believe the LSC is the so-called Sabin strain although Sabin does not admit that this is the strain he put in the vaccine. He claimed to have given it some additional passages and that his strain was different" (Schaeffer, CDC-OH). From Washington, C. P. Li asked the Pfizer Company to help him secure strains of Type I virus isolated at Tulane University, which had not been passed in tissue culture more than two or three times. "I intend to attempt to develop a live vaccine still using the monkey skin technique," he said (Li to John Fox, November 3, 1955, RG 88, 74-8, Box 1, WNRC).

41. In 1948 WHO established its Influenza Information Service, a worldwide coordinated system of laboratories that sought out new strains of influenza in the hope that a mutant capable of causing a pandemic would be detected and a vaccine developed in time. This might prevent a recurrence of the disaster of 1918, when Spanish flu killed millions of people around the world, including approximately half a million in the United States alone.

42. Langmuir, "Surveillance of Communicable Diseases of National Importance," p. 188.

43. Ibid.

44. Langmuir, telephone interview, February 3, 1989.

45. Two EIS officers, D. A. Henderson and Fred Dunn, put out the report.

46. Alexander Langmuir, Mario Pizzi, William Y. Trotter, and Frederick L. Dunn, "Asian Influenza Surveillance," *PHR* 73 (February 1958): 115; William Y. Trotter, Frederick L. Dunn, Robert H. Drachman, D. A. Henderson, Mario Pizzi, and Alexander Langmuir, "Asian Influenza in the United States, 1957–1958," *American Journal of Hygiene* 70 (1959): 37–38.

47. Arthur M. Silverstein has an excellent short account of the changing character of the influenza virus in *Pure Politics & Impure Science: The Swine Flu Affair* (Baltimore: Johns Hopkins Press, 1981), ch 6. The possibility of an influenza pandemic had long been kept in mind. There was much discussion in

the 1950s about influenza coming in waves, Type A making its appearance every two years, Type B every four years. The theory seemed to fit as far back as 1918. In the 1940s, when he was a member of the Army's Commission on Acute Respiratory Disease, Langmuir and his colleagues wrote a paper entitled the "Periodicity of Influenza," and although he dismissed it as "pious pompous poppycock" almost forty years later, he was not surprised when the long-expected variant of the A strain appeared in 1957. See Langmuir, "Territory of Epidemiology," pp. 353–54. For an account of the dramatic influenza epidemic of 1918, see Alfred W. Crosby, *Epidemic and Peace, 1918* (Westport, Conn.: Greenwood Press, 1976).

48. Trotter et al., "Asian Influenza in the United States, 1957–1958," p. 34; *Atlanta Constitution,* August 20, October 24, and December 11 and 26, 1957.

49. Trotter et al., "Asian Influenza in the United States," pp. 35–36.

50. Jensen came to Montgomery from the University of Michigan, where he had worked for years with Dr. Thomas Francis, Jr., the nation's leading authority on influenza. Francis initiated influenza studies in the United States in 1934. In Michigan, Jensen and his colleagues studied the antigenic relationships among influenza viruses. It was this work that showed the rapid changes in the influenza virus that dictated almost annual changes in the vaccine. A brief account of Francis's work with influenza is in his obituary, *New York Times,* October 2, 1969, p. 47. For Jensen's work, see *Alabama Journal,* January 16, 1958.

51. *Scope Weekly,* November 20, 1957.

52. Bruce H. Dull, CDC-OH, March 19, 1984. In 1957 there were few guidelines protecting the rights of human subjects, but there was strong emphasis on volunteerism. In the prison tests, Dull followed rigid security procedures; all needles and syringes were counted before prison officials. Once he and fellow EIS officer, William Neill, had several hundred blood samples in a cardboard box so big it took two of them to carry it. As they waited for one security gate to be opened, Neill tapped on the box and said in a loud voice, "Don't worry, we'll have you out of here in no time, Little Joe."

53. *San Francisco Chronicle,* September 23, 1957; *Washington Post and Times Herald,* October 10, 1957; *Wall Street Journal,* October 1, 1957.

54. *Atlanta Journal,* September 7, 1957; *Atlanta Journal-Constitution,* September 29, 1957; *Scope Weekly,* September 25 and December 16, 1957.

55. Langmuir, "Epidemiology of Asian Influenza," pp. 7–9; Langmuir, "Surveillance of Communicable Diseases of National Importance," p. 189.

56. *Atlanta Journal,* October 28, 1957, January 16, 1958; *New York Times,* September 27, 1957, p. 21.

57. Benison, *Tom Rivers,* p. 555.

CHAPTER 6

1. CDC, *Proceedings of the Biennial Staff Conference, March 25–29, 1957,* pp. A–1, 8–9, RG 90, 65A870, Box 1.

2. Robert Anderson, CDC-OH, audiotape, June 3, 1982.

3. William C. Watson, CDC-OH, September 25, 1985.

4. Watson, author interview, May 5, 1987, Atlanta.

5. Sidney Olansky, CDC-OH, June 5, 1985. Initially the VDRL laboratory was put on Staten Island because of easy access to clinical material, but as the scope of the venereal disease program widened, the decision was made to move it to a more central location.

6. Olansky, CDC-OH; CDC, *Report of Activities, July 1956–June 1957* [Atlanta, 1957], p. 46.

7. Alan M. Brandt, *No Magic Bullet: A Social History of Venereal Disease in the United States since 1880* (New York: Oxford University Press, 1985), pp. 143–44.

8. Watson, CDC-OH.

9. Mountin quoted in Thomas Parran, "A Career in Public Health," *PHR* 67 (October 1952): 937.

10. Watson, CDC-OH. The fact that PHAs worked mainly with blacks did not mean that syphilis was absent from the white population. It was probably underreported. Elizabeth Fee has observed that a "social silence" surrounded the problem of syphilis in Baltimore in the 1920s. "Patients did not talk about their diseases, physicians did not report them, the health department did not publicize them, and the newspapers never mentioned them. The diseases were thus largely invisible" (Fee, "Sin versus Science: Venereal Disease in Twentieth-Century Baltimore," in *AIDS: The Burdens of History*, ed. Elizabeth Fee and Daniel M. Fox [Berkeley: University of California Press, 1988], p. 124).

11. Windell R. Bradford, author interview, October 2, 1987, Atlanta.

12. The most complete study of the Tuskegee experiment is James H. Jones, *Bad Blood: The Tuskegee Syphilis Experiment—A Tragedy of Race and Medicine* (New York: Free Press, 1981). The Tuskegee project had not been kept secret. Reports of findings appeared regularly. See, for example, J. K. Shafer, Lida J. Usilton, and Geraldine A. Gleeson, "Untreated Syphilis in the Male Negro: A Prospective Study of the Effect on Life Expectancy," *Milbank Memorial Fund Quarterly* 32 (July 1954): 262–73. The article was published simultaneously in the July 1954 issue of *PHR*.

13. *New Orleans Times-Picayune*, March 20, 1957; *Washington Daily News*, March 21, 1957.

14. *Gainesville* [Ga.] *Daily Times*, March 7, 1957; *Chicago American*, April 5, 1960; *Chicago Daily Tribune*, April 6, 1960.

15. Langmuir to E. Russell Alexander, February 18, 1959, RG 90, 62A726, Box 4; *Scope Weekly*, August 5, 1959; Symposium on Present Status of Poliomyelitis and Poliomyelitis Immunization, AMA, November 30, 1960, Atlanta.

16. Other members of the commitee were Drs. David Bodian, W. McD. Hammon, Joseph L. Melnick, John R. Paul, and Roderick Murray (chairman).

17. Minutes, branch staff meeting, November 17, 1958, RG 90, 65A870, Box 1.

18. Leroy E. Burney, "Current Status of Live Poliovirus Vaccine," *JAMA*, December 18, 1959 (MS copy), RG 90, 63A789, Box 2.

19. Albert Sabin to Langmuir, November 30, 1959, RG 90, 63A789, Box 2; minutes, branch chiefs staff meeting, April 11, 1960, in ibid.

20. Langmuir to chief, CDC, April 15, 1960, RG 90, 63A789, Box 2.

21. *Atlanta Journal,* January 23 and 24, 1961; *Atlanta Constitution,* January 24, 1961; *Medical Tribune,* February 13, 1961.

22. "Babies and Breadwinners" campaign, 2d progress report, April 26, 1961, CDC archives; *Journal of the American Osteopathic Association,* April 1961, clipping, Scrapbook 4.

23. Michael Gregg, author interview, July 15, 1987.

24. Mildred M. Galton to chief, microbiology section [CDC], October 23, 1957, RG 90, 65A870, Box 1.

25. James Steele, CDC-OH, audiotapes, May 29 and June 17, 1981; videotape, 1986; William Cherry, CDC-OH, 1982; Alan Donaldson to chief, CDC, February 8, 1957, RG 90, 65A870, Box 1.

26. Langmuir, author interview, April 9, 1987; Sencer, author interview, December 27, 1988.

27. Minutes, branch staff meeting, September 24, 1958, RG 90, 65A879, Box 1; *Washington Morning Star,* September 24, 1958.

28. *Atlanta Journal-Constitution,* November 30, 1958.

29. Ralph Hogan, CDC-OH; William Ewing, CDC-OH, May 1985. The first edition of the Edwards and Ewing book, published by Burgess Publishing Company, appeared in 1955, the second in 1962, and the third in 1972. The first had 179 pages; the fourth, 536 pages.

30. Marion Brooke, CDC-OH; Albert H. Coons to H. K. Wood, January 20, 1958, copy in RG 90, 62A726, Box 4.

31. William Cherry, CDC-OH; *Scope Weekly,* January 1, 1958; Donald S. Martin to Alan W. Donaldson (with Hogan and Kokko notes), July 6, 1956, RG 90, 62A726, Box 4.

32. Donaldson quoted in *Scope Weekly,* January 1, 1958. The FA technique consists of spreading material suspected of containing a given pathogenic organism on a slide, covering the smear with a drop of known antibody solution that has previously been tagged with fluorescein, washing to remove excess antibody solution, and examination of the smear under ultraviolet light by means of a microscope provided with special optical equipment. See "Fluorescein-Tagged Antibody Technique for Rapid Identification of the Pathogenic Organisms" (MS), RG 90, 62A726, Box 4. Numerous papers have appeared in the scientific literature on FA work at CDC. The first was Morris Goldman, "Use of Fluorescein-tagged Antibody to Identify Cultures of *Endamoeba histolytica* and *Endamoeba coli,*" *American Journal of Hygiene* 59 (May 1954): 318–25.

33. Robert J. Anderson, "Communicable Disease Control" (report for Bayne-Jones Committee [1958]), RG 90, 63A789, Box 1; Fleming quoted in *Science News Letter,* July 18, 1959; Technology Branch, Fiscal Year 1959 budget justification, RG 90, 62A716, Box 4.

34. Examples of press coverage of FA technique are found in the *Washington Post,* February 22, 1959; Alice Lake, "Tracking Killer Germs," *Saturday*

Evening Post, October 13, 1962; Willard Neal, "Medical Detectives Attack the Virus Mysteries," *Atlanta Journal and Constitution Magazine,* August 30, 1959.

35. R. J. Anderson to chief, BSS, April 7, 1958, RG 90, 65A870, Box 1.

36. "Meeting of Subcommittee on Staphylococcal-Streptococcal Infections, June 4, 1957," RG 90, 65A870, Box 1. Phage typing was originated by two London bacteriologists, G. S. Wilson and J. D. Atkinson. Bacteria may be identified through the use of bacteriophages or phages—viruses that attack bacteria—which are so highly specific that they allow for "fingerprinting" the various staph types. Each phage would destroy a particular type of staphylococcus. The organism to be identified is streaked on a glass dish marked off with a grid pattern of twenty-five squares, one for each of the standard phage types. Wherever the staph colony is dissolved, its identity is established. The most frequent strain found in hospitals was 42B/52/80/81, or 80/81 for short.

37. Langmuir to chief, CDC, February 28, 1958, RG 90, 65A870, Box 1; *New York Times,* March 22, 1958.

38. "Summary of Recommendations of the National Conference on Hospital-Acquired Staphylococcal Diseases," RG 90, 65A870, Box 1.

39. Minutes, executive staff meeting, September 23, 1958, RG 90, 65A870, Box 1; Simmons, author interview, October 6, 1987.

40. Only the headquarters for TB research remained in Washington. The tuberculosis laboratory was already in Atlanta, having moved several years earlier primarily because 10,000 square feet of space was available at Lawson General Hospital, room enough for laboratories, offices, and 10,000 guinea pigs. Those in Washington practically commuted to Chamblee to oversee the work.

41. Phyllis Edwards, CDC-OH, 1982; Robert Anderson, CDC-OH; Ted Bauer, CDC-OH. For a brief account of the successful battle against tuberculosis, see "Centennial: Koch's Discovery of Tubercle Bacillus," *MMWR,* 31 (March 19, 1982): 121–23.

42. Borches quoted in *Atlanta Journal-Constitution,* September 1, 1958.

43. *Atlanta Constitution,* July 1, 1958; Scheele quoted in *Centerpiece* 4 (July 1950).

44. Glenn S. Usher, "Epidemic Aid Mission to East Pakistan, Communicable Disease Center," May to July 1958, RG 90, 65A870, Box 1; Philip Brachman, author interview, May 7, 1987; Bruce H. Dull, CDC-OH, March 19, 1984.

CHAPTER 7

1. The political transformation of the Public Health Service in the 1950s is traced in Mullan, *Plagues and Politics,* ch. 6. Annual appropriations for the PHS quadrupled during the Eisenhower years to $840 million, much of it going to NIH. When Dr. James Shannon became NIH director in 1955, its budget was $100 million; two years later it was $200 million. See Shorter, *Health Century,* p. 72.

2. "Proposed Construction of Communicable Disease Center Building near Atlanta, Georgia," Agenda, 51st Annual Conference of the Surgeon General, December 8–11, 1952, RG 90, 74A1539, Box 5.

3. Story recounted in Theodore Bauer, CDC-OH.

4. *Atlanta Constitution,* July 22, 1955; November 16, 1956.

5. Robert J. Anderson, CDC-OH, September 25, 1984; Anderson, CDC-OH, audiotape, June 3, 1982.

6. *Atlanta Constitution,* February 15, 1957; March 22, 1957.

7. John Fogarty to President Eisenhower, January 2, 1958, RG 90, 65A870, Box 1.

8. Theodore Bauer, CDC-OH.

9. William Watson, author interview, May 5, 1987, Atlanta. Fogarty treated budget requests from NIH the same way. Dr. William Henry Sebrell, director of NIH from 1948 to 1955, recalled testifying before the House subcommittee: "My testimony . . . consisted essentially of being asked how much more did we need. Fogarty would ask the question . . . 'We understand that you are only allowed to ask for so much; if you didn't have that prohibition, how much would you ask for? How much can you effectively use?'" (Sebrell, interview with Albert Siepert and William T. Carrigan, December 8–9, 1970, NIH/NLM Oral History Project, NLM, p. 152).

10. Robert Anderson, CDC-OH.

11. James Goddard, CDC-OH, August 15, 1985; Anderson, CDC-OH, audiotape; Watson, author interview, May 5, 1987; Fogarty obituary, *New York Times,* January 11, 1967, p. 25. Mary Lasker's influence was phenomenal. It was she who proposed the creation of a Heart Institute at NIH. Dr. Leonard Scheele, then assistant chief of the Cancer Institute, wrote the bill, got it checked by several of his superiors on a Saturday, and on Sunday presented it to Mrs. Lasker, who got it introduced in Congress on Monday. By Friday, the Heart Institute bill had been approved by the House and Senate and was ready for the president's signature. (Scheele, interview, March 22, 1963, in George Rosen Oral History Project, 1962–64, NLM, pp. 29–30.)

12. Robert J. Anderson, CDC-OH; Michael Gregg, author interview, July 15, 1987; Philip Brachman, author interview, May 7, 1987; Boisfeuillet Jones, author interview, October 1, 1987.

13. Robert J. Anderson, CDC-OH, audiotape, videotape; William Watson, author interview, May 8, 1987.

14. Robert J. Anderson, CDC-OH.

15. The impact of air-conditioning on southern life is described in Raymond Arsenault, "The Long Hot Summer: The Air Conditioner and Southern Culture," *Journal of Southern History* 50 (November 1984): 597–628.

16. Earl Arnold, CDC-OH; Marion Brooke, CDC-OH; Earl Arnold to chief, facilities planning office, June 27, 1960; Donald S. Martin to chief, CDC, May 2, 1960; "Preliminary Evaluation of Space Requests," June 1960, all RG 90, 63A789, Box 1; Theodore J. Bauer, chief, BSS, executive memorandum, October 2, 1961, in CDC Scrapbook 4.

17. Anderson, CDC-OH, videotape, audiotape.

18. S. W. Simmons to chief, CDC, February 1, 1960; Smith to [Simmons], August 18, 1960; Ross W. Buck to chief, CDC, March 28, 1960; Walter L. Wiegner to Buck, June 27, 1960, all RG 90, 63A789, Box 1.

19. Mae Melvin, CDC-OH; William Ewing, CDC-OH.

20. Earl Arnold, CDC-OH; Jim Paine to the author, March 24, 1987; *Atlanta Journal,* July 18, 1960.

21. John Fogarty, "Remarks" at dedication of CDC, RG 90, 65A165, Box 1.

CHAPTER 8

1. Minutes, branch chiefs staff meeting, October 17, 1960, RG 90, 63A789, Box 2.

2. Bruce Dull, CDC-OH; Dull, author interview, September 28, 1987; David Sencer, CDC-OH, April 19, 1983; Langmuir, interview in "Leaders in American Medicine," NLM.

3. Michael Gregg, author interview, July 15, 1987; David Sencer, CDC-OH, April 19, 1983.

4. *MMWR* 10 (January 13, 1961): 2; Gregg, author interview; Sencer, CDC-OH; Bruce Dull, CDC-OH, March 19, 1984.

5. James Goddard, CDC-OH, August 15, 1985; Langmuir, interview in "Leaders in American Medicine," NLM.

6. Alan Donaldson to A. P. Almond, October 20, 1960; RG 90, 63A789, Box 1; asst. chief, Technology Branch, to deputy chief, CDC, November 29, 1960, ibid. Draft, "Justification for Construction of New Building for the Savannah Laboratories," RG 90, 75A1154, Box 1; *Atlanta Journal,* May 15, 16, 1961.

7. Langmuir, author interview; Sencer, CDC-OH.

8. William Watson, author interview, May 8, 1987, Atlanta. The city's black newspaper, the *Atlanta Daily World,* duly noted CDC's progress in race relations: a black college graduate was a technician at the center, and a black high school graduate, hired as a janitor, was being trained to become a technician after scoring well on an examination (*Atlanta Daily World,* October 31, 1961).

9. William Darrow, author interview, May 14, 1987; *Atlanta Constitution,* May 9, 1962; *Atlanta Journal,* May 12, 1962.

10. Darrow, author interview; Watson, author interview, May 5, 1987, Atlanta.

11. HEW, PHS, *The Eradication of Syphilis: A Task Force Report to the Surgeon General, Public Health Service on Syphilis Control in the United States* (Washington, D.C.: GPO, 1962), pp. 3, 10, 30. The other members of the Task Force were Arthur C. Curtis, M.D., Department of Dermatology, College of Medicine, University of Michigan; A. L. Gray, M.D., executive officer, Mississippi State Board of Health; Benno E. Kuechle, vice president, Employers Mutual of Wausau, Wisconsin; and T. Lefoy Richman, projects coordinator, National Commission on Community Health Services, New York City.

12. CDC, *The Year in Review, 1962: The Venereal Disease Branch* (Atlanta, 1962), p. 4.

13. *Medical Tribune,* January 25 and 28, February 1, 1963.

14. Brown quoted in *Medical Tribune,* April 8, 1964. *Antibiotic News,* December 14, 1966.

15. "CDC Report of Activities, FY 1964" (MS, CDC archives), pp. 250–54.

16. *Atlanta Journal,* December 15, 1965; *Atlanta Constitution,* April 26, 1967; *Medical World News,* September 22, 1967; Sencer, author interview, December 27, 1988, Atlanta.

17. David Sencer, CDC-OH.

18. Ibid.; Fogarty quoted by Bill Watson, author interview, May 8, 1987.

19. *Medical Tribune,* February 27–28, 1965; "CDC Report of Activities, FY 1964," pp. 1–3; Sencer, CDC-OH, April 19, 1983.

20. S. W. Simmons, "The Urgent Need for Expansion of Research and Development in Support of the Aedes Aegypti Eradication Program" (February 23, 1966, CDC archives). Simmons suggested an ovi-trap that neither killed nor caught mosquitoes. This trap, a shiny black jar with a paddle, attracted the female mosquitoes by its scent and color. If eggs were laid there, investigators sprayed the area for mosquitoes.

21. *U.S. Medicine,* November 15, 1968; "Surveillance of Dengue in the Americas: A Report to the Director, PAHO," 16 January 1970, RG 90, 73A1051, Box 3.

22. "The U.S. Position for XIX Meeting of Directing Council, PAHO, and Regional Committee of WHO, Sept.–Oct. 1969," RG 90, 73A1051, Box 3; "Summary of *Aedes aegypti* Meeting, El Paso, Texas, Sept. 11, 1969," ibid., Box 2.

23. *Atlanta Journal,* May 15, 1969.

CHAPTER 9

1. James Goddard, interview by James Harvey Young, April–June 1969 (Special Collections, Robert F. Woodruff Library, Emory University, Atlanta), pp. 123–25. Hereafter Goddard-Young transcript.

2. Goddard's experience in the PHS was quite varied. In Denver he headed the federal employee health service and started the government's first executive health program. In North Carolina he drove a semitrailer to cotton mill villages and took ten thousand chest X-rays for a tuberculosis survey. In New York he developed a driver research and testing center. Goddard-Young transcript, pp. 29, 36–37, 63–64.

3. James Goddard, CDC-OH, August 15, 1985; Goddard-Young transcript, pp. 36–37; *Drug News Weekly,* January 17, 1966.

4. Hugh Park, "Around Town," *Atlanta Journal,* undated clipping, CDC Scrapbook 3.

5. Goddard, CDC-OH. The exchange between Goddard and Langmuir probably occurred when the budget for 1966 was presented. The EIS had seventy-two officers that year as compared with thirty-four in 1965. In 1966 the Epidemiology Branch renewed its old, but somewhat neglected, policy of assigning EIS officers to the states through its new Division of Field Services. This was done in connection with the immunization campaign (see chapter 10).

6. Park, "Around Town" (cited n. 4 above); Philip Brachman, author interview, May 7, 1987, Atlanta.

7. Langmuir to chief, CDC, September 27, 1961, RG 90, 64A809, Box 3; *New York Herald Tribune,* June 21, 1961; Martin Favero, author interview, October 2, 1987, Atlanta.

8. James L. Goddard, "Control of Infectious and Serum Hepatitis" (MS), RG 90, 64A809, Box 1.

9. Alexander Langmuir, interview with Harlan Phillips, March 25, 1964, George Rosen Oral History Project, NLM, p. 55. In the late 1960s, Dr. Baruch S. Blumberg of NIH, working with serum from Australian aborigines, isolated the Australian antigen of the hepatitis B virus. CDC's hepatitis work leaped forward (see chapter 17).

10. *New York Times,* April 9, 1967; *Medical Tribune,* April 8, 1964; February 25–26, 1967.

11. Brachman, author interview; Andrew Sparks, "He's the Nation's Top Germ Detective," *Atlanta Journal-Constitution Magazine,* December 19, 1965. Boring was chief of the epidemic aids laboratory section.

12. *Veterinary Dispatch,* August–September 1964; *Atlanta Journal,* August 6, 1964; *Medical World News,* September 11, 1964; *Houston Post,* July 9, 1965; "CDC Report of Activities, FY 1965" (MS, CDC archives), p. 30.

13. CDC, *Report of Activities, 1961* (Atlanta: GPO, 1961), p. 68; *1963,* pp. 197–200; *1964,* pp. 230–33; *Lab World,* July 1964, p. 706; Dixie Snider and John Seggerson, author interview, October 9, 1987, Atlanta. When the federal tuberculosis program was created in 1944, there was no treatment for the disease except surgery, isolation, bed rest, sunshine, juice, and vitamins. Chest surgeons of the future developed their technique in sometimes gruesome operations on tuberculosis patients. Beginning in the late 1940s, and continuing into the next decade, streptomycin and isoniazid proved the effectiveness of chemotherapy, and drug trials showed which techniques worked best. These were the first controlled chemotherapy trials ever done. Cancer studies followed methods developed in the TB program.

14. The journal article announcing this success is a modern classic. See Charles C. Shepard, "The Experimental Disease That Follows the Injection of Human Leprosy Bacilli into Foot-Pads of Mice," *Journal of Experimental Medicine* 112 (September 1960): 445–54.

15. Joseph McDade, author interview, May 12, 1987, Atlanta; McDade, "Tribute to Charles Shepard" (June 4, 1985), CDC-OH; Fred Murphy, author interview, May 12, 1987, Atlanta.

16. Fred Clark quoted in McDade, "Tribute to Charles Shepard."

17. David Sencer, author interview, April 6, 1988, Boston.

18. Goddard, CDC-OH; John F. Winn to John Bagby, April 30, 1965, RG 90, 69A388, Box 6; *Medical Tribune,* July 2–3, 1966; CDC, *Report of Activities, 1962* (Atlanta, 1962), p. 35; Goddard-Young transcript, p. 165.

19. Maya Pines, "Danger in Our Medical Labs," *Harper's* 227 (October 1963): 84–85; "Administration of National Laboratory Improvement Program" (position paper, September 15, 1966), RG 90, 71A284, Box 3. CDC's

earlier programs in laboratory improvement included the VDRL test for diagnosis of syphilis; a microbiology-improvement program, directed mainly at state- and city-operated laboratories; and a program in clinical chemistry and hematology, directed towards hospital and research labs. Though they were seldom used, the National Laboratory Improvement Program could impose sanctions against private laboratories.

20. Donald S. Martin to chief, CDC, December 19, 1961, RG 90, 65A165, Box 1; George B. Tremmell, memorandum of record, February 13, 1962, ibid.; Katherine Barnwell, "Show How You Can Get Diseases," *Atlanta Journal-Constitution Magazine,* September 11, 1960; Willard Neal, "Atlanta the Hollywood of Health Movies," ibid., July 26, 1964.

21. David Sencer, CDC-OH; *Medical Tribune,* May 25–26, 1965; James Lieberman to chief, CDC, November 28, 1966, RG 90, 71A284, Box 4. Steele kept Lieberman out of the commissioned corps as a veterinarian because the veterinary school from which he graduated was not accredited. After earning a Master of Public Health degree, Lieberman was commissioned as a sanitarian.

22. Langmuir, George Rosen transcript, NLM, p. 51; Langmuir, interview in "Leaders in American Medicine," NLM; Godfrey Oakley, author interview, September 29, 1987.

23. Goddard, CDC-OH; Sencer, CDC-OH, April 19, 1983. According to Carl Tyler, Langmuir's decision to begin family-planning work at CDC began after he was offered a chance to join the Population Council, a New York–based organization originally funded by the Rockefeller and Ford Foundations. The council wanted Langmuir to develop an international cadre of science-based population experts who would be to family-planning and population what the EIS was to the practice of epidemiology in the United States. Langmuir felt, however, that the Population Council was not as committed to the project as he was. "So if they could not do it right, he would come back to Atlanta and show them how it should be done" (Tyler, author interview, May 22, 1987).

24. Langmuir to J. Lyle Conrad, June 12, 1987, copy in author's files; Conrad, author interview, July 8, 1987.

25. Goddard-Young transcript, p. 153.

26. Ibid.

27. Goddard, CDC-OH.

28. Hugh Park, "Around Town," *Atlanta Journal-Constitution,* May 17, 1964.

29. Goddard, CDC-OH.

30. Goddard-Young transcript, p. 132.

31. Sencer, CDC-OH; Goddard, CDC-OH.

CHAPTER 10

1. Minutes, branch chiefs staff meeting, June 19, 1961, RG 90, 64A809, Box 2.

2. C. A. Smith, memorandum of record, June 14, 1961, RG 90, 64A809,

Box 2; [David Sencer?], "Testimony before Roberts Committee, March 27, 1961" (MS), RG 90, 64A809, Box 1; Sencer to Dr. James Lang, Division of Health Mobilization, October 16, 1961, ibid., Box 3; Sencer quoted in *Atlanta Journal*, September 29, 1961.

3. Windell Bradford, author interview, October 2, 1987.

4. Alexander Langmuir to Lyle Conrad, June 13, 1987, copy in author's files.

5. The NIH microbiologist Bernice Eddy found cancer-causing viruses in monkey cells from which the polio vaccine was grown. Her boss, Joseph Smadel, at first dismissed these as "lumps." See Shorter, *Health Century*, p. 197.

6. *New York Times*, March 13, 1961; *Wall Street Journal*, August 14, 1961.

7. Luther Terry to H. W. Blades, president, Wyeth Labs, December 5, 1961, RG 90, 64A809, Box 1.

8. C. A. Smith to surgeon general, June 7, 1961; David Sencer, memorandum for the record, June 13, 1961, RG 90, 64A809, Box 1; Smith to John R. Paul, June 19, 1961, ibid., Box 2; *Newsweek*, July 3, 1961. The routine laboratory evidence on the "normal" incidence of polio viruses in the population was also generated at CDC. For months before the Atlanta epidemic, the CDC lab had collected rectal swabs from healthy preschool children in six American cities and isolated and identified the enteroviruses. "Report from Enterovirus Unit of Laboratory Branch, CDC, Jan. 1961," RG 90, 64A804, Box 2.

9. [George Stenhouse], "Summary, Tri-County Vaccine Program," September 27, 1961, RG 90, 64A809, Box 1. As the designated center for polio control, CDC served as the vaccine bank. The frozen vaccine was shipped within twenty-four hours wherever it was needed without charge.

10. David Sencer, CDC-OH; [Sencer] "Immunization Campaign" (MS), RG 90, 64A809, Box 1. President Kennedy's message to Congress was printed in full in the *New York Times*, February 18, 1962, p. 16.

11. Sencer, CDC-OH; Stewart quoted in *New York Times*, March 2, 1962, p. 31.

12. *Atlanta Journal*, December 14, 1963; *Medical Tribune*, December 27, 1963; Goddard quoted in *Medical World News*, September 27, 1963.

13. Donald A. Henderson, John J. Witte, Leo Morris, and Alexander D. Langmuir, "Paralytic Disease Associated with Oral Polio Vaccines," *JAMA* 90 (October 5, 1964): 41, 43.

14. Ibid., p. 48

15. Minutes, Advisory Council on Immunization Practices, July 17–18, 1964, RG 90, 75A69, Box 1.

16. Langmuir, interview in "Leaders in American Medicine," NLM; Albert Sabin to James Goddard, July 25, 1964, RG 90, 75A69, Box 1.

17. Gordon C. Brown to D. A. Henderson, July 31, 1964, RG 90, 75A69, Box 1.

18. A. L. Gray to Henderson, July 27, 1964; Langmuir to William McD. Hammon, August 17, 1964; David Bodian to Langmuir, August 21, 1964, RG 90, 75A69, Box 1.

19. Bruce Dull, CDC-OH; minutes, ACIP meeting, May 25–26, 1964, RG 90, 75A69, Box 1. There were an estimated 1,800,000 cases of rubella in 1964, the largest rubella epidemic since 1935 and possibly the worst in history. The only known prophylaxis at that time was gamma globulin. Rubella is a major cause of birth defects if it strikes women in the first trimester of pregnancy.

20. Dull, author interview.

21. CDC, *Report of Activities, 1962,* p. 25; *1964,* p. 20.

22. Alexander Langmuir, Donald A. Henderson, and Robert E. Serfling, "The Epidemiological Basis for the Control of Influenza," *American Journal of Public Health* 54 (April 1964): 570.

23. *Medical Tribune,* December 15, 1963, April 11–12, 1964; Roger Honkanen, "Flu Stays a Jump Ahead of Vaccines," *Atlanta Journal-Constitution Magazine,* December 1, 1963.

24. *New Orleans Times-Picayune,* May 26, 1965; *New Orleans States-Item,* May 26, 1965.

CHAPTER 11

1. Sencer to Otis L. Anderson, telegram, March 4, 1966, RG 90, 69A388, Box 6.

2. Sencer, author interview, April 6, 1988.

3. Sencer, CDC-OH; Sencer, author interview.

4. Lyle Conrad, author interview, October 5, 1987, Atlanta.

5. Michael Gregg, author interview, July 15, 1987, Atlanta; Dennis Tolsma, author interview, October 8, 1987, Atlanta.

6. The other centers in the newly recognized PHS were the National Institutes of Health, Bureau of Health Services, Bureau of Health Manpower, and National Institute of Mental Health.

7. Jennie Jacobs Kronfeld and Marcia Lynn Whicker, *U.S. National Health Policy: An Analysis of the Federal Role* (New York: Praeger, 1984), p. 79; *Medical World News,* January 27, 1967; Mullan, *Plagues and Politics,* p. 158; Sencer, CDC-OH. The new PHS structure had three agencies that reported to Lee: the omnibus Health Services and Mental Health Administration (HSMHA), FDA, and NIH.

8. Following the example of those who worked for the Atlanta institution at the time, I shall also use the initials CDC rather than the formally correct NCDC.

9. Minutes, staff services staff meeting, September 11, 1968, RG 90, 71A284, Box 3; Sencer, author interview.

10. Sencer, CDC-OH.

11. Sencer, CDC-OH; Simmons, CDC-OH; "Justification for Nomination of Wayland J. Hayes, Jr., for Distinguished Service Medal" [1968], RG 90, 71A831, Box 6; CDC, *Pesticides and Public Health* (Atlanta: NCDC, 1967).

12. Simmons, CDC-OH; Sencer, author interview.

13. David Sencer, "Address at Dedication of Fort Collins Facility, Sept. 29, 1967" (MS, CDC archives); Sencer, author interview.

14. Advisory Committee on Foreign Quarantine, "Report to the Surgeon

General," RG 90, 83-0079; Leo J. Gehrig, deputy surgeon general, to associate chief for program, BSS, November 22, 1966, ibid.

15. Sencer, author interview; Sencer, CDC-OH.

16. Sencer, author interview; Watson, author interview, May 8, 1987, Atlanta; Gregg, author interview.

17. Langmuir quoted in "Trapping Communicable Disease at Its Source," *Medical World News,* October 20, 1967 (reprint); Carl Tyler, author interview, May 22, 1987, Atlanta.

18. Godfrey Oakley, author interview, September 29, 1987, Atlanta.

19. Dixie Snider and John Seggerson, author interview, October 9, 1987; *Medical Tribune,* April 9–10, 1966.

20. *Wall Street Journal,* June 18, 1968.

21. *Medical World News,* August 8, November 21, 1969.

22. Walter Dowdle, author interview, October 7, 1987, Atlanta. The paper reporting results of this work is Walter R. Dowdle, André J. Nahmias, Rebecca W. Harwell, and Frank P. Pauls, "Association of Antigenic Type of *Herpesvirus hominis* with Site of Viral Recovery," *Journal of Immunology* 99 (1967): 974–80.

23. President Johnson quoted in the *Washington Post,* August 6, 1965; John R. Bagby, Jr., to chief, Office of Planning and Analysis, BSS, August 12, 1965, RG 90, 69A388, Box 6.

24. Cong. Joel T. Broyhill (Va.), "Rat Control Bill," *Congressional Record,* June 20, 1967, p. 19549.

25. Richard Prindle to surgeon general, November 18, 1967, RG 90, 71A831, Box 6; Sencer, author interview; Donald Millar, author interview, October 13, 1987, Atlanta.

26. Unsigned handwritten note, "Poor People's File," RG 90, 72A66, Box 3.

27. *Medical World News,* September 27, 1968, p. 11.

28. "What the 'Hong Kong Flu' Has Taught the Experts," *JAMA* 207 (March 17, 1969): 2016–17, 2026; "Mysterious Behavior of 'Hong Kong' Influenza Still Stumps Epidemiologists," *JAMA* 210 (March 10, 1969): 1006–7.

29. *Wall Street Journal,* May 16, 1969; *Atlanta Constitution,* October 9, 1969; William Cherry, CDC-OH.

30. CDC, *A Report on Laboratory Performance and Methods of Improvement* (Atlanta: CDC, 1966), Cong. Fogarty to Sec. Gardner, July 28, 1966, and report of committee, pp. 1–15; Brooke quoted, *Medical Tribune,* January 22–23, 1966.

31. Herbert Alden, letter to editor, *Atlanta Constitution,* February 18, 1967; David Sencer, "For NCDC," *U.S. Medicine,* January 15, 1968; *Newark Evening News,* October 11, 1967; Sencer, CDC-OH.

CHAPTER 12

1. Goddard quoted in the *New Orleans States-Item,* May 25, 1965.

2. Philip J. Landrigan, "Measles Surveillance in the United States, 1971," in *Communicable Disease Control Conference, Houston, Texas, March 13–16, 1972* (Atlanta: CDC, 1972), p. 71.

3. Langmuir to Conrad, June 12, 1987, copy in author's files; Conrad, author interview, July 3, 1987.

4. Langmuir to Conrad, June 12, 1987; Robert Freckleton and Langmuir to PHS regional health directors, February 28, 1966, RG 90, 69A388, Box 6. The 1966 and 1967 classes were the largest EIS ever had. David Sencer remembers the decision to increase the class size to put extra epidemiologists in the field differently. The mechanism to make grants to the states for immunization allowed for personnel to be provided in lieu of cash. Growth of the EIS was so rapid that "they did not get good supervision and the retention rate dropped during that period. Langmuir said that it was marvelous to have all these people, but if you look at that cluster of people who went through at that time, more went into private practice and did not stay in public health" (Sencer, author interview, April 6, 1988, Boston).

5. John F. Enders to Sencer, March 11, 1966; Sencer to Enders, March 17, 1966; L. M. Pane to S. T. Henshall (president of Merck Sharpe & Dohme), January 10, 1966, copy; "Addendum to Protocol for Study of Standardized Dosage of Measles Immune Globulin, March 26, 1966." All in RG 90, 69A388, Box 6.

6. David J. Sencer, H. Bruce Dull, and Alexander D. Langmuir, "Epidemiologic Basis for Eradication of Measles in 1967," *PHR* 82 (March 1967): 254, 256.

7. A. W. Hedrick, "The Corrected Average Attack Rate from Measles among City Children," *American Journal of Hygiene* 11 (May 1930): 576–600.

8. Sencer et al., "Epidemiologic Basis for Eradication of Measles in 1967," pp. 255–56.

9. David Sencer, "Measles Spread Proves Strong Effort Needed," *U.S. Medicine,* January 15, 1968; *Newsweek,* March 20, 1967; *Medical Tribune,* November 16, 1966; *Medical World News,* April 14, 1967. In regard to the immunization campaign, the AMA was on the "horns of a dilemma. They could not say no" (Goddard, CDC-OH).

10. NCDC, *The National Communicable Disease Center* (pamphlet, n.p. [Atlanta], n.d.); *Medical World News,* June 2, 1967; *Atlanta Constitution,* August 15, 1966; *Atlanta Journal,* undated clipping, CDC Scrapbook 5.

11. Sargent Shriver to Surgeon General Stewart, January 16, 1967; RG 90, 70A1209, Box 9; F. Robert Freckleton to chief, CDC (n.d.), RG 90, 69A388, Box 6; Sencer, "Measles Spread."

12. [NCDC], *Measles Surveillance Workbook* [Atlanta, 1967], p. 24; Sencer, "Measles Spread."

13. *Atlanta Journal,* October 16, 1968; *Medical World News,* February 2, 1968.

14. *Medical World News,* November 29, 1968; Conrad, author interview; Alan Hinman, author interview, October 2, 1987, Atlanta.

15. National Rubella Immunization Program, progress report, December 12, 1969, RG 90, 72A1147, Box 2; Immunization Project Grants, 1969–70, ibid.; Mauldin and Cavanaugh quoted in *Medical World News,* October 10, 1969.

16. *Medical World News,* July 19, 1970.

17. Philip J. Landrigan and J. Lyle Conrad, "Current Status of Measles in the United States," *Journal of Infectious Diseases* 124 (December 1971): 620–22; Conrad, author interview.

18. Langmuir, "Territory of Epidemiology," p. 355.

CHAPTER 13

1. Michael Crichton, *The Andromeda Strain* (New York: Knopf, 1969).

2. One veteran had plague, the first imported case in forty years; several had leprosy; another had meliodosis, a disease so rare that it had been reported only six times before in the Western Hemisphere.

3. CDC, *Report of Activities, 1963,* p. 10; John Noble, author interview, April 8, 1988, Boston. Hemorrhagic smallpox was identified by an NIH scientist, Dr. Karl Johnson, who later joined CDC's staff.

4. Boisfeuillet Jones, "CDC and Emory: The Early Years," Joseph Mountin Lecture, 1983, CDC, CDC-OH; *Atlanta Constitution,* July 7, 1970.

5. *Medical Tribune,* July 24, 1967; NCDC, "Briefing Notes" ([1969], CDC archives); Harold Martin, "Mystery of Malaria," *Atlanta Constitution,* September 10, 1969.

6. "PAHO Seminars on Malaria, 1964–1965" (CDC archives), p. 6; *Malaria Manual for U.S. Operations Missions,* ibid.; Donald R. Johnson, "Status of Malaria Eradication in India—1965," *Mosquito News* 25 (December 1956): 361–74.

7. Justin M. Andrews, "Perspective on Malaria Today," *JAMA* 184 (June 15, 1963): 875.

8. William H. Stewart to David E. Bell, May 27, 1964, RG 90, 69A388, Box 6; Donald S. Martin to Sencer, February 7, 1966, ibid.; Martin to John R. Bagby, February 24, 1966, CDC archives.

9. *Medical Tribune,* August 14, 17, 1967.

10. Sencer to surgeon general, September 7, 1966, RG 90, 68A388, Box 6.

11. Donald R. Johnson, "Report of WHO, PAHO, UNICEF/AID/PHS Annual Malaria Eradication Conference, Oct. 26–27, 1966" (CDC archives).

12. Sencer, author interview; Robert Kaiser, memo, August 7, 1967, RG 90, 71A284, Box 4; Sencer to surgeon general, February 6, 1967, 71A831, Box 6.

13. Sencer, author interview; Billy Griggs, author interview, September 24, 1987, Atlanta. CDC was involved with six countries in Central America, three in South America, one in the Caribbean, one in Africa, and seven in Asia. Griggs compared CDC's dilemma to the failure of a full-time maid to live up to a guest's expectations: there is little the guest can do about it.

14. John R. Bagby, Jr. to Dr. Lee M. Howard, War on Hunger, AID, September 13, 1968, RG 90, 71A284, Box 4.

15. Sencer, author interview; Griggs, author interview.

16. Martha Jane Petersen, *Villa International Atlanta: First 20 Years* (pamphlet: n.p., n.d.); *Christian Observer*, August 5, 1970.

17. Sencer, CDC-OH.

18. *Atlanta Constitution*, March 26, 1964; *Arizona Republic*, December 5, 1966.

19. Hugh Park, "Around Town," *Atlanta Journal*, December 9, 1965.

20. S. W. Simmons, CDC-OH; Martin Favero, author interview, October 2, 1987, Atlanta.

21. Sencer, CDC-OH.

22. *Medical World News*, July 11, 1969, pp. 32–34.

23. Sencer, CDC-OH; Walter Dowdle, author interview, October 7, 1987, Atlanta.

CHAPTER 14

1. J. Donald Millar, author interview, October 13, 1987, Atlanta; J. Michael Lane, author interview, September 24, 1987, Atlanta; Horace G. Ogden, *CDC and the Smallpox Crusade* ([Washington, D.C.]: CDC, 1987), pp. 13–14; Farr quoted in D. A. Henderson, "Smallpox Eradication," *PHR* 95 (September–October 1980): 425.

2. Ogden, *CDC and the Smallpox Crusade*, pp. 16–18; D. A. Henderson, "The Eradication of Smallpox," *Scientific American* 235 (October 1976): 28.

3. "Miracle in Tonga" (CDC videotape [1965?]).

4. Ogden, *CDC and the Smallpox Crusade*, pp. 17–18.

5. J. Donald Millar, "Seasons in the Sun," Joseph Mountin Lecture, October 27, 1986, CDC-OH (mimeographed, transcript in author's file), pp. 15–16.

6. Ogden, *CDC and the Smallpox Crusade*, pp. 21–23.

7. "Report: Togo Measles Vaccination Activities, 1965" (MS), RG 90, 70A1209, Box 9. The term had two Land Rovers and a Peugeot station wagon; six jet injector guns; a freezer and two refrigerators for vaccine; syringes and needles; pressure cookers for sterilizing instruments; and record-keeping equipment. Every week they got a week's supply of the perishable vaccine from the freezer in Lome, a hundred miles south of their headquarters, and kept it cold in butane gas and kerosene refrigerators. The largest number of vaccinations they gave in a single day was 1,129—not all that many considering the theoretical possibilities of the jet injector; the fewest was 11.

8. Millar, "Seasons in the Sun," pp. 14–15.

9. D. A. Henderson to "Professor," December 2, 1965; Henderson, "Program for Measles-Smallpox Vaccination for West Africa," RG 90, 69A388, Box 6.

10. *Weekly Compilation of Presidential Documents* [November ?, 1965]; unidentified clipping, RG 90, 69A388, Box 6; D. A. Henderson, "Disease Eradication: Dream or Illusion," Joseph Mountin Lecture, October 26, 1987, CDC, CDC-OH.

11. Henderson was accompanied by Dr. Henry Gelfand, of CDC's staff; Dr. Warren Winkelstein, a consultant; and Dr. Clayton Curtis, medical director of the African Bureau of AID.

12. Ogden, *CDC and the Smallpox Crusade*, pp. 19–20, 26–27.

13. Henderson to chief, CDC, January 6, 1966, RG 90, 69A388, Box 6.

14. D. A. Henderson, "Smallpox Eradication," *PHR* 95 (September–October 1980): 425.

15. Billy Griggs, author interview, September 24, 1987, Atlanta; Don Millar, author interview, October 13, 1987, Atlanta; Don Hopkins, author interview, July 23, 1987, Atlanta.

16. Ogden, *CDC and the Smallpox Crusade*, pp. 30–31; Millar, "Seasons in the Sun," p. 18.

17. Millar, "Seasons in the Sun"; Millar, author interview; Ogden, *CDC and the Smallpox Crusade*, p. 29.

18. Millar, "Seasons in the Sun," p. 3; Henderson, "Eradication of Smallpox," p. 30.

19. Donald R. Hopkins, *Princes and Peasants: Smallpox in History* (Chicago: University of Chicago Press, 1983), pp. 202–3.

20. Ogden, *CDC and the Smallpox Crusade*, p. 45; *JAMA* 203 (February 26, 1968): 22.

21. Lane, author interview.

22. Henderson, "Eradication of Smallpox," p. 29; F. Fenner, D. A. Henderson, I. Airta, Z. Jezak, and I. D. Ladny, *Smallpox and Its Eradication* (Geneva: WHO, 1988), p. 885.

23. "Studies of Smallpox Vaccination Employing Bifurcated Needle" (MS), RG 90, 75A69, Box 5.

24. William Foege, CDC-OH, May 13, 1985.

25. Lane, author interview; Sencer, CDC-OH; William Foege, "Smallpox, Gandhi, and CDC," Joseph Mountin Lecture, October 26, 1984, CDC, CDC-OH.

26. Foege to D. A. Henderson, September 10, 1967, RG 90, 78A0119, Box 1.

27. They were Nigeria, Togo, Dahomey, Mali, Upper Volta, Niger, and Guinea. Millar, "Seasons in the Sun," p. 25.

28. Ibid., p. 26.

29. Ibid., p. 28; *The Word* 1 (January–February 1970): 4; Phil Garner, "Dread Disease Nears Extinction," *Atlanta Journal-Constitution Magazine*, April 14, 1974. Sencer, Millar and James Hicks, the administrative officer for the regional office in Lagos, were in Boubon where Hicks and Millar got certificates for their "exemplary assistance provided since the beginning of the campaign." Hicks gave the Africans all the credit. "We didn't [just] go in and do it for them," he said.

30. "Smallpox Eradication / Measles Control Program" (undated memo), RG 90, 75A1730, Box 6; Lane, author interview; Millar, "Seasons in the Sun," pp. 27–28.

31. Lane, author interview; William Foege, "Status of Smallpox Vaccination in the United States," in *Communicable Disease Control Conference, Houston, Texas, March 13–16, 1972*, p. 88. The argument may be followed in J. M. Lane and J. D. Millar, "Routine Childhood Vaccination against Smallpox

Reconsidered," *NEJM* 281 (November 27, 1969): 1220–24, and "Physicians Debate Routine Smallpox Vaccinations," *JAMA* 210 (November 10, 1969): 999–1000.

32. D. A. Henderson to Foege, May 25, 1972, RG 90, 75A12730, Box 6; Lane quoted, *Atlanta Constitution,* July 18, 1974.

33. Foege, CDC-OH.

34. Foege to Sencer, December 28, 1974, RG 90, 78A42, Box 8.

35. *New Delhi Statesman,* February 13, 1975; *Times of India,* undated clipping, RG 90, 78A42, Box 8.

36. Lawrence K. Altman, "Global War on Smallpox Expected to Be Won in '76," *New York Times,* September 23, 1975; Henderson, "Eradication of Smallpox," p. 33.

37. Ogden, *CDC and the Smallpox Crusade,* pp. 92–109, passim; Hopkins, *Princes and Peasants,* p. 310.

38. James H. Nakano, "The Role of CDC in the Global Eradication of Smallpox" (MS, author's files).

39. Sencer, author interview.

CHAPTER 15

1. *MMWR* 16 (September 9, 1967): 301–2.

2. Chief, foreign quarantine program, "Unknown Disease in Germany Due to Contact with African Green Monkeys" (MS, October 27, 1967), RG 90, 72A66, Box 3.

3. *Atlanta Constitution,* April 18, 1968; *Medical World News,* August 15, 1969.

4. John R. Bagby to asst. sec., comptroller, HEW, January 24, 1968; Ross W. Buck to director, Division of Buildings and Facilities, PHS, January 31, 1968, RG 90, 71A284, Box 4. In 1948, NIH constructed Building 7 as a maximum security laboratory for infectious-disease research and dedicated it as a "Memorial Laboratory" to PHS investigators who had died from laboratory-acquired infections. It had biological containment cabinets and negative air pressure, but it may not have provided adequate security for the Marburg virus.

5. Karl Johnson, author interview, May 26, 1988, Atlanta; *The Word* 1 (October–November 1969): 1.

6. Conrad, author interview, October 5, 1987. A lively account of the appearance of Lassa fever in Nigeria and its subsequent history is John G. Fuller, *Fever! The Hunt for a New Killer Virus* (New York: Reader's Digest Press, 1974).

7. *MMWR* 18 (August 23, 1969): 293.

8. Conrad, author interview; Johnson, author interview; *Dateline: CDC* 9 (January 1977): 1.

9. Conrad, author interview.

10. Johnson, author interview.

11. Ibid. The other CDC staff members involved in the investigation in

Zaire and Sudan were Drs. Joseph McCormick, Michael White, Stan Foster, David Hayman, and Donald Francis.

12. Joseph McCormick, author interview, October 13, 1987, Atlanta; Johnson, author interview.

13. Conrad, author interview.

14. McCormick, author interview.

CHAPTER 16

1. *The Word* 1 (April–June 1970): 1.

2. *Atlanta Constitution,* May 7, 1969; *Atlanta Journal,* May 8, 1969; Reg Murphy, *Atlanta Journal-Constitution,* July 6, 1969.

3. "Historical Development of the Ten-State Nutrition Survey 1968–1970" (MS), RG 90, 75A1730, Box 6; Watson, author interview, May 8, 1987, Atlanta. The states included in the survey were Texas, Louisiana, New York, Massachusetts, Kentucky, West Virginia, Michigan, Washington, California, and South Carolina.

4. Dennis Tolsma, author interview, October 8, 1987, Atlanta.

5. David Sencer, author interview, April 6, 1988, Boston.

6. HEW, *Highlights, Ten-State Nutrition Survey, 1968–1970* (Atlanta [1972]), DHEW Publication (HSM) 72-8134, passim.

7. Milton Z. Nichaman to director, CDC, February 1, 1973, RG 90, 86-0048, Box 5. States included in the study were Arizona, Kentucky, Tennessee, Washington, and Louisiana.

8. CDC, *Nutrition Surveillance Annual Summary,* (Atlanta, 1975), passim. The best indication of recent undernutrition is the relation of weight to height; that for long-term undernutrition, the relation of height to age. Hemogloblin levels determined which groups had potential nutritional problems.

9. Nichaman to director, CDC, April 21, 1971; Foege to Jeffrey W. House, February 4, 1971, RG 90, 75A1730, Box 6.

10. Howard A. Schneider to Cong. Paul G. Rogers, March 28, 1973; Sencer to asst. sec. for health, August 13, 1973, RG 90, 86-0048, Box 5.

11. Sencer, memo to all CDC employees, November 30, 1971, RG 90, 75A1730, Box 6.

12. James Patterson, *The Dread Disease: Cancer and Modern American Culture* (Cambridge, Mass.: Harvard University Press, 1987), pp. 205–10, 216. William H. Sebrell says that NIH had the data on cancer and cigarette smoking while he was NIH director in the early 1950s. He wanted to release some of the information, but Surgeon General Scheele would not permit it. Scheele's position was that the data were not conclusive. Sebrell, NIH/NLM Oral History project, pp. 147–48.

13. Sencer, memorandum for the record, August 5, 1974; Sencer to Terrence J. Boyle, December 11, 1974, RG 90, 86-0048, Box 5.

14. Jennie Jacobs Kronenfeld and Marcia Lynn Whicker, *U.S. National Health Policy: An Analysis of the Federal Role* (New York: Praeger, 1984), p. 79; Don Millar, author interview; Sencer, CDC-OH.

15. Bill Watson, author interview, June 23, 1987. The National Institute of

Environmental Health Sciences, part of NIH, was established at Research Tri-angle Park, North Carolina, in 1969. Its foremost accomplishment was to confirm the link between asbestos and cancer.

16. U.S. House, Committee on Government Operations, *Control of Toxic Substances in the Workplace,* Hearing, May 11, 12, and 18, 1976 (Washington, D.C.: GPO, 1976), testimony of John F. Finklea, p. 64 (Y4.G74/7:T66/2).

17. Don Millar, author interview.

18. [Horace G. Ogden], *Health Promotions and Education at CDC* ([1987], mimeographed), pp. 1–18; copy in author's files.

19. Horace G. Ogden, "Health Education: A Federal Overview," *PHR* 91 (May–June 1976): 203–4; Sencer, CDC-OH; Watson, author interview, May 8, 1987.

20. Watson, author interview.

CHAPTER 17

1. Millar, "Seasons in the Sun," p. 5; Millar, author interview, October 13, 1987. Millar became director of CDC's Division of State and Community Services.

2. Secretary, HEW, to the president, November 24, 1971, copy, RG 90, 75A1730, Box 6.

3. J. D. Millar, "Current Status of Venereal Disease and Venereal Disease Control," in *Communicable Disease Control Conference, Houston, Texas, March 13–16, 1972,* pp. 6, 11.

4. Jones, *Bad Blood,* pp. 1, 11–12, 190–96.

5. Sencer, author interview, April 6, 1988, Boston.

6. Venereal Disease Branch, State and Community Services Division, "Background Paper on Tuskegee Study" (MS, CDC archives). Thirteen articles on the study had been published since 1936.

7. Jones, *Bad Blood,* pp. 206–11.

8. Sencer, author interview.

9. Jones, *Bad Blood,* pp. 215–17.

10. Alan M. Brandt, "Racism and Research: The Case of the Tuskegee Syphilis Study," *Hastings Center Report* 8 (December 1978): 27.

11. T. G. Benedek, "The 'Tuskegee Study' of Syphilis: An Analysis of Moral versus Methodologic Aspects," *Journal of Chronic Diseases* 31 (January 1978): 47–48.

12. Albert Balows, author interview, October 14, 1987, Atlanta.

13. Dixie Snider and John Seggerson, author interview, October 9, 1987, Atlanta; Sencer quoted in *Atlanta Constitution,* July 1, 1969.

14. Richard A. Garibaldi, Michael B. Gregg, Ronald Drusin, and Phyllis Edwards, "Preliminary Report: Hepatitis Associated with Isoniazid Chemopro-phylaxis, Washington, D.C." (January 18, 1971), RG 90, 75A1730, Box 6; Phyllis Q. Edwards (1982), CDC-OH.

15. *The Word 5* (September 1973): 1; Millar, author interview.

16. Because lead interferes with the ability of the red blood cells to carry oxygen, the danger to health is great. Among other effects are muscular weak-ness and lowered intelligence.

17. "Review Statement, Lead in Automotive Emissions" (Nov. 7, 1975), RG 90, 78A0117, Box 1; Millar, author interview; Vernon Houk, author interview, October 13, 1987, Atlanta.

18. Millar, author interview; Sencer, author interview.

19. Michael Gregg, author interview, July 15, 1987; Stephen C. Hadler, author interview, October 1, 1987.

20. Blumberg's detection of the Australian antigen was reported in the *New York Times,* October 19, 1966, pp. 1, 65. He won the Nobel Prize for this work in 1976.

21. Martin Favero, author interview, October 2, 1987. The joint venture of CDC and NIH in hepatitis research would not have surprised Justin Andrews, former director of CDC and director of NIAID at the time of his death in 1967. Andrews predicted it in 1964. Through its contacts with the states, CDC had a means of getting information from the whole country, NIH had the funds and facilities. The combination should lead to a "tremendous expansion of programs" (Andrews, interview, July 27, 1964, NIH/PHS Oral History Project, NLM, pp. 14–15).

22. Alexander Langmuir expressed the same idea in 1964. He told Harlan Phillips: "We give the maximum to service, and then we find all sorts of wonderful things that nobody else knows about, and we convert these into our research activities. It's quite a different approach, and it has paid off. It has given us a uniqueness that no other group has because we are there" (Langmuir, George Rosen Oral History Project, NLM, p. 51).

23. Favero, author interview; Michael Gregg, author interview. CDC's inhouse publication described the hepatitis A virus as looking like very small tennis balls surrounded by halos of antibody particles. See *Dateline: CDC* 6 (November 1974): 1.

24. William Foege to Dr. Richard M. Krause, April 19, 1978, RG 90, 80-0047, Box 1; Sencer, CDC-OH.

25. Marcus M. Key to asst. sec. of labor, OSHA, March 11, 1974, RG 90, 86-0048, Box 5.

26. Theodore I. Kloth, "Sahel Nutrition Survey" (MS), RG 90, 86-0048, Box 5; "Nepal Nutrition Status Survey," January–May 1975 (MS), pp. 1–2, RG 90, 78A42, Box 8.

27. W. E. van Heyningen and John R. Seal, *Cholera: The American Scientific Experience, 1947–1980* (Boulder, Colo.: Westview Press, 1983), pp. 114–15, 230–31. William Foege, author interview, October 12, 1987, Atlanta.

28. S. H. Clarke, "Weekly Report to Caspar Weinberger, May 8, 1975," RG 90, 77A-0101; *Dateline: CDC* 8 (January 1976): 1.

CHAPTER 18

1. Between 1971 and 1974, the number of cases of measles in the United States dropped from 74,000 to 22,000. There were slightly more cases in 1975 (24,000).

2. "Forum on Swine Flu with David Sencer, J. Donald Millar, Windell Bradford, William Watson, and Donald Berreth, Sept. 30, 1983," CDC-OH. Hereafter, "Swine Flu Forum."

3. Michael Gregg, author interview, July 15, 1987; "Swine Flu Forum."

4. *MMWR* 25 (February 20, 1976): 47.

5. "Meeting on Influenza at BoB/FDA, Feb. 27, 1976" (for the record, March 1, 1976), RG 90, 78A42, Box 6.

6. Charles H. Hobe, Jr., and Michael A. W. Hattwick, "Limiting the Effects of Influenza Epidemics," *Postgraduate Medicine* 58 (December 1975): 59–63; Arthur M. Silverstein, *Pure Politics & Impure Science: The Swine Flu Affair* (Baltimore: Johns Hopkins University Press, 1981), pp. 50–59.

7. "Swine Flu Forum"; Richard E. Neustadt and Harvey Fineberg, *The Epidemic That Never Was: Policy-Making & the Swine Flu Affair* (New York: Vintage Books, 1983), pp. 27–28. The Neustadt and Fineberg book is one of two that deal extensively with the politics of the swine flu immunization campaign. *Epidemic That Never Was* is critical of CDC and Sencer. Silverstein, *Pure Politics & Impure Science*, cited in n. 6 above, is more sympathetic to CDC's role.

8. CDC, summary minutes of meeting, March 10, 1976, ACIP, RG 90, 78A42, Box 6.

9. Walter Dowdle, author interview, October 7, 1987; "Swine Flu Forum." The "Action Memorandum" is reprinted in Neustadt and Fineberg, *Epidemic That Never Was*, pp. 198–206.

10. "Swine Flu Forum."

11. Neustadt and Fineberg, *Epidemic That Never Was*, p. 35.

12. Albert B. Sabin to Sencer, March 23, 1976, RG 90, 78A42, Box 6.

13. "Swine Flu Forum."

14. Donald Millar, author interview, October 13, 1987.

15. Goldfield, quoted in Neustadt and Fineberg, *Epidemic That Never Was*, p. 61.

16. Sencer, author interview; James P. Pilliod to Sencer, April 4, 1976, RG 90, 78A42, Box 6; Alexander, quoted in Neustadt and Fineberg, *Epidemic That Never Was*, p. 60.

17. "Swine Flu Forum."

18. Ibid.; Millar, author interview.

19. "Swine Flu Forum."

20. Ibid.; *Newsday*, August 7, 1976; U.S. House, Committee on Interstate and Foreign Commerce, *"Legionnaire's Disease,"* Hearing, November 23 and 24, 1976, Serial No. 94-159, (Washington, D.C.: GPO, 1977), testimony of David Sencer, pp. 93–135 (Y4.In8/4:94-159).

21. Sencer, CDC-OH; "Swine Flu Forum"; *Dateline: CDC* 8 (August 1976): 2.

22. *New York Times*, August 8, 1976.

23. *Medical Tribune*, September 8, 1976; *New York Times*, September 15, 1976, editorial.

24. *Washington Post*, November 29, 1976; *Atlanta Constitution*, August 7,

1976; October 28, 1976; *New York Times,* October 29, 1976; "Swine Flu Forum."

25. *Philadelphia Daily News,* September 10, 1976.

26. Sencer testimony cited in n. 20 above; UPI wire story, November 24, 1976.

27. Silverstein, *Pure Politics and Impure Science,* p. 116.

28. Lawrence Schonberger, author interview, October 7, 1987, Atlanta.

29. Foege, "Smallpox, Gandhi, and CDC."

30. Foege quoted, *Atlanta Journal,* January 3, 1977.

31. Joseph McDade, author interview, May 12, 1987, Atlanta. A detailed and lively account of McDade's triumph is Donald C. Drake, "Twists, Turns, and Eureka! The Legion Bug," *Philadelphia Inquirer,* July 17, 1977.

32. Sencer, CDC-OH; "Follow-up on Respiratory Illness—Philadelphia," *MMWR,* special issue, 26 (January 18, 1977): 9–11.

CHAPTER 19

1. David Sencer, CDC-OH.

2. Transcript, Califano press conference, February 8, 1977, pp. 14–15, RG 90, 80-0047, Box 1. A copy of the Sencer petition is in CDC archives.

3. Walter Dowdle, author interview; Karl Johnson, author interview; "[Lab Deaths] Task Force Report," RG 90, 79-0045.

4. Lawrence Schonberger, author interview; Dowdle, author interview.

5. Neustadt and Fineberg, *Epidemic That Never Was,* pp. xxvi, 23. The volume cited is the expanded version of the original report published by Random House in 1981.

6. Robert D. Bahn, review of *The Swine Flu Affair: Decision-Making on a Slippery Disease,* by Richard Neustadt, *Political Science Quarterly* 94 (Winter 1979–80): 680–81.

7. Millar, author interview.

8. Joseph McDade, author interview.

9. Albert Balows, author interview.

10. Unidentified MS forwarded to Bill [Foege ?], [November 1977?], RG 90, 84-0024, Box 3; McDade quoted in *Atlanta Constitution,* October 14, 1977.

11. U.S. Senate, Committee on Human Resources, *Legionnaires' Disease, 1977,* Hearing, November 9, 1977 (Washington, D.C.: GPO, 1978), testimony of William Foege, pp. 47–48 (Y4.H88:L52/3/977).

12. Ibid., testimony of Leonard Bachman, pp. 66–67; comment by Senator Kennedy, p. 67; Dowdle, author interview; *Atlanta Constitution,* November 10, 1977. Senator Kennedy may have made the Nobel Prize remark as he left the Hearing for another appointment. It does not appear in the official record.

13. Phil Patton, "What Dr. Runsdorf Knows (and the Government Doesn't) about Legionnaires' Disease," *New York,* January 19, 1979; Lawrence K. Altman, letter, *NEJM* 298 (April 13, 1978): 851; *National Enquirer,* December 6, 1977; Edward H. Kass, "Legionnaires' Disease," *NEJM* 297 (December 1, 1977): 1229–30; "Sec. Califano to All CDC Employees," December 14, 1977, RG 90, 84-0024, Box 3.

14. William Foege, handwritten notes in program for International Symposium on Legionnaires' Disease, November 13–15, 1978, Atlanta, RG 90, 84-
0024, Box 3.

CHAPTER 20

1. *Dateline: CDC* 9 (March 1977): 1.
2. Foege, author interview, October 12, 1987; Michael Gregg, author interview, July 15, 1987.
3. William Foege and William Watson, June 4, 1984, CDC-OH (hereafter
Foege-Watson).
4. Ibid.
5. Quoted in Neustadt and Fineberg, *Epidemic That Never Was,* p. 130.
6. Foege-Watson; Foege, author interview; J. Lyle Conrad, author interview, July 8, 1987. The senators most sympathetic to CDC were Sam Nunn,
Dale Bumpers, Ted Kennedy, and Mark Hatfield.
7. Letter file, RG 90, 79-0045, Box 3.
8. They represented the American Medical Association, the American Public Health Association, consumers, and health departments.
9. Millar, author interview; [CDC] Programs and Policies Advisory Committee, *Recommendations for a National Strategy for Disease Prevention* [At-
lanta, 1978], pp. 5–10.
10. Programs and Policies Advisory Committee, *Recommendations,* pp.
11–13, 48.
11. Dennis Tolsma, author interview, October 8, 1987.
12. PHS, *Healthy People: The Surgeon General's Report on Health Promotion and Disease Prevention* (Washington, D.C.: GPO, 1979), pp. viii–ix.
Specifically, the report called for a 35 percent reduction in infant mortality
(fewer than 9 deaths per 1,000 live births); a 20 percent reduction in deaths of
children aged 1 to 14 (to fewer than 34 per 100,000); a 20 percent reduction of
deaths among adolescents and young adults to age 24 (fewer than 93 per
100,000); a 25 percent reduction in deaths among the 25 to 64 age group (fewer
than 400 per 100,000), and a reduction of 20 percent in the number of days of
illness among those over 64 (fewer than thirty days per year).
13. *Promoting Health / Preventing Disease: Objectives for the Nation*
(Washington, D.C.: GPO, 1980). The list of goals was compiled at a conference
in Atlanta in June 1979 by a large group of experts from academia, public
health, and private practice. Some of these 226 goals were within sight by early
1990, but many were not. Among the "likely to be met" goals were reduction
in gonorrhea and gonococcal pelvic inflammatory disease. "Unlikely to be met"
was the reduction in syphilis; in 1988 the rates were the highest in forty years.
Among the biggest disappointments was reduction in infant mortality. After
two decades of consistent improvement in levels of infant mortality, progress
slowed substantially during the 1980s in the United States (which ranks nineteenth among industrialized nations in this respect). See "Progress toward
Achieving the 1990 Objectives for the Nation for Sexually Transmitted Diseases," *MMWR* 39 (February 2, 1990): 53–57; "National Infant Mortality

Surveillance," Summary No. 3, *MMWR Surveillance Summaries* 38 (December 1989): 1–9.

14. Daniel S. Greenberg, "Carter's Purge: The Califano File," *NEJM* 301 (August 23, 1979): 451–52.

15. *MMWR* 28 (July 6, 1979): 301–4; "Injury Control Initiative" (November 7, 1979), RG 90, 82-0107, Box 3.

16. Foege-Watson, CDC-OH; Alice Ring, author interview, October 14, 1987, Atlanta. Dr. Donald Fredrickson resigned as NIH director in 1981; he was not ousted by the administration.

17. Foege, author interview. In a quarter century, he saw the number of countries with infant mortality rates of 15 percent drop from fifty-nine to eleven, the number of countries with a life expectancy of less than forty years go from thirty-four to two.

18. "Recommendations on International Health Priorities for CDC" (October 14, 1976), RG 90, 79-0045, Box 3.

19. U.S. House, Committee on International Relations, *Underdevelopment in Africa,* Hearing, September 7, 8, 15, and 20, 1977, (Washington, D.C.: GPO, 1978), testimony of William Foege, pp. 57–63 (Y4.In8/16:Af8/7).

20. Donald R. Hopkins to William Foege, June 21, 1979, RG 90, 82-0107, Box 5; Philip Brachman, interview, May 7, 1987.

21. William Foege to the secretary, August 10, 1979; Califano to James T. McIntyre, Jr., August 2, 1979, RG 90, 86-0109, Box 1.

22. A detailed account of the Kampuchean relief program is CDC, *Emergency Refugee Health-Care: A Chronicle of Experience in the Khmer Assistance Operation, 1979–1980* (n.p., n.d. [Atlanta, 1983]).

23. Sacid Xasan Muse to Wolf Bulle, March 26, 1981, RG 90, 85-0109, Box 2.

CHAPTER 21

1. *New York Times,* December 10, 1976, pt. 2, p. 7; Conrad, author interview, July 8, 1987.

2. Alan R. Hinman, author interview, October 2, 1987. It was at the Senate hearings that the first immunization conference was announced. The previous spring some congressmen had suggested that immunization against polio, measles, and other diseases might be combined with swine flu immunization to reach more people and save money. For reasons both scientific and logistical, the attempt was not made. See *New York Times,* April 1, 1976, p. 62.

3. Hinman, author interview.

4. *New York Times,* April 6, 1977, pp. 1, 17.

5. Foege-Watson, May 13, 1985.

6. Secretary Califano's first attempt to get money for the initiative was to use the $30 to $35 million left over from the swine flu program, but he ran into a bureaucratic obstacle: money from one fund could not be swapped to another. Columnist James Reston called this "zero-based stupidity" (clipping, undated column [1977?], RG 90, 82-1050, Box 3).

7. Hinman, author interview; Foege-Watson; *Dateline: CDC* 9 (November–December 1977): 1.

8. Joseph Califano, "Remarks," National Immunization Conference, December 12, 1978, RG 90, 82-0107, Box 3.

9. Hinman, author interview.

10. Hinman to Foege, December 8, 1978; Hinman, "Measles" (MS), RG 90, 84-0024, Box 3.

11. Hinman, author interview; William Foege, "Uses of Epidemiology in the Development of Health Policy," *PHR* 99 (May–June 1984): 235. A convenient summary of the problems in measles control is Alan R. Hinman, A. David Brandling-Bennett, and Phillip I. Nieburg, "The Opportunity and Obligation to Eliminate Measles from the United States," *JAMA* 242 (September 14, 1979): 1157–62.

12. Foege to secretary, HEW, March 20, 1979, RG 90, 82-0107, Box 3; Foege-Watson.

13. John K. Iglehart, "A Conversation with Dr. Theodore Cooper," *Milbank Memorial Fund Quarterly* 55 (Summer 1977): 357–58; Foege-Watson. Foege thought the problem might be solved if an exclusion from the required vaccinations at school entry were given for philosophical reasons. Parents would be forced to make a decision: "When polio rates were down to 60 to 65 perent it was not because 35 percent of parents were saying, 'We want our children to have polio,' but because they had never been forced to make a decision" (Foege, author interview).

14. Alan Hinman prefers the term *elimination* to *eradication*. "Eradication represents interruption of transmission, elimination of an agent from an area so that the risk of reintroduction is so low that you can stop preventive measures. Elimination is a step short of that: interruption of transmission from a given area, so that there is no naturally occurring disease there. But there is still a significant enough risk of importation to require maintenance of immunization" (Hinman, author interview).

15. Hinman, author interview; Foege, "The Global Elimination of Measles," *PHR* 97 (September–October 1982): 405. The upsurge of measles in the United States in 1990 testifies to the difficulty of measles control.

16. U.S. Senate, Committee on Labor and Human Resources, *Immunization and Preventive Medicine, 1982,* Hearing, May 7, 1982 (Washington, D.C.: GPO, 1982), testimony of William Foege, pp. 26–27 (Y4.L11/4:Im6/2/982).

CHAPTER 22

1. By May 1977 *The Last Chance Diet* had sold 75,000 hardcover copies and 1.3 million in paperback. Dr. Linn opened two offices in Pennsylvania, and one each in Delaware, New York City, and Washington, D.C., where the diet was so popular guests took it with them to luncheon and dinner parties and ate nothing at all. *New York Times,* May 18, 1977, pt. 3, pp. 1, 9.

2. U.S. House, Committee on Interstate and Foreign Commerce, *Liquid Protein Diets,* Hearing, December 28, 1977, Serial No. 95-83 (Washington, D.C.: GPO, 1978), testimony of William Foege, pp. 2–10 (Y4.In8/4:95-83); *New York Times,* December 19, 1977, p. 14; *New York,* January 30, clipping, RG 90, 84-0025, Box 3.

3. Lawrence Schonberger, author interview, October 7, 1987; *MMWR* 29 (July 11, 1980): 321–22; *MMWR* 29 (November 7, 1980): 532–39.

4. Foege-Watson; *MMWR* 31 (February 12, 1982): 56; *MMWR* 31 (June 11, 1982): 289–90.

5. Walter Dowdle, author interview; Schonberger, author interview; Foege-Watson.

6. President's Commission on the Accident at Three Mile Island, testimony of William Foege (MS), August 17, 1979, RG 90, 82-0107, Box 5; Marilyn K. Goldhaber et al., "The Three Mile Island Population Registry," *PHR* 98 (November–December 1983): 604.

7. Kathleen Kreiss, Philip T. Landrigan, Clark W. Heath, John Liddle, and David D. Bayse to director, CDC, March 16, 1978, RG 90, 82-0107, Box 3; *Atlanta Constitution,* December 29, 1982.

8. Thomas H. Maugh II, "An Environmental Time Bomb Gone Off," *Science* 204 (May 25, 1979): 820.

9. Gina Bari Kolata, "Love Canal False Alarm Caused by Botched Study," *Science* 208 (June 13, 1980): 1239–42; Constance Holden, "Love Canal Residents under Stress," ibid., pp. 1242–44. Two officials who brought the EPA report to the city were held hostage for several hours, because "they would have been torn apart" if they had been let out the front door.

10. Draft, Foege's remarks on toxic wastes, June 4, 1980, RG 90, 82-0151, Box 4.

11. Arthur D. Bloom to Foege, July 24, 1980, RG 90, 83-0014, Box 1.

12. Phil Taylor to Foege, July 22, 1980, RG 90, 83-0014, Box 1.

13. Foege to asst. sec. for health, December 29, 1980, RG 90, 84-0024, Box 2; Vernon Houk, author interview, October 13, 1987.

14. *New York Times,* December 25, 1982, p. 6, December 27, p. 14, and December 30, p. 1; *Atlanta Journal Constitution,* December 25 and 28, 1982.

15. Houk, author interview; Dowdle, author interview. A detailed account of the Agent Orange studies is Michael Gough, *Dioxin, Agent Orange: The Facts* (New York: Plenum Press, 1986), chs. 5, 6. The Agent Orange issue refused to die; it was still a lively and controversial issue in 1990.

16. Godfrey Oakley, author interview, September 29, 1987; *MMWR* 28 (August 3, 1979): 358.

17. Schonberger, author interview; "Public Health Service Accomplishments, 1977–1979" (MS), p. 22, RG 90, 82-0197, Box 5; Balder K. Nottay, Olan M. Kew, Milford H. Hatch, John T. Heyward, and John F. Obijeski, "Molecular Variation of Type I Vaccine-Related and Wild Polioviruses during Replication in Humans," *Virology* 108 (January 30, 1981): 405–23.

18. "Toxic Shock Syndrome—United States," *MMWR* 29 (May 23, 1980): 229–30.

19. "Follow-up on Toxic Shock Syndrome—United States," *MMWR* 29 (June 27, 1980): 297–99.

20. Foege-Watson.

21. Maria E. Donawa, George R. Schmid, and Michael T. Osterholm, "Toxic Shock Syndrome: Chronology of State and Federal Epidemiologic Stud-

ies and Regulatory Decision-Making," *PHR* 99 (July–August 1984): 342–50; "Follow-up on Toxic Shock Syndrome," *MMWR* 29 (September 19, 1980): 441–45.

22. *Los Angeles Times,* March 22, 1981.

23. "Mt. St. Helens Volcano Reports, June–August 1980," RG 90, 84-0024, Box 2; Yvonne Horn, "St. Helens Fallout: Sifting for Health Hazards," *Impact,* September 26, 1980, p. 12.

24. Jeffrey Koplan, author interview, October 2, 1987, Atlanta.

CHAPTER 23

1. Michael Lane, author interview, September 24, 1987; Foege-Watson.

2. Philip Brachman to Walter Dowdle, August 12, 1980, RG 90, 83-0014, Box 1; Karl Johnson, author interview, May 26, 1988.

3. Lane, author interview.

4. Roslyn Robinson to Foege, November 26, 1979, April 18, 1980, RG 90, 87-0087, Box 2; Michael Gregg, author interview, July 15, 1987.

5. William Foege, author interview, October 12, 1987; Martin Favero, author interview, October 2, 1987.

6. Mark Hollis, June 24, 1985, CDC-OH.

7. Ellen Wormser to Peter Gness, January 3, 1980; Hod Ogden, "Background Comment" (MS, February 14, 1980); Julius B. Richmond, memorandum for secretary, HEW, March 11, 1980, all in RG 90, 87-0077, Box 2.

8. Foege to asst. sec. for health, April 23, 1980, RG 90, 87-0077, Box 2.

9. Dennis Tolsma, author interview, October 8, 1987.

10. See Willard Cates, Jr., H. W. Ory, R. W. Rochet, and Carl W. Tyler, Jr., "The Intrauterine Device and Deaths from Spontaneous Abortion," *NEJM* 295 (November 18, 1976): 1155–59; CDC, "Oral Contraceptive Use and the Risk of Ovarian Cancer: Cancer and Steroid Hormone Study," *JAMA* 249 (March 25, 1983): 1596–99; CDC, "Oral Contraceptive Use and the Risk of Endometrial Cancer: Cancer and Steroid Hormone Study," ibid., pp. 1600–1604.

11. An exception was sexually transmitted diseases (STD) in the Center for Prevention Services.

12. Donald Millar, author interview, October 13, 1987; Vernon Houk, author interview, October 13, 1987; Godfrey Oakley, author interview, September 29, 1987.

13. Millar, author interview.

14. AFGE Local 42, press release, September 9, 1981, RG 90, 85-0110, Box 4.

15. Millar, author interview.

16. "Leading Work-Related Diseases and Injuries—United States," *MMWR* 32 (January 21, 1983): 24–26. The ten leading causes of occupational illness identified by the NIOSH staff are occupational lung disease, musculoskeletal injuries, occupational cancers, severe occupational traumatic injuries, occupational cardiovascular disease, disorders of reproduction, neurotoxic dis-

orders, noise-induced hearing loss, dermatological conditions, and psychological disorders.

17. Millar, author interview.

18. Favero, author interview; Stephen Hadler, author interview, October 1, 1987, Atlanta.

19. Karen Davis, "Reagan Administration Health Policy," *Journal of Public Health Policy* 2 (December 1981): 317.

20. Foege-Watson. The new Viral and Rickettsial Diseases Laboratory was dedicated in October 1988.

CHAPTER 24

1. James W. Curran, author interview, June 23, 1987, Atlanta; Randy Shilts, *And the Band Played On: Politics, People and the AIDS Epidemic* (New York: St. Martin's Press, 1987), pp. 54, 61, 66.

2. Even when demand was relatively high, pentamidine was not profitable enough for the manufacturer, May & Baker, to get it licensed. Hence, its distribution through CDC. Pentamidine was largely replaced by trimethoprim-sulfamethozole (TMP/SMX) in 1974.

3. "*Pneumocystis* Pneumonia—Los Angeles," *MMWR* 30 (June 5, 1981): 250–51; Shilts, *Band Played On*, p. 62.

4. "Kaposi's Sarcoma and *Pneumocystis* Pneumonia among Homosexual Men—New York City and California," *MMWR* 30 (July 3, 1981): 305–7.

5. Michael Lane, author interview, March 2, 1987, Atlanta.

6. CDC Task Force on Kaposi's Sarcoma and Opportunistic Infections, "Epidemiological Aspects of the Current Outbreak of Kaposi's Sarcoma and Opportunistic Infections," *NEJM* 306 (January 28, 1982): 248.

7. Harold Jaffe, author interview, April 30, 1987, Atlanta.

8. Besides Drs. Curran, Jaffe, and Guinan, they were Drs. Harry Haverkos, Alexander Kelter, Martha Rogers, and William Darrow.

9. Paul Weisner, author interview, March 2, 1987, Atlanta; Lane, author interview; Curran, author interview.

10. Lane, author interview.

11. Mullan, *Plagues and Politics,* p. 201.

12. Curran; author interview; Jaffe, author interview.

13. Jaffe, author interview. The detailed reports of the control studies are Harold W. Jaffe et al., "National Case-Control Study of Kaposi's Sarcoma and *Pneumocystis carinii* Pneumonia in Homosexual Men: Part 1, Epidemiologic Results," *Annals of Internal Medicine* 99 (August 1983): 145–51; Martha F. Rogers et al., ". . . Part 2: Laboratory Results," ibid., pp. 151–57.

14. Weisner, author interview. The first hepatitis B vaccine trials were conducted by Dr. Wolf Szmuness of the New York Blood Center, and results were announced in the fall of 1981. CDC's long-planned vaccine trials began after those in New York. They were delayed because government lawyers were concerned about problems of liability.

15. Shilts, *Band Played On,* p. 73.

16. CDC Task Force, "Epidemiological Aspects of . . . Kaposi's Sarcoma and Opportunistic Infections," pp. 251–52.

17. William Darrow, author interview, May 14, 1987, Atlanta; "A Cluster of Kaposi's Sarcoma and *Pneumocystis carinii* Pneumonia among Homosexual Male Residents of Los Angeles and Orange Counties, California," *MMWR* 31 (June 18, 1982): 305–7.

18. U.S. House, Committee on Energy and Commerce, *Kaposi's Sarcoma and Related Opportunistic Infections,* Hearing, April 13, 1983, Serial No. 97-125 (Washington, D.C.: GPO, 1982), testimony of James W. Curran, pp. 13–22 (Y4.En2/3:97-125).

19. Waxman quoted in Shilts, *Band Played On,* pp. 143–44.

20. Gerald M. Oppenheimer, "In the Eye of the Storm: The Epidemiological Construction of AIDS," in *AIDS: The Burdens of History,* ed. Fee and Fox, pp. 268, 277, 279.

21. Anthony S. Fauci, editorial, *Annals of Internal Medicine* 98 (June 1982): 777–79.

22. Spira quoted in Jean A. Marx, "New Disease Boggles Medical Community," *Science* 217 (August 1982): 619.

23. Bruce Evatt, author interview, April 29, 1987, Atlanta; Foege quoted by Jaffe, author interview.

24. Curran, author interview; Shilts, *Band Played On,* pp. 167–68.

25. Curran, author interview; "Opportunistic Infections and Kaposi's Sarcoma among Haitians in the United States," *MMWR* 31 (July 9, 1982): 353–54; "*Pneumocystis carinii* Pneumonia among Persons with Hemophilia A," *MMWR* 31 (July 16, 1982): 365–67.

26. Shilts, *Band Played On,* pp. 169–71; [CDC Public Affairs Office], "AIDS Chronology" (MS, n.d.), entry for July 17, 1982, copy in author's files.

27. Curran, author interview.

28. "Update on Acquired Immune Deficiency Syndrome (AIDS) among Patients with Hemophilia A," *MMWR,* 31 (December 10, 1982): 644–46, 652; "Possible Transfusion-Associated Acquired Immune Deficiency Syndrome (AIDS)—California," ibid.: 652–54; "Unexplained Immunodeficiency and Opportunistic Infections in Infants—New York, New Jersey, California," *MMWR* 31 (December 17, 1982): 665–67.

29. Harold Jaffe, author interview.

30. "When the AIDS crisis appeared, the blood bankers' inclination was essentially to deny that it was a major threat to blood safety. Special donor-screening procedures were ineffective and disruptive in their view. Attempts to implement them would only call attention to the disease's link to transfusion," observes Harvey M. Sapolsky in "AIDS, Blood Banking, and the Bonds of Community," *Dædalus* 118 (Summer 1989): 151.

31. Evatt, author interview.

32. *Newsweek,* December 27, 1982.

33. Neustadt and Fineberg, *Epidemic That Never Was,* pp. 130–31.

34. "Prevention of Acquired Immune Deficiency Syndrome (AIDS): Report

of Inter-Agency Recommendations," *MMWR* 32 (March 4, 1983): 101–3; Evatt, author interview.

35. Walter R. Dowdle, "The Epidemiology of AIDS," *PHR* 98 (July–August 1983): 310.

36. More than pride was involved. A large amount of money was also at stake in the form of patent rights to the AIDS antibody test.

37. Fred Murphy, author interview. Nothing is entirely without risk. The antibody test has inherent limitations, and there is some risk of AIDS transmission through blood transfusions. A rate of one in a million was cited at first. By 1989, the risk was listed at between one in 10,000 and one in 100,000, with some researchers citing one in 5,000. This means between 35 and 700 new AIDS cases each year among the 3.5 million patients who receive transfusions. Sapolsky, "AIDS, Blood Banking, and the Bonds of Community," p. 153.

38. Evatt, author interview; Stephen McDougal, author interview, May 13, 1987, Atlanta.

39. McDougal, author interview.

40. A convenient summary of CDC's role in AIDS epidemiology is William L. Heyward and James W. Curran, "The Epidemiology of AIDS in the U.S.," *Scientific American* 259 (October 1988): 72–81.

41. Joseph McCormick, author interview, October 13, 1987, Atlanta.

42. "The Real Epidemic: Fear and Despair," *Time,* July 4, 1983, pp. 56–58.

43. Charles E. Rosenberg, "What Is an Epidemic? AIDS in Historical Perspective," *Dædalus* 118 (Spring 1989): 1–17.

A Bibliographical Note

ORIGINAL SOURCES

This study is based primarily on the official records of the Centers for Disease Control in Atlanta and on oral history. Thousands of boxes from CDC are at the Atlanta Federal Records Center, East Point, Georgia. Most of those selected for this study are from the office of the director (before 1967, chief) on the premise that these would give a broader overview than records from individual units. In addition to these materials, CDC's small archival collection, kept in Building 1, 1600 Clifton Road, was also useful. This consists of four filing cabinets of uncatalogued miscellaneous documents, photographs, manuscripts, and occasionally a letter.

Several years ago an oral history collection was begun at CDC. The videotapes are usually half an hour to an hour in length, but some are much longer. The audiotapes vary widely in length, and all are quite fragile. Videotapes of the Joseph Mountin Lecture Series and other special events at CDC are also in this collection. No transcripts have been made. Personal interviews with members of CDC's staff, past and present, supplemented this material. Extensive abstracts of both the CDC collection and the personal interviews are in the author's files.

Additional oral history material is found in two files at the National Library of Medicine (NLM), Bethesda, Maryland: the Oral History Project of the National Institutes of Health/National Library of Medicine (NIH/NLM), and the George Rosen Oral History Project (1962–64). Material relating to CDC in the NIH/NLM collection includes interviews with Justin Andrews, Rolla E. Dyer, and William H. Sebrell. From the George Rosen collection, the most important interviews are with Victor H. Haas, Mark D. Hollis, Alexander D. Langmuir, Leonard A. Scheele, and Norman H. Topping. Transcripts are available for most of these. Also at NLM is a videotaped interview with Langmuir, conducted in 1979, for the "Leaders in American Medicine" series of the Alpha

Omega Alpha honor medical society. A transcript of several long interviews of James Goddard by James Harvey Young (April–June 1969) is in Special Collections, Robert F. Woodruff Library, Emory University, Atlanta, and at NLM.

Important material on the Cutter incident is in the files of NIH, the Food and Drug Administration (FDA), and the Bureau of State Services (BSS) at the Washington National Records Center (WNRC), Suitland, Maryland. From NIH, see RG 90, 64A875, Boxes 1–4; from BSS, RG 90, 60A560, Box 44, and 60A527, Box 4; from FDA, RG 88, 74-9, Box 1. Access may be obtained under the Freedom of Information Act.

CDC staff members are the authors of hundreds of journal articles, often cited in the notes. A convenient collection of Joseph Mountin's work is *Selected Papers by Joseph W. Mountin, M.D.* (n.p.: Joseph W. Mountin Memorial Committee, 1956). Also useful are these publications of CDC: The annual reports (1946–), variously named; *Morbidity and Mortality Weekly Reports* (1961–); and in-house journals, *The Word* (1969–73) and *Dateline: CDC* (1974–). CDC has reprinted articles by David Sencer on CDC activities that appeared annually in *U.S. Medicine* (January 15, 1968–January 15, 1975).

SECONDARY SOURCES
(SPECIFIC TO CDC)

CDC has six very large scrapbooks of newspaper clippings dating from 1946 to the late 1960s. After that time, clippings were stored in the Public Affairs Office. Some dealing with a discrete subject (swine flu, for example) are filed together; most have been put on microfilm in chronological order. There is no index. All of the newspaper citations, except those from the *New York Times*, are from these collections.

Dramatic accounts of the work of the EIS by Berton Roueché appeared in the *New Yorker* periodically, beginning in 1957. Many of these accounts have been reprinted in the following collections of Roueché's work: *The Incurable Wound and Further Narratives of Medical Detection* (Boston: Little, Brown, 1957). *A Man Named Hoffman and Other Narratives of Medical Detection* (Boston: Little, Brown, 1958); *The Orange Men* (Boston: Little, Brown, 1971); *The Disease Detectives, I* (New York: Times Books, 1980); and *The Disease Detectives, II* (New York: E. P. Dutton, 1984).

Other accounts of the disease detectives are John G. Fuller, *Fever! The Hunt for a New Killer Virus* (New York: Reader's Digest Press, 1974); Jules Archer, *Epidemic! The Story of the Disease Detectives* (New York: Harcourt Brace Jovanovich, 1977); and Gerald Astor, *The Disease Detectives: Deadly Medical Mysteries and the People Who Solved Them* (New York: New American Library, 1984).

For CDC's involvement with specific diseases, see:

SMALLPOX CRUSADE. Horace G. Ogden, *CDC and the Smallpox Crusade*, HHS Pub. No. (CDC) 87-8400 (Washington, D.C.: CDC, 1987); F. Fenner, D. A. Henderson, I. Arita, Z. Jezek, and I. D. Ladny, *Smallpox and Its Eradication* (Geneva: World Health Organization, 1988).

TUSKEGEE EXPERIMENT. James H. Jones, *Bad Blood: The Tuskegee Syphilis Experiment* (New York: Free Press, 1981; Allan M. Brandt, "Racism and Research: The Case of the Tuskegee Syphilis Study," *Hastings Center Report* 8 (December 1978): 21–29; T. G. Benedek, "The 'Tuskegee Study' of Syphilis: Analysis of Moral versus Methodologic Aspects," *Journal of Chronic Diseases* 31 (January 1978): 35–50.

SWINE FLU. Richard E. Neustadt and Harvey V. Fineberg, *The Epidemic That Never Was: Policy Making and the Swine Flu Affair* (New York: Vintage Books, 1983); Arthur M. Silverstein, *Pure Politics and Impure Science: The Swine Flu Affair* (Baltimore: Johns Hopkins University Press, 1981); Arthur J. Viseltear, "A Short Political History of the 1976 Swine Influenza Legislation," in *History, Science, and Politics: Influenza in America, 1918–1976,* ed. June E. Osborn (New York: Prodist, 1977).

LEGIONNAIRES' DISEASE. Gordon Thomas and Max Morgan-Witts, *Anatomy of an Epidemic* (Garden City, N.Y.: Doubleday, 1982).

AIDS. Randy Shilts, *And the Band Played On: Politics, People and the AIDS Epidemic* (New York: St. Martin's Press, 1987); Gerald M. Oppenheimer, "In the Eye of the Storm: The Epidemiological Construction of AIDS," in *AIDS: The Burdens of History,* ed. Elizabeth Fee and Daniel M. Fox (Berkeley: University of California Press, 1988); Harvey M. Sapolsky, "AIDS, Blood Banking, and the Bonds of Community," *Dædalus* 118 (Summer 1989): 145–63; William L. Heyward and James W. Curran, "The Epidemiology of AIDS in the U.S.," *Scientific American* 259 (October 1988): 72–81.

GENERAL WORKS

Benison, Saul. *Tom Rivers: Reflections on a Life in Medicine and Science.* Cambridge, Mass.: MIT Press, 1967.

Brandt, Allan M. *No Magic Bullet: A Social History of Venereal Disease in the United States since 1880.* New York: Oxford University Press, 1985.

Carson, Rachel. *Silent Spring.* Boston: Houghton Mifflin, 1962, 1987.

Carter, Richard. *Breakthrough: Saga of Jonas Salk.* New York: Trident Press, 1966.

Cassedy, James H. *Demography in Early America: Beginnings of the Statistical Mind, 1600–1800.* Cambridge, Mass.: Harvard University Press, 1969.

———. *American Medicine and Statistical Thinking, 1800–1860.* Cambridge, Mass.: Harvard University Press, 1984.

Crosby, Alfred W., Jr. *Epidemic and Peace, 1918.* Westport, Conn.: Greenwood Press, 1976.

Dowling, Harry F. *Fighting Infection: Conquests of the Twentieth Century.* Cambridge, Mass.: MIT Press, 1977.

Dubos, René. *The Dreams of Reason: Science and Utopias.* New York: Columbia University Press, 1961.

———. *Man Adapting.* New Haven: Yale University Press, 1965.

Dunlap, Thomas R. *DDT: Scientists, Citizens & Public Policy.* Princeton, N.J.: Princeton University Press, 1981.

Duffy, John. *The Sanitarians: A History of American Public Health*. Urbana and Chicago: University of Illinois Press, 1990.

Fee, Elizabeth. *Disease and Discovery: A History of the Johns Hopkins School of Hygiene and Public Health, 1916–1939*. Baltimore: Johns Hopkins University Press, 1987.

Furman, Bess. *A Profile of the United States Public Health Service, 1798–1948*. Washington, D.C.: n.p., n.d.

Gough, Michael. *Dioxin, Agent Orange: The Facts*. New York: Plenum Press, 1986.

Hamilton, Virginia Van der Veer. *Lister Hill: Statesman from the South*. Chapel Hill: University of North Carolina Press, 1987.

Harden, Victoria. *Inventing the NIH: Federal Biomedical Research Policy, 1887–1937*. Baltimore: Johns Hopkins University Press, 1986.

Hopkins, Donald R. *Princes and Peasants: Smallpox in History*. Chicago: University of Chicago Press, 1983.

Katz, Alfred H., and Jean S. Felton, eds. *Health and Community: Readings in the Philosophy and Sciences of Public Health*. New York: Free Press, 1984.

Klein, Aaron E. *Trial by Fury: The Polio Vaccine Controversy*. New York: Charles Scribner's Sons, 1972.

Kronfeld, Jennie Jacobs, and Marcia Lynn Whicker. *U.S. National Health Policy: An Analysis of the Federal Role*. New York: Praeger, 1984.

Last, John M., ed. *Maxcy-Rosenau, Public Health and Preventive Medicine*. 12th ed. New York: Appleton, Century-Crofts, 1986.

Mullan, Fitzhugh. *Plagues and Politics: The Story of the United States Public Health Service*. New York: Basic Books, 1989.

Parran, Thomas. *Shadow on the Land: Syphilis*. New York: Reynal & Hitchcock, 1937.

Patterson, James T. *The Dread Disease: Cancer and Modern American Culture*. Cambridge, Mass.: Harvard University Press, 1987.

Paul, John R. *History of Poliomyelitis*. New Haven: Yale University Press, 1971.

Rosen, George. *Preventive Medicine in the United States, 1900–1975: Trends and Interpretations*. New York: Science History Publications, 1975.

Shorter, Edward. *The Health Century*. New York: Doubleday, 1987.

Smillie, Wilson G. *Public Health: Its Promise for the Future*. New York: Macmillan, 1955.

Starr, Paul. *The Social Transformation of American Medicine*. New York: Basic Books, 1982.

U.S. Surgeon General's Advisory Committee on Smoking and Health. *Smoking and Health: Report of the Advisory Committee to the Surgeon General of the Public Health Service*. PHS Pub. No. 1103. Washington, D.C.: GPO, 1964.

Van Heynigen, W. E., and John R. Seal. *Cholera: The American Scientific Experience, 1947–1980*. Boulder, Colo.: Westview Press, 1983.

Williams, Ralph C. *The United States Public Health Service, 1798–1950*. Washington, D.C.: Commissioned Officers Association of United States Public Health Service, 1951.

Zinsser, Hans. *Rats, Lice and History*. Boston: Little, Brown, 1935.

Index

Compositor:	Braun-Brumfield, Inc.
Text:	10/13 Sabon
Display:	Sabon
Printer and Binder:	Braun-Brumfield, Inc.